Introduction to Nonparametric Statistics for the Biological Sciences Using R

Thomas W. MacFarland • Jan M. Yates

Introduction to Nonparametric Statistics for the Biological Sciences Using R

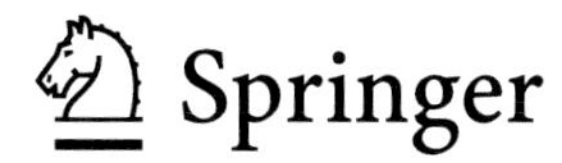

Springer

Thomas W. MacFarland
Office of Institutional Effectiveness
Nova Southeastern University
Fort Lauderdale, FL, USA

Jan M. Yates
Abraham S. Fischler College of Education
Nova Southeastern University
Fort Lauderdale, FL, USA

ISBN 978-3-319-30633-9 ISBN 978-3-319-30634-6 (eBook)
DOI 10.1007/978-3-319-30634-6

Library of Congress Control Number: 2016934853

Printed on acid-free paper

This Springer imprint is published by Springer Nature
The registered company is Springer International Publishing AG Switzerland

Preface

This text is about the use of nonparametric statistics for the biological sciences and the use of R to support data organization, statistical analyses, and the production of both simple and publishable graphics. Nonparametric techniques have a role in the biological sciences, and R is uniquely positioned to support the actions needed to accommodate biological data and subsequent hypothesis-testing and graphical presentation.

Introduction to Nonparametric Statistics for the Biological Sciences Using R begins with a general discussion of data, specifically the four commonly listed data types: nominal, ordinal, interval, and ratio. This discussion is critical to this text given the frequent use of nominal and ordinal data using nonparametric statistics. The beginning presentation then moves to an introductory display of R, with a caution that far more detail in the use of R and specifically R syntax is covered in later chapters.

The remaining chapters are largely self-contained lessons that cover the following individual nonparametric tests, listed here in the order of presentation in the book:

- Sign Test
- Chi-square
- Mann-Whitney U Test
- Wilcoxon Matched-Pairs Signed-Ranks Test
- Kruskal-Wallis H-Test for Oneway Analysis of Variance (ANOVA) by Ranks
- Friedman Twoway Analysis of Variance (ANOVA) by Ranks
- Spearman's Rank-Difference Coefficient of Correlation
- Binomial Test
- Walsh Test for Two Related Samples of Interval Data
- Kolmogorov-Smirnov (K-S) Two-Sample Test
- Binomial Logistic Regression

A common approach is used for each nonparametric analysis, promoting a consistent and thorough attempt at analyses: background on the lesson, the importing of data into R, data organization and presentation of the Code Book, initial visualization of the data, descriptive analysis of the data, the statistical analysis, and interpretation of outcomes in a formal summary. Most chapters have additional lessons, listed in an addendum, and many chapters have multiple addenda.

This text should help beginning students and researchers consider the use of nonparametric approaches to analyses in the biological sciences. With R used as a platform for presentation, the diligent reader will develop a reasonable level of expertise with the R language, aided by the clearly shown syntax in an easy-to-read fixed format font.

Additionally, all datasets are available on the publisher's Web page for this text. Each dataset is presented in .csv (i.e., comma-separated values) file format, facilitating simple use and universal availability, regardless of selected operating system and computing platform. The subject matter for these datasets is fairly general and should apply as useful examples to all disciplines in the biological sciences.

A parametric approach to biologically oriented statistical analyses is frequently seen in the literature. However, as presented throughout this text, a nonparametric approach should also receive consideration when there are concerns about scale, distribution, and representation. That is to say, nonparametric statistics provide a useful purpose for inferential analyses when data (1) do not meet the purported precision of an interval scale, (2) there are serious concerns about extreme deviation from normal distribution, and (3) there is considerable difference in the number of subjects for each breakout group.

Consider the importance of each condition from the three conditions listed above and why a nonparametric approach should be considered, either as an exploratory approach to statistical testing, a final approach to statistical testing, or at least as a confirming approach to statistical testing.

- **Scale:** Many nonparametric analyses are based on ranked data, where the scale used to define data may not be as precise as desired. Given the realities of field work in the biological sciences, there are many times when it is not possible to obtain a precise measure (i.e., a measure that uses a scale that is both reliable and valid). Instead, field staff may only be able to obtain measures such as (1) large, medium, or small; (2) successful or not successful; etc. When precise measures are lacking, data that are instead ranked can be applied to good effect through the use of nonparametric analyses.
- **Distribution:** As many biologically focused research projects are put into place, it often becomes only too evident that the sample in question not only does not follow normal distribution patterns for selected variables, but the measurements do not even begin to approximate any semblance of normal distribution. Nonparametric techniques are extremely valuable when distribution patterns come into question, since many nonparametric tests are based on the use of ranks and are distribution-free (i.e., selected nonparametric tests are often quite appropriate even when data from the sample do not meet expected distribution patterns typically associated with a normally distributed population).

- **Representation:** There are many situations when there are extreme differences in the number and corresponding percent of total for breakout groups when samples are drawn from a population. Consider the representation of blood types. In the United States, there is extreme variation in the expected representation of blood type, such that O-positive is an expected blood type for nearly 40 % of the population, whereas AB-negative is a rare blood type and is observed for only 1 %, or less, of the population. This difference in representation by blood type is so extreme that comparisons of some measured variable by the two blood types would be greatly compromised in most cases, unless a nonparametric approach was used for later inferential analyses.

Although many nonparametric analyses were developed back when nearly all analyses were attempted using paper and pencil, it is now common to use a computer-mediated approach with contemporary statistical analysis software. This text is based on the use of R for this purpose. The R programming language is freely available open source software that it is now among the top 10 programs for worldwide use. R has gained wide acceptance due to its flexibility for data organization and data management, statistical analysis, and production of graphical images portraying relationships between and among data.

The comparative advantage of R is not only its functionality, which is also found to a degree in other computer-based programs; but, instead, the comparative advantage of R is the user community, where interested individuals can develop and use functions that operate on data for specific purposes and these actions are self-initiated, with no interference by a manager-led development team or marketing staff members. With R, a researcher has control over the data in ways that cannot be equaled when using commercial software that can be limiting to the imagination.

However, a limited degree of functionality is available when R is first downloaded. The extreme functionality comes from the more than 5000 packages available to the worldwide R community, with many packages having 25, 50, 100, or more functions. Again, the R data-centric environment is free and the R software is open source, such that the use of R is only limited by vision and skills. Functions developed by others are made freely available and the functions can be modified as desired.

Fort Lauderdale, FL, USA

Thomas W. MacFarland
Jan M. Yates

Contents

List of Figures

Chapter 1
Nonparametric Statistics for the Biological Sciences

Abstract Nonparametric statistics provide a useful purpose for inferential analyses when data: (1) do not meet the purported precision of an interval scale, (2) there are serious concerns about extreme deviation from normal distribution, and (3) there is considerable difference in the number of subjects for each breakout group. It is not totally uncommon to hear terms such as ranking tests and distribution-free tests to describe the inferential tests associated with nonparametric statistics, due to the use of nominal and ordinal data and data that may not meet the desired assumption of normal distribution (i.e., bell-shaped curve). Although those who work in the biological sciences would ideally like to have precise measurement for their data, to have data that follow normal distribution patterns, and to have adequately-sized samples for all breakout groups, only too often these three desires are not met. Nonparametric statistics and the many inferential tests associated with nonparametric statistics provide a valuable set of options on how these data can be used to good effect. Following along with these aspirations, the R environment and the many external packages associated with R offer many practical applications that support inferential tests associated with nonparametric statistics.

Keywords Anderson-Darling test • Bar plot (stacked, side-by-side) • Box plot • Central tendency • Code book • Continuous scale • Density plot • Distribution-free • Dotplot • Frequency distribution • Histogram • Interval • Mean • Median • Mode • Nominal • Nonparametric • Normal distribution • Ordinal • Parametric • Quantile-Quantile (QQ, Q-Q) • Ranking • Ratio • Violin plot

1.1 Background on This Lesson

The purpose of this set of lessons is to provide guidance on how R is used for nonparametric data analysis:

- To introduce when nonparametric approaches to data analysis are appropriate.
- To introduce the leading nonparametric tests commonly used in biostatistics and how R is used to generate appropriate statistics for each test.

T.W. MacFarland, J.M. Yates, *Introduction to Nonparametric Statistics for the Biological Sciences Using R*, DOI 10.1007/978-3-319-30631-6_1

- To introduce common graphics (i.e., figures) typically associated with nonparametric data analysis and how R is used to generate appropriate graphics in support of each dataset.

The **primary purpose of this introductory lesson** is to provide guidance on how R is used to distinguish between data that could be classified as nonparametric as opposed to data that could be classified as parametric. Saying that immediately brings to question the meaning of nonparametric data and as a counterpart, the meaning of parametric data, with both approaches to data classification covered extensively in this lesson.

The **secondary purpose of this introductory lesson** is to introduce R syntax and to provide an advance organizer on how R is used to organize data, prepare statistical analyses, and generate quality graphical images. For this introductory lesson merely give broad attention to R syntax and focus only on the concepts associated with data distribution and outcomes from provided samples. The many packages, functions, and arguments associated with R are covered in detail in later lessons.

1.2 Data Types

At the broadest level and as will be demonstrated in this lesson, nonparametric data are often considered *distribution-free* data. That is to say, there is no anticipated or expected pattern to how nonparametric data are distributed. Accordingly, the converse is that for parametric data there is some type of distribution pattern, where the data typically have some degree of expected semblance to the normal curve.

Data can take many forms. The number of common snapping turtles (*Chelydra serpentina*) in a freshwater pond is one type of datum—a simple headcount. The mean weight of these turtles is an entirely different type of datum—a mathematical average based upon measured weights: the Sum of All Weights divided by the Number of All Subjects Weighed equals Mean Weight. Yet, a headcount of snapping turtles and the mean weight of snapping turtles would both be associated with a research study into the ecology of fresh water ponds.

Given this simple example of counts v measurements, it is best to consider how data can be conceptualized from different perspectives. One way to view data is to differentiate between **nonparametric data** and **parametric data**:

- Nonparametric data are data that are either **counted** or **ranked**.
  - Counted Data—An actual headcount of the number of snapping turtles sunning on the shoreline of a freshwater pond during a warm spring afternoon is an example of a nonparametric datum.
  - Ranked Data—Due to potential injury from handling a snapping turtle (i.e., injury to both the specimen as well as the handler) to gain information on length or weight, it may be necessary to establish protocols so that adult snapping turtles are visually ranked (i.e., categorized) as large, medium, or

small, with no effort to actually capture specimens and, in turn, obtain more precise measurements. This ranking is another example of a nonparametric datum.

- Parametric data are data that are **measured**.
  - Typical parametric biological data would include a wide variety of measurements, such as: height or length of a subject in either inches or centimeters, weight of a subject in either pounds or kilograms, or Systolic Blood Pressure (SBP) while at rest with millimeters of mercury (mm Hg) used as a measure of pressure.
  - A typical measurement of parametric biological data may include proxy measurements such as dry weight of scat, width of claw marks on tree bark, estimated weight of eaten prey, etc.

The difference between nonparametric data and parametric data need not be confusing, although it often is for those who are only beginning biological research careers. If a datum was either counted or ranked, then it is common to view the datum as a nonparametric datum. At the broadest level, if a datum was somehow measured (recognizing that all measurements may not be as precise as desired, but that is a separate issue to this discussion) then the datum may be a parametric datum. Selection of tests for statistical analysis and the ability to select the appropriate test are an important reason for learning how to differentiate between nonparametric data and parametric data.

Given all of this attention to data and differences between nonparametric data and parametric data, consider how it is generally agreed that there are four levels of data measurement, often viewed using the acronym NOIR: (1) nominal, (2) ordinal, (3) interval, and (4) ratio.

1.2.1 Nominal Data

Nominal (i.e., named) data are **counted** and are conveniently placed into predefined categories. A common example is to consider gender and to count the number of females and males in a sample. Assuming that each subject from a sample can only be either female or male at the time the sample is examined, the concept of female and correspondingly the number of female subjects is a nominal datum. Following along with this approach, the concept of male and, correspondingly, the number of male subjects is also a nominal datum. Note how there is no measurement of gender other than to assign a headcount number for those subjects who are considered female and a corresponding headcount number for those subjects who are considered male.

1.2.2 *Ordinal Data*

Ordinal (i.e., ordered) data are **ranked** data that represent some type of predefined hierarchy. As such, ordinal data show some attempt at measurement and allow greater inference than data associated with the nominal scale. To return to the previous example on weights of biological specimens, imagine that in an inventory of adult snapping turtles the sample consisted of six adult specimens and that the previously mentioned ordering scheme were used to assign size as a proxy for weight and length:

- Specimen 201504121001 Size = Large
- Specimen 201504121002 Size = Medium
- Specimen 201504121003 Size = Medium
- Specimen 201504121004 Size = Small
- Specimen 201504121005 Size = Large
- Specimen 201504121006 Size = Small

Further assume that established protocols and training were used to make size-type assignments by field researchers. Although these measures for size (e.g., large, medium, small) certainly do not have the precision of weights gained from a calibrated scale or length gained from a calibrated ruler, if the sample of six snapping turtles were representative of the overall population then this sample certainly provides a general sense of size for the population. The data could then be used to prepare frequency distributions, bar charts, etc., of size, with size serving as a proxy measure of weight and length.

1.2.3 *Interval Data*

Interval (i.e., degree of difference) data are **measured in equal units (i.e., intervals)**. Consider systolic blood pressure (SBP) of adult male subjects. SBP readings of 118, 122, and 126 could conceivably be three possible measures on an interval scale, measured as mm Hg SBP using a sphygmomanometer.[1] If indeed the scale is interval, then it is known that the degree of difference between 118 and 120 is equal to the degree of difference between 122 and 124 or the degree of difference between 126 and 128. There is a degree of precision to an interval scale that is not found with a less precise scale, such as an ordinal ranking-type scale that only uses low, average, or high to describe SBP. In turn, it is possible to make greater inference with interval data than is possible when using nominal data and interval data.

[1]By long-standing convention regarding blood pressure measurements and the use of non-digital sphygmomanometers, it is common to express mm Hg SBP readings as even numbers, only.

1.2.4 *Ratio Data*

Ratio (i.e., some type of mathematical comparison) data have the characteristics of interval data, but ratio data also have two other very important characteristics:

- Ratio data have a true and unique value for **zero** (i.e., the Kelvin scale has an absolute zero temperature).
- Ratio data are **real numbers** and they can be subjected to standard mathematical procedures (e.g., addition, subtraction, multiplication, division). Because of this characteristic, ratio data can be expressed in ratio form. With ratio data, you can assume that a measured value of 50 is truly twice the measure of 25, whatever the measure represents (e.g., length, width, temperature, hours, etc.).

1.3 How R Syntax, R Output, and Graphics Show in This Text

As a guide to the way the R syntax, R output, and graphics shown immediately below and throughout this text are organized, R syntax used for input is shown within a green frame and R output is shown within a red frame:

```
R syntax shows in this green frame.
```

```
R output shows in the red frame.
```

This simple technique should make it fairly easy to distinguish between input and output without the need for an excessive display of screen snapshots. A simple display is shown immediately below of R syntax as input and the resulting R output:

```
2 + 2

TestScores <- c(98, 75, 83, 92, 94, 79, 71, 83)

median(TestScores)
mean(TestScores)
sd(TestScores)
length(TestScores)
```

```
> 2 + 2
[1] 4
>
> TestScores <- c(98, 75, 83, 92, 94, 79, 71, 83)
>
> median(TestScores)
[1] 83
> mean(TestScores)
[1] 84.375
```

```
> sd(TestScores)
[1] 9.530965
> length(TestScores)
[1] 8
```

All R syntax shows in this text, but to keep the length to a reasonable number of pages, only selected output shows. Of course, all output can be generated merely by using the data and R syntax associated with this text.[2]

In the same way that all output does not show in this text, only selected figures show. Again, use the data and R syntax to practice and generate the figures. Remember that par(ask=TRUE) is used to manage the screen, to show one figure at a time.

1.4 Graphical Presentation of Populations

Along with an expectation of increased precision of measurement, with both interval and ratio measures, there is also an expectation that interval data and ratio data for a population and subsequently a sample from a population follow some degree of normal distribution. A visual display of data may not fully equate to a perfect bell-shaped curve, but there should be at least some degree of adherence to this model. Otherwise, if data are distribution-free and do not follow an expected degree of distribution of values, then it may be desirable to think of nonparametric statistics as an alternate to the use of parametric statistics.

With this general information on the different types of data and the possible impact that data types have on selected statistical tests, think about the practical implications of data for the biological sciences regarding how data are viewed. From this comparison consider how the following conditions impact later decisions:

- Precision of data measurement
- Distribution patterns
- Sample size (i.e. representation: Is the sample representative of the population?)

Even with recognition that there is always the possibility of outliers (i.e., extreme values that are not errors), do the data follow along theoretical limits and normal distribution patterns? When data do not follow a pattern of normal distribution, it is common to use a nonparametric approach to later statistical analyses or to at least consider the use of a nonparametric approach to statistical analyses. Initial bias toward data and data types must be avoided.

For example, imagine that adult males are measured for height. A few adult males may be approximately 60 inches or less, and equally, a few adult males may be 80 inches or more. However, most adult males will be about 70 inches, within some

[2] All .csv datasets are posted on the publisher's Web page devoted to this text.

degree of variance. If the sample were representative of the overall population a graphical distribution of the data will follow along a normal curve. To demonstrate this concept, look at the two samples (the samples are generated using rnorm() and runif(), R-based functions) on the height of adult males, where one sample follows along a normal distribution pattern and the other sample fails to exhibit a normal distribution pattern.

1.4.1 Samples that Exhibit Normal Distribution

With R, use the rnorm() function and appropriate arguments to create an object variable that displays normal distribution for a sample of 10,000 subjects, representing the height (inches) of adult males. Use rnorm() function arguments so that the sample represents the height of 10,000 subjects (adult males) with mean = 70 inches and standard deviation = 5 inches.[3] Display descriptive statistics, a histogram, and a density plot of the sample. Although R syntax in an interactive fashion is used in this lesson, the immediate concern is on the concepts associated with nonparametric data compared to parametric data. Adequate documentation is used with the R syntax shown below and far more detail on the use of R syntax is explained in later lessons. Again, for this lesson, focus on the concepts of data distribution, sample size, nonparametric v parametric data, etc., and avoid undue concern about the R syntax which is explained in detail later.

The initial R syntax used for each lesson shows immediately below, as Housekeeping. This R syntax will remove unwanted files from any prior work, declare the working directory, etc. This startup R syntax is then followed by the R syntax directly associated with this part of the lesson (Fig. 1.1).

```
###############################################################
# Housekeeping                               Use for All Analyses    #
###############################################################
date()              # Current system time and date.
R.version.string    # R version and version release date.
ls()                # List all objects in the working
                    # directory.
rm(list = ls())     # CAUTION: Remove all files in the working
                    # directory. If this action is not desired,
                    # use the rm() function one-by-one to remove
                    # the objects that are not needed.
ls.str()            # List all objects, with finite detail.
getwd()             # Identify the current working directory.
setwd("F:/R_Nonparametric")
                    # Set to a new working directory.
                    # Note the single forward slash and double
```

[3] It is common to see the use of uppercase and lowercase for terms, such as mean = 123 or Mean = 123, when used in a narrative presentation. Both approaches are used in this text.

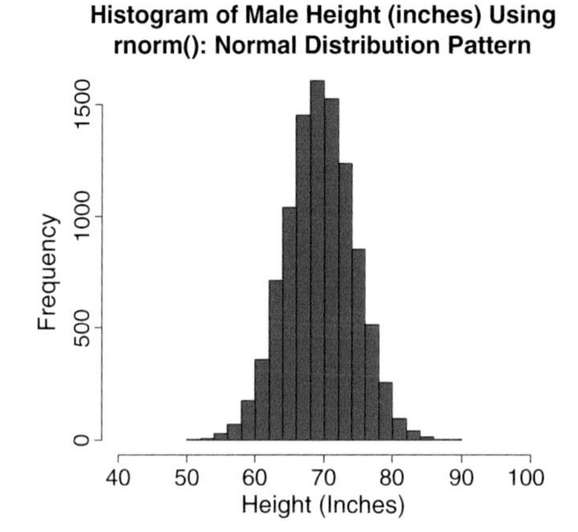

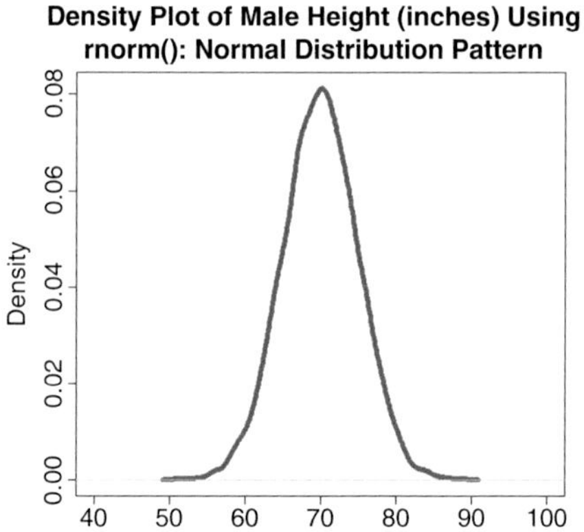

Fig. 1.1 Histogram and density plot: normal distribution

```
                     # quotes.
                     # This new directory should be the directory
                     # where the data file is located, otherwise
                     # the data file will not be found.
getwd()              # Confirm the working directory.
list.files()         # List files at the PC directory.
################################################################
```

```
MHeight_rnorm <- round(rnorm(10000, mean=70, sd=5))
  # Create an object called MHeight_rnorm, which consists of
  # 10,000 random subjects, with mean equal to 70 inches and
  # standard deviation equal to 5 inches.  The object variable
  # MHeight_rnorm represents a theoretical representation of
  # heights for adult males, measured in inches.  Note how the
  # round() function was also used, so that whole numbers are
  # generated, only.
  #
  # When using the rnorm() function and the runif() function,
  # be sure to note how the actual values generated will change
  # with each use.

head(MHeight_rnorm)      # First line(s) of data
tail(MHeight_rnorm)      # Last line(s) of data
summary(MHeight_rnorm)   # Summary
mean(MHeight_rnorm)      # Mean
sd(MHeight_rnorm)        # SD
median(MHeight_rnorm)    # Median

par(ask=TRUE)             # Side-by-Side Histogram
par(mfrow=c(1,2))         # and Density Plot
hist(MHeight_rnorm,       # Histogram function
  breaks=25,              # Adequate bins
  col="red",              # Color
  font=2,                 # Bold
```

```
  font.lab=2,            # Bold labels
  cex.axis=1.25,         # Large axis
  main="Histogram of Male Height (inches) Using
  rnorm(): Normal Distribution Pattern",
  xlab="Height (Inches)",# Label text
  xlim=c(40,100))        # Axis limits
plot(density(MHeight_rnorm), lwd=6, col="red",
  font=2, font.lab=2, cex.axis=1.25,
  main="Density Plot of Male Height (inches) Using
  rnorm(): Normal Distribution Pattern",
  xlab="Height (Inches)", xlim=c(40,100))
  # Note above and throughout these lessons that
  # the function par(ask=TRUE) is used to freeze
  # the screen, making it necessary to either
  # press or click the Enter key, which gives
  # more control over screen actions.
  #
  # The parameters in par(mfrow=c(1,2)) are used
  # so that output of the hist() function and
  # output of the plot() function would occupy
  # one row and two columns, placing the two
  # figures side-by-side and in turn allow easy
  # comparison.
```

1.4.2 Samples That Fail to Exhibit Normal Distribution

With R, use the runif() function and appropriate arguments to create an object variable that populates a sample with random numbers—ignoring any attempt to have normal distribution. Again, there will be 10,000 subjects (adult males) in this sample but observe the descriptive statistics, histogram, and density plot for this sample of random adult male heights, all falling within the limits set using runif() function arguments: minimum = 55 inches and maximum = 85 inches, or about + and − three standard deviations from mean = 70 inches and standard deviation = 5 inches. Once again, focus on the concept of distribution patterns. The documentation provided, along with the R syntax, should be useful. These functions and arguments will be explained in far greater detail in later lessons (Fig. 1.2).

```
MHeight_runif <- round(runif(10000, min=55, max=85))
  # Create an object called MHeight_runif, which consists of
  # 10,000 random subjects.  The minimum value will be 55
  # inches and  the maximum value will be 85 inches.  Note how
  # these limits are in general parity of + and - three
  # standard deviations of the above example, where the mean
  # was 70 inches and standard deviation was 5 inches (e.g.,
  # 70 - (5 inches per SD * 3 SDs) = 55 and 70 + (5 inches per
  # SD * 3 SDs) = 85).  The object MHeight_runif represents a
  # theoretical representation of heights for adult males, but
  # by no means a normal distribution that is based on a set
```

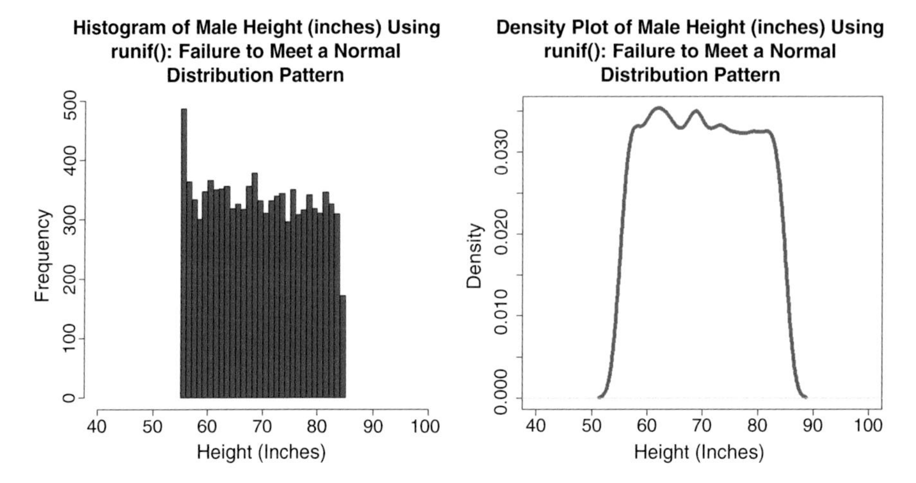

Fig. 1.2 Histogram and density plot: failure to meet normal distribution

```
# mean and a set standard deviation.  Again, the round()
# function was used, so that whole numbers are generated,
# only.
#
# When using the rnorm() function and the runif() function,
# be sure to note how the actual values generated will change
# with each use.
```

```
head(MHeight_runif)      # First line(s) of data
tail(MHeight_runif)      # Last line(s) of data
summary(MHeight_runif)   # Summary
mean(MHeight_runif)      # Mean
sd(MHeight_runif)        # SD
median(MHeight_runif)    # Median

par(ask=TRUE)             # Side-by-Side Histogram
par(mfrow=c(1,2))         # and Density Plot
hist(MHeight_runif,       # Histogram function
  breaks=25,              # Adequate bins
  col="red",              # Color
  font=2,                 # Bold
  font.lab=2,             # Bold labels
  cex.axis=1.25,          # Large axis
  main="Histogram of Male Height (inches) Using
  runif():  Failure to Meet a Normal
  Distribution Pattern",
  xlab="Height (Inches)",# Label text
  xlim=c(40,100))         # Axis limits
plot(density(MHeight_runif), lwd=6, col="red",
  font=2, font.lab=2, cex.axis=1.25,
  main="Density Plot of Male Height (inches) Using
  runif():  Failure to Meet a Normal
```

```
Distribution Pattern",
xlab="Height (Inches)", xlim=c(40,100))
# Note above and throughout these lessons that
# the function par(ask=TRUE) is used to freeze
# the screen, making it necessary to either hit
# or click the Enter key, which gives more
# control over screen actions.
#
# The parameters in par(mfrow=c(1,2)) are used
# so that output of the hist() function and
# output of the plot() function would occupy
# one row and two columns, placing the two
# figures side-by-side and in turn allow easy
# comparison.
```

Although the samples found in object MHeight_rnorm and object MHeight_runif both share the same general descriptive statistics, with a Mean of about 70 inches and a Median of about 70 inches, there are vast differences between object MHeight_rnorm and object MHeight_runif in terms of distribution patterns:

- Data for the sample MHeight_rnorm tend to follow a normal distribution pattern, as exhibited in the accompanying histogram and density plot.
- Data for the sample MHeight_runif do not follow along a normal distribution pattern, as exhibited in the accompanying histogram and density plot.

Accordingly, it is suggested that the use of a nonparametric approach would be the most appropriate way to address any statistical analyses or tests using the MHeight_runif sample. There is simply no assumption of normal distribution for the MHeight_runif dataset.

1.5 R and Nonparametric Analyses

1.5.1 Precision of Scales: Ordinal vs Interval

Ideally, researchers in the biological sciences would work only with data that meet desired levels of measurement. As an example using forage crops, due to economic pressures it is no longer acceptable to measure yields for alfalfa (*Medicago sativa*) in whole numbers, such as 4 or 5 tons of alfalfa per acre. Cost-accounting of modern agri-business practices now demands more precision, such as measuring alfalfa yields as 4.25 tons per acre, 4.95 tons per acre, 5.15 tons per acre, etc. Even more precision should accompany these weight measures, such as moisture content of hay when put into storage, an empirical measure for condition of the hay, total digestible nutrients (TDN), crude protein (CP), etc. Using the many tools available today this type of measured precision can be obtained.

1.5.2 Deviation from Normal Distribution

Although extreme precision may be desired, there are times when researchers in the biological sciences do not have the ability to obtain desired levels of measurement, due to a variety of reasons including limited budgets, time constraints, possible harm if specimens were collected, etc. Consider a situation where an insect pest represents a major threat to crop production and the role of Integrated Pest Management (IPM) team members (i.e., scouts) for data collection regarding the crop and pest presence.

For this example, assume that an insect pest has the potential to soon damage a specific crop and that in response to this potential damage, some type of treatment was applied to 15 different research plots:

- Some plots (N = 8) received a biological treatment, to minimize insect damage.
- Some plots (N = 7) received a chemical treatment, to minimize insect damage.

Approximately 3 days after treatment, when it is judged safe to walk in the chemically-treated plots,[4] IPM team members went into the 15 different plots and made quick assessments of damage from the infestation, largely to determine effectiveness of the different treatments and to also determine if follow-up treatments are needed. Due to the need for a possible quick same-day application of a second treatment (instead of the regular practice of counting the specific number of destructive insects per square meter at five random locations in each plot) IPM protocols were used that call for rapid damage assessment, using a simple three-tiered scale for crop damage: (1) Minimal Damage, (2) Moderate Damage, and (3) Extreme Damage. Although this type of measure lacks precision, assume that the IPM scouts have had proper training and that they closely follow the protocols associated with this type of rapid crop assessment.

Again, although this three-tiered scale is appropriate given the need for rapid response to a known threat of insect infestation, it certainly lacks precision. Given this background, look at the way R is used to organize the data for monitoring 15 separate plots of insect infestation after treatment, both biological treatment and chemical-based treatment.

Use R in an interactive mode to create the data, placing values into three separate object variables: Plot, Treated, and Damage. In later lessons separate spreadsheet-based datasets will be imported into R, but for these introductory examples data are created in an interactive fashion.

```
Plot <- c("A", "B", "C", "D", "E",
          "F", "G", "H", "I", "J",
          "K", "L", "M", "N", "O")
  # Create a character-based object vector

class(Plot)         # Determine class
```

[4]The word *plot* is frequently used in agriculture to refer to a small section of a field. Do not confuse the term plot, used in this context, with the R plot() function.

```
str(Plot)              # Determine structure
Plot                   # Show all values

Treated <- c(2, 2, 1, 1, 2,
             1, 2, 1, 1, 2,
             1, 2, 2, 1, 1)
  # Create a numeric-based object vector:
  # 1 = Biological and 2 = Chemical

class(Treated)         # Determine class
str(Treated)           # Determine structure
Treated                # Show all values

Damage <- c(2, 1, 3, 2, 2,
            2, 1, 3, 3, 2,
            2, 1, 2, 2, 3)
  # Create a numeric-based object vector:
  # 1 = Minimal, 2 = Moderate, 3 = Extreme

class(Damage)          # Determine class
str(Damage)            # Determine structure
Damage                 # Show all values
```

Use R in an interactive fashion to join the three separate object variables (e.g., Plot, Treated, and Damage) into a single object. By default, the constructed object will initially be a matrix.

```
Report <- cbind(Plot, Treated, Damage)
  # Use the cbind() function to join Plot,
  # Treated, and Damage into a matrix (by
  # default), with the data placed into
  # columns.

class(Report)          # Determine class

str(Report)            # Determine structure
Report                 # Show all data
```

For many purposes, it is often best to use data that are organized as a dataframe and not a matrix. Use R in an interactive fashion to coerce the matrix (i.e., Report) into a dataframe (i.e., Report.df). Although it is not required, as a good programming practice note below how **.df** is used as part of the object name, to provide adequate documentation that the object is a dataframe.

```
Report.df <- data.frame(Report)
  # Transform the data in object variable
  # Report into a dataframe, and call the
  # new object Report.df.

class(Report.df)       # Determine class
str(Report.df)         # Determine structure
Report.df              # Show all data
```

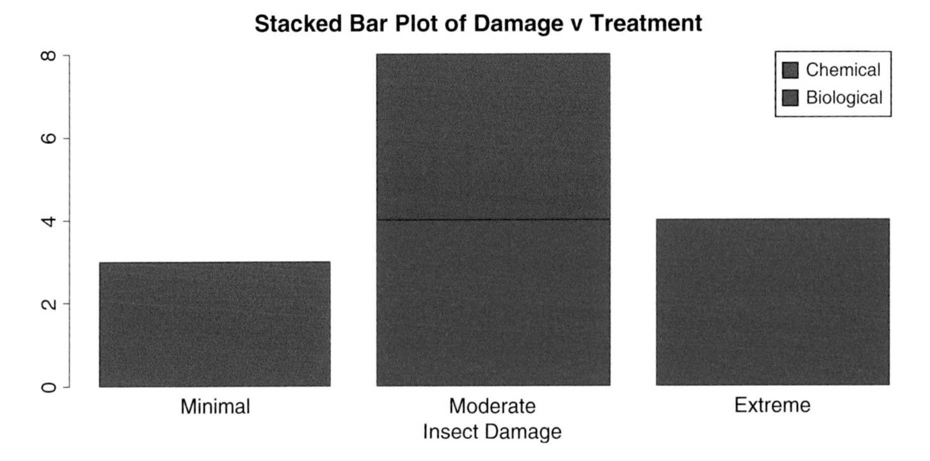

Fig. 1.3 Stacked bar plot of two object variables

```
   Plot Treated Damage
1     A       2      2
2     B       2      1
3     C       1      3
4     D       1      2
5     E       2      2
6     F       1      2
7     G       2      1
8     H       1      3
9     I       1      3
10    J       2      2
11    K       1      2
12    L       2      1
13    M       2      2
14    N       1      2
15    O       1      3
```

At this point, note how R was used in an interactive fashion so that data were put into three separate object variables, and these three objects were then joined together, initially as a matrix with three columns. The matrix was then put into dataframe format. The next set of actions will provide labels and final desired format for each object variable, to improve how output shows when text and graphical images are generated.

Note also how formal notation is used, where the name for the dataframe and the name for the object variable are both used with the $ sign serving as a separator between the two, such as Report.df$Plot, Report.df$Treated, and Report.df$Damage, etc. This type of nomenclature may be somewhat verbose, but it can be used to avoid later problems when there might otherwise be a conflict in how object variables are named and used (Fig. 1.3).

```
Report.df$Plot <- factor(Report.df$Plot,
  labels=c("Plot A", "Plot B", "Plot C",
           "Plot D", "Plot E", "Plot F",
           "Plot G", "Plot H", "Plot I",
           "Plot J", "Plot K", "Plot L",
           "Plot M", "Plot N", "Plot O"))
  # Coerce object variable Report.df$Plot
  # into a factor and assign labels

class(Report.df$Plot)          # Determine class
str(Report.df$Plot)            # Determine structure
summary(Report.df$Plot)        # Summary
Report.df$Plot                 # Show all data
par(ask=TRUE)
barplot(table(Report.df$Plot), col=rainbow(15),
  main="Barplot of Report.df$Plot", font=2)
  # Use the table() function to determine frequency
  # distribution and then prepare a simple barplot of
  # that outcome, for quality assurance purposes.
  #
  # There are 15 values for Report.df$Plot so note
  # how each value was assigned a unique color, based
  # on the way col=rainbow(15) was used.
  #
  # Along with a descriptive title, the figure was
  # enhanced with bold text by using font=2.

Report.df$Treated <- factor(Report.df$Treated,
  labels=c("Biological", "Chemical"))
  # Coerce object variable Report.df$Treated into
  # a factor and assign labels

class(Report.df$Treated)       # Determine class
str(Report.df$Treated)         # Determine structure
summary(Report.df$Treated)     # Summary
Report.df$Treated              # Show all data
par(ask=TRUE)
barplot(table(Report.df$Treated), col=rainbow(2),
  main="Barplot of Report.df$Treated", font=2)
  # Use the table() function to determine frequency
  # distribution and then prepare a simple barplot of
  # that outcome, for quality assurance purposes.
  #
  # There are 2 values for Report.df$Treated so note
  # how each value was assigned a unique color, based
  # on the way col=rainbow(2) was used.

Report.df$Damage  <- factor(Report.df$Damage,
  labels=c("Minimal", "Moderate",  "Extreme"))
  # Coerce object variable Report.df$Damage into
  # factor and assign labels

class(Report.df$Damage)        # Determine class
```

```
str(Report.df$Damage)         # Determine structure
summary(Report.df$Damage)     # Summary
Report.df$Damage              # Show all data
par(ask=TRUE)
barplot(table(Report.df$Damage), col=rainbow(3),
  main="Barplot of Report.df$Damage", font=2 )
  # Use the table() function to determine frequency
  # distribution and then prepare a simple barplot of
  # that outcome, for quality assurance purposes.
  #
  # There are 3 values for Report.df$Damage so note
  # how each value was assigned a unique color, based
  # on the way col=rainbow(3) was used.
```

With each object variable appropriately organized and assigned labels, perform a few quality assurance actions against the entire dataframe (i.e., Report.df).

```
class(Report.df)              # Determine class
str(Report.df)                # Determine structure
summary(Report.df)            # Summary
```

```
      Plot          Treated        Damage
 Plot A :1   Biological:8   Minimal :3
 Plot B :1   Chemical  :7   Moderate:8
 Plot C :1                  Extreme :4
 Plot D :1
 Plot E :1
 Plot F :1
```

Use R-based assignment to create a new object (i.e., DamageTreatment). The object DamageTreatment will be the output of applying the table() function against a crosstabulation of the object variables Report.df$Treated and Report.df$Damage.

```
DamageTreatment <- table(Report.df$Treated, Report.df$Damage)
ftable(DamageTreatment)                      # Table output
xtabs(~Treated+Damage, data=Report.df)       # Table output
summary(DamageTreatment)                     # Summary

par(ask=TRUE)
barplot(DamageTreatment, xlab="Insect Damage",
  col=c("blue","red"), legend=rownames(DamageTreatment),
  main="Stacked Bar Plot of Damage v Treatment",
  beside=FALSE, font.lab=2, font.axis=2, cex.axis=1.25)
  # Create a barplot of DamageTreatment, the crosstab of
  # Report.df$Treated and Report.df$Damage.
  #
  # Use appropriate arguments to add color, a legend, a
  # main title, bold fonts, and large print.  Use the
  # argument beside=FALSE to make a stacked barplot instead
  # of a side-by-side barplot.
```

The emphasis in this early lesson is on measurement, not R syntax. When viewing the example, the codes (e.g., Minimal, Moderate, and Extreme) used to indicate insect damage after treatment represent a degree of measurement, but certainly not a precise degree of measurement. Consider how a plot marked as Minimal, with just a slight increase in damage, could be classified as Moderate. Or, a plot marked as Extreme could have near total destruction of the crop, whereas another plot marked Extreme could have been just slightly more damaged than a field marked with Moderate damage.

Given this degree of precision, or more appropriately—lack of precision, the data associated with the object variable Report.df$Damage are ordinal and not interval. That is to say, there is certainly an ordering to the data: Extreme represents more damage than Moderate and Moderate represents more damage than Minimal. Even so, the data are ordered, only. Given only this degree of measurement, using an ordinal scale and not an interval scale, it would be appropriate to use nonparametric techniques with any analyses involving Report.df$Damage.

As a reminder about the nature of data in this sample, the data associated with objects Report.df$Plot and Report.df$Treated represent headcounts in this example. The 15 plots linked to Report.df$Plot merely have 15 different names, and there is no suggestion that there is any ordered value to the 15 plots (i.e., Report.df$Plot). Equally, the same can be said for data associated with Report.df$Treated, where two terms are used to express the type of treatment, biological or chemical. There is no suggestion that there is any degree of ordering to the treatments (Report.df$Treated) used in this example.

1.5.3 Sample Size and Possible Issues with Representation

It is common for beginning researchers to worry about sample size so much that unfortunately the issue of sample *representation* of the overall population is given inadequate attention. Sample size is important and small samples should be carefully examined to determine if nonparametric or parametric approaches should be considered for later statistical analyses. However, a small sample by itself is not the immediate concern—the main concern should always be to question if the sample is representative of the population. A theoretical example will provide a broad demonstration of how sample size may impact selected approach (nonparametric or parametric), and a second example will offer a more real-world example of how sample size needs consideration.

1.5.3.1 Example 1: Theoretical Example of Attention to Sample Size

Consider an example involving Systolic Blood Pressure (SBP) that will explore how sample size brings to question whether data should be viewed as either nonparametric or parametric. In this example the focus is on sample size and a set of sample object vectors that increasingly decrease in size. Notice how the rnorm() function is used to create a dataset and that arguments associated with the rnorm() function are used to establish the N, mean, and standard deviation of the dataset.

To demonstrate this example look at a set of six object variables where each object variable has Mean = 120 and Standard Deviation = 10. However, the sample size decreases from 1,000,000 to eventually 10—yet again, each object variable is assigned Mean = 120 and Standard Deviation = 10.

The emphasis in this example will be on the visual images since ostensibly each object variable has the same mean and standard deviation.

```
SBP_1000000 <- round(rnorm(1000000, mean=120, sd=10))
SBP_100000  <- round(rnorm(100000, mean=120, sd=10))
SBP_10000   <- round(rnorm(10000, mean=120, sd=10))
SBP_1000    <- round(rnorm(1000, mean=120, sd=10))
SBP_100     <- round(rnorm(100, mean=120, sd=10))
SBP_10      <- round(rnorm(10, mean=120, sd=10))

mean(SBP_1000000); sd(SBP_1000000); length(SBP_1000000)
mean(SBP_100000); sd(SBP_100000); length(SBP_100000)
mean(SBP_10000); sd(SBP_10000); length(SBP_10000)
mean(SBP_1000); sd(SBP_1000); length(SBP_1000)
mean(SBP_100); sd(SBP_100); length(SBP_100)
mean(SBP_10); sd(SBP_10); length(SBP_10)
  # Confirm descriptive statistics (Mean and SD) and
  # observe how length (e.g., N) declines.  Note how
  # Mean and SD are somewhat variable as length
  # declines.  This observation will also show when
  # the density plots and histograms are prepared for
  # each theoretical distribution.
```

Prepare highly-embellished graphical images of how data are distributed. Place these images into a single presentation: density plot and histogram. A set of par() function arguments, used at a global level, will enhance presentation of these images. Remember that this R-based syntax is described in far more detail in later lessons.

```
savefont      <- par(font=2)        # Bold
savelwd       <- par(lwd=4)         # Line Width
savecol       <- par(col="red")     # Color
savecex.lab   <- par(cex.lab=1.25)  # Label Size
savecex.axis  <- par(cex.axis=1.25) # Axis Size
savefont.lab  <- par(font.lab=2)    # Label Bold
savefont.axis <- par(font.axis=2)   # Axis Bold
par(ask=TRUE)                   # Side-by-Side
par(mfrow=c(3,2))               # Density Plots
plot(density(SBP_1000000)) # N = 1000000
plot(density(SBP_100000))  # N = 100000
plot(density(SBP_10000))   # N = 10000
plot(density(SBP_1000))    # N = 1000
plot(density(SBP_100))     # N = 100
plot(density(SBP_10))      # N = 10
```

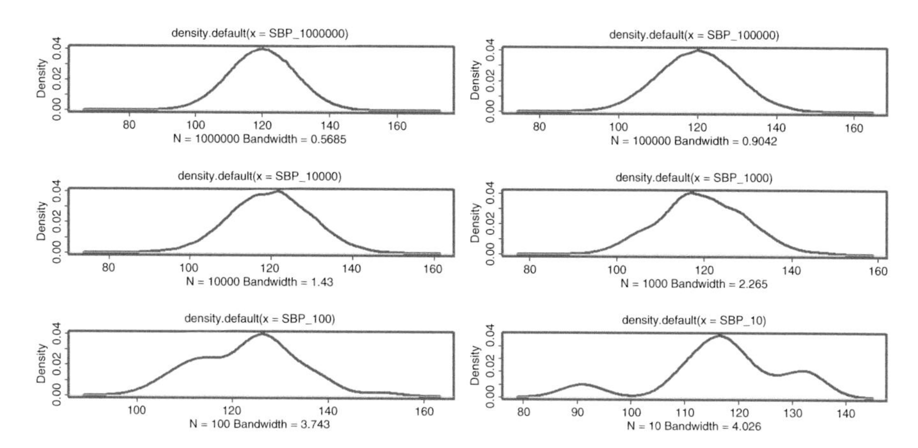

Fig. 1.4 Multiple density plots

```
par(savefont); par(savelwd); par(savecol);
par(savecex.lab); par(savecex.axis);
par(savefont.lab); par(savefont.axis)
```

Notice how there is a semblance of normal distribution until the last few density plots, where the number of subjects in the sample declines greatly. For object variable SBP_10, with only ten values, there is simply no demonstration of normal distribution. It would be unwise to use a parametric analysis that demands normal distribution. This is an example of where a nonparametric approach would be best for any analyses involving SBP_10, all due to failure to see normal distribution with such a small sample size (Fig. 1.4).

A histogram of data distribution for each Systolic Blood Pressure (SBP) sample may be a better graphic if the density plot is currently an unfamiliar graphical tool.

```
savefont      <- par(font=2)         # Bold
savelwd       <- par(lwd=4)          # Line Width
savecex.lab   <- par(cex.lab=1.25)   # Label Size
savecex.axis  <- par(cex.axis=1.25)  # Axis Size
savefont.lab  <- par(font.lab=2)     # Label Bold
savefont.axis <- par(font.axis=2)    # Axis Bold
par(ask=TRUE)                      # Side-by-Side
par(mfrow=c(3,2))                  # Histograms
hist(SBP_1000000, col="red", xlim=c(0,200)) # N = 1000000
hist(SBP_100000, col="red", xlim=c(0,200))  # N = 100000
hist(SBP_10000, col="red", xlim=c(0,200))   # N = 10000
hist(SBP_1000, col="red", xlim=c(0,200))    # N = 1000
hist(SBP_100, col="red", xlim=c(0,200))     # N = 100
hist(SBP_10, col="red", xlim=c(0,200))      # N = 10
par(savefont); par(savelwd);
par(savecex.lab); par(savecex.axis);
par(savefont.lab); par(savefont.axis)
```

Similar to what was displayed in the density plots, look at the way the distribution pattern begins to degrade when the sample size (i.e., N, or length() using R syntax) gets exceedingly small. Even at N = 100 there is some semblance of normal distribution. However, with an exceptionally small sample size, as seen with SBP_10, it is simply not possible to say that the data for this sample (i.e., SBP_10) exhibit normal distribution, at least using a visual display of the data.

1.5.3.2 Example 2: Real-World Example of Attention to Sample Size

Sample size needs to be considered when exploring data and possibly later when deciding that a sample does not warrant a parametric approach to data analysis, such that a nonparametric approach may be the more appropriate selection. However, sample size alone is not the one-and-only determining issue. A small dataset could easily show normal distribution and a large dataset could equally fail to achieve normal distribution. Sample size, alone, is not the determining factor to automatically decide if data are best viewed as either nonparametric or parametric.

Consider the two similar sample datasets shown below, with each dataset consisting of nine numeric values. The values represent subject weights (pounds). Each dataset has nine values, but one dataset (Class_A) exhibits a semblance of normal distribution and the other dataset (Class_B) does not exhibit normal distribution. Again, representation of the dataset (typically, displayed as a histogram or density plot) must be considered along with sample size.

Imagine a class (e.g., Class_A) of Grade 7 students (typically 11, 12, or 13 years old), where there are only nine students in the class. Each student was weighed (pounds, not kilograms), and the weights are expressed below using R syntax:

```
Class_A <- c(105, 109, 100, 113, 120, 108, 111, 117, 121)
  # Create a numeric-based object vector

median(Class_A)                   # Median
mean(Class_A)                     # Mean
sd(Class_A)                       # Standard Deviation
summary(Class_A)                  # Summary
```

Now, imagine another class (e.g., Class_B) of nine students that somehow had the same weights for the first seven (of the nine) students in Class_A, but see how the descriptive statistics change when the weights for Class_B Student 8 and Class_B Student 9 are different from the weights for Class_A Student 8 and Class_A Student 9. Again, only two students (e.g., Class_B Student 8 and Class_B Student 9) had different weights than their counterparts in Class_A.

```
Class_B <- c(105, 109, 100, 113, 120, 108, 111, 187, 221)
  # Create a numeric-based object vector

median(Class_B)              # Median
mean(Class_B)                # Mean
sd(Class_B)                  # Standard Deviation
summary(Class_B)             # Summary
```

A side-by-side graphical image of density plots for Class_A and Class_B will show data distribution patterns for students in these two classes.

```
savefont      <- par(font=2)         # Bold
savelwd       <- par(lwd=4)          # Line Width
savecol       <- par(col="red")      # Color
savecex.lab   <- par(cex.lab=1.25)   # Label Size
savecex.axis  <- par(cex.axis=1.25)  # Axis Size
savefont.lab  <- par(font.lab=2)     # Label Bold
savefont.axis <- par(font.axis=2)    # Axis Bold
par(ask=TRUE)            # Side-by-Side Density Plots
par(mfrow=c(1,2))        # of Class_A and Class_B
plot(density(Class_A))
plot(density(Class_B))
par(savefont); par(savelwd); par(savecol);
par(savecex.lab); par(savecex.axis);
par(savefont.lab); par(savefont.axis)
```

With a somewhat different emphasis on graphical presentation, a set of side-by-side dotcharts provides another view of data distribution.

```
savefont      <- par(font=2)         # Bold
savelwd       <- par(lwd=2)          # Line Width
savecol       <- par(col="red")      # Color
savefont.lab  <- par(font.lab=2)     # Label Bold
savefont.axis <- par(font.axis=2)    # Axis Bold
par(ask=TRUE)            # Side-by-Side Density Plots
par(mfrow=c(1,2))        # of Class_A and Class_B
dotchart(Class_A,
  main="Dotchart Class A Weights",   # Main title
  xlab="Weight (Pounds)",            # X axis label
  ylab="Subject",                    # Y axis label
  xlim=c(0,250),                     # X axis limits
  pch=19,                            # Dot type (solid circle)
  col=(1:9),                         # Color sequence
  cex=1.25)                          # Font size
dotchart(Class_B, main="Dotchart Class B Weights",
  xlab="Weight (Pounds)", ylab="Subject", xlim=c(0,250),
  pch=19, col=(1:9), cex=1.25)
par(savefont); par(savelwd); par(savecol); par(savefont.lab);
par(savefont.axis)
```

If the vertical presentation of a dotchart is hard to follow then consider the use of a stripchart to show the same data for Class_A and Class_B.

```
savefont      <- par(font=2)        # Bold
savelwd       <- par(lwd=2)         # Line Width
savecol       <- par(col="red")     # Color
savefont.lab  <- par(font.lab=2)    # Label Bold
savefont.axis <- par(font.axis=2)   # Axis Bold
par(ask=TRUE)          # Side-by-Side Density Plots
par(mfrow=c(1,2))      # of Class_A and Class_B
stripchart(Class_A,
  main="Stripchart Class A Weights",# Main title
  xlab="Weight (Pounds)",           # X axis label
  xlim=c(0,250),                    # X axis limits
  pch=19,                           # Symbol
  cex=1.10)                         # Font size
stripchart(Class_B, main="Stripchart Class B Weights",
  xlab="Weight (Pounds)", xlim=c(0,250), pch=19, cex=1.10)
par(savefont); par(savelwd); par(savecol); par(savefont.lab);
par(savefont.axis)
```

Regarding descriptive statistics for subjects from both groups, the median weight was 111 pounds for subjects in both Class_A and Class_B. In contrast, the mean weight for subjects in Class_A was 111.5556 pounds, and the mean weight for subjects in Class_B was 130.4444 pounds.

- Of course, the median weight is based on a ranking of the data, with the median representing a midpoint. In this example, the midpoint is the same for both Class_A and Class_B.
- In contrast, the mean weight represents an arithmetic average. The arithmetic average changed greatly when weight for Class_B Student 8 and Class_B Student 9 was substituted for the weight of Class_A Student 8 and Class_A Student 9.

```
Class_A; median(Class_A); mean(Class_A); sd(Class_A)
```

```
[1] 105 109 100 113 120 108 111 117 121
[1] 111
[1] 111.5556
[1] 6.966188
```

```
Class_B; median(Class_B); mean(Class_B); sd(Class_B)
```

```
[1] 105 109 100 113 120 108 111 187 221
[1] 111
[1] 130.4444
[1] 42.9072
```

Considering the large difference in mean weights for students from both classes, recall that the only change in this simple example was the weight for two students. A weight of 187 pounds for Class_B Student 8 seems somewhat high, but it is perhaps not totally unexpected for a Grade 7 student ranging in age from 11 to 13 years old. However, did Class_B Student 9 really weight 221 pounds? Is this value an outlier or is this value an error, either due to an initial error in data collection when field notes were prepared or a later error during data entry? Although uncommon, it is possible that an 11–13 year old Grade 7 student could weight 221 pounds. Of course, an error of some type could also be the reason for this value—an incorrect value if that were the case. The diligent researcher will go back to the original source of data and either confirm or discount the presence of outliers or, if needed, identify the error source and make corrections.

Assume that the data for both Class_A and Class_B are correct. If that were the case, would it be appropriate to use a Student's t-Test for Independent Samples to compare weights for Class_A to Class_B, to see if there were a statistically significant difference (`p <= 0.05`) in weights between the two classes? Ideally, a test of this type might assume that the two samples (e.g., Class_A weights and Class_B weights) are taken from the same population, but that assumption could easily be disputed in this example after looking at the Class_A and Class_B side-by-side density plots, dotcharts, and stripcharts.

- Going back to the advance organizer mentioned at the beginning of this lesson, it could be stated that the weights for Class_A follow an acceptable normal distribution pattern and that the data are parametric even though the sample is somewhat small (i.e., N = 9). As a fairly broad statement, there are parameters for the Class_A data and these parameters are visually evident in a density plot.
- However, there may be a question if the data for Class_B follow an acceptable normal distribution pattern. The extreme variance in data for Class_B are such that it could be declared that the data for Class_B are nonparametric. They do not follow set (i.e., expected) parameters.

This simple example is presented within the context of an exceptionally small (e.g., Class_A N = 9 and Class_B N = 9) sample for each of the two object variables. Sample size (either small or large) by itself is not enough to declare if data meet the assumptions needed for parametric analysis. It is generally best to graphically display the data, regardless of sample size, to view representation.

1.6 Definition of Nonparametric Analysis

Given this discussion about nonparametric statistics and sample datasets that may benefit from a nonparametric approach to inferential analysis, nonparametric statistics provide a useful purpose for when data meet certain conditions:

- Consider a nonparametric approach to statistical analysis when data do not meet the precision of an interval scale and instead data are viewed from a nominal or ordinal perspective.
- Consider a nonparametric approach to statistical analysis when there are serious concerns about extreme deviation from normal distribution.

- Consider a nonparametric approach to statistical analysis when there is considerable difference in the number of subjects for each breakout group.

Given these different considerations, it is evident that there is no single visual test to determine if data meet the assumptions needed to use analyses that depend on a parametric approach to data analysis. It is perhaps best to say that nonparametric statistics takes into account those analyses where there are no (or at least fewer) assumptions about data distribution patterns (i.e., normal distribution) and the subsequent impact of distribution patterns on parameters typically associated with the mean and either variance or standard deviation. As often found in the literature, nonparametric analyses are based on the assumption that data are distribution free.

Given this definition and from a practical viewpoint, nonparametric analyses are often associated with either beginning exploratory analyses or ending confirmatory analyses. More importantly, nonparametric analyses are often used when there may be questions whether data meet the assumptions need for parametric analysis. An experienced researcher may want to subject a dataset to both nonparametric and parametric analyses, to: (1) first explore the data and (2) later confirm outcomes using a different view of the data.

Consider another simple example, either of subject weights or subject Systolic Blood Pressure (SBP). Instruments and protocols exist such that it is generally a reasonable task to obtain reliable and valid measures for either weight or SBP. For either weight or SBP, imagine that the data show a semblance of normal distribution, but there is some observed deviation away from a normal distribution pattern:

- How much deviation from normal distribution can a researcher accept before a parametric approach is considered inappropriate and a nonparametric approach is a more prudent choice? This question can be applied as general exploratory analyses are approached or it can be applied as a confirming activity.
- For day-to-day research, as opposed to the simple examples shown in this introductory lesson, data do not come pre-labeled as either nonparametric or parametric. Many actions, perhaps involving the preparation of both descriptive statistics and graphical presentations, are needed before a judgment of this type can be made with any degree of assurance. Even then, peers may have other views and these other views should be considered as part of an interactive and collaborative decision-making process.

Nonparametric statistics have an important role in biostatistics in that they provide a set of tools for when data do not follow any reasonable interpretation of normal distribution, for whatever reason (i.e., extreme values or sample size) and therefore assumptions about distribution cannot be accepted. A nonparametric approach to data analysis should never be viewed as a second choice. Instead, a nonparametric approach to data analysis should be viewed along a continuum of acceptable choices, with the best choice based on data characteristics and research needs.

1.7 Statistical Tests and Graphics Associated with Normal Distribution

In this lesson, the emphasis has been on a visual display of distribution patterns. The use of density plots, histograms, dot charts, and strip charts are all certainly useful and they are excellent tools for presenting overall distribution of selected datasets. A general sense of data distribution is gained from these visual observations and consequently some degree of judgment is made regarding analysis of the data from a nonparametric perspective or from a parametric perspective.

Going beyond visual inspection, be sure to always consider the many statistics directly associated with data distribution:

- Mode
- Median
- Mean (Arithmetic Mean, Geometric Mean, and Harmonic Mean)
- Variance
- Standard Deviation
- Minimum, Maximum, and Range
- Skewness
- Kurtosis

There is at least one R-based function in support of each of these statistics and there are often multiple functions for each type of analysis, with these many functions found in different R-based packages.[5]

There are also a few statistical tests, also supported by R, that provide some degree of empirical estimate of normal distribution and these include:

- Anderson-Darling Test for Normality
- Kolmogorov-Smirnov Test
- Lilliefors (Kolmogorov-Smirnov) Test for Normality
- Shapiro-Wilk Normality Test

For this discussion, consider two separate datasets: X_rnorm and X_runif. These two datasets are created in a manner similar to what was seen at the beginning of this lesson. For each, the dataset will be created using R in an interactive fashion, the dataset will be presented visually, and then the many statistics associated with distribution patterns and mentioned immediately above will be presented. The specialized tests, such as the Anderson-Darling Test for Normality, the Lilliefors (Kolmogorov-Smirnov) Test for Normality, and the Shapiro-Wilk Normality Test have some value and explicit detail on how each test is used in R is available

[5]As open-source software, a comparative advantage of R over proprietary software is that the user community contributes to development of the software. A limited degree of functionality is available when R software is first downloaded. The extreme functionality comes from the more than 5000 packages available to the R community, with most packages having 25, 50, 100, or more functions. These packages are easily and freely obtained, from host sites throughout the world.

by using the R help(function_name) function (e.g., help(mean), help(median), help(sd), etc.).[6]

Some of the R syntax used below calls for the use of functions found in external R-based packages. When R is first downloaded a large set of base functions is immediately available. However, there are thousands (perhaps 5000 or more) external R-based packages that have functions that provide opportunities for analysis and graphical presentation far beyond what is available when the base R package is downloaded. Note below how these packages are obtained, how they are named, and how they are used. As a general comment, it is the availability of these thousands of R-based packages and functions that makes R a superior environment for data analysis and graphical presentation.

```
install.packages("nortest")
library(nortest)              # Load the nortest package.
help(package=nortest)         # Show the information page.
sessionInfo()                 # Confirm all attached packages.
# Select the most local mirror site using Set CRAN mirror.

install.packages("asbio")
library(asbio)                # Load the asbio package.
help(package=asbio)           # Show the information page.
sessionInfo()                 # Confirm all attached packages.
# Select the most local mirror site using Set CRAN mirror.

install.packages("psych")
library(psych)                # Load the psych package.
help(package=psych)           # Show the information page.
sessionInfo()                 # Confirm all attached packages.
# Select the most local mirror site using Set CRAN mirror.
```

Create a Dataset That Should Ostensibly Show Normal Distribution

```
X_rnorm <- round(rnorm(5000, mean=100, sd=5))
  # Create an object called X_rnorm, which consists of 5,000
  # random subjects, with mean equal to 100 and standard
  # deviation equal to 5.  The object X_rnorm represents a
  # theoretical set of otherwise unnamed measurements.  Note
  # how the round() function was also used, so that whole
  # numbers are generated, only.
  #
  # When using the rnorm() function and the runif() function,
  # be sure to note how the actual values generated will change
  # with each use.
```

[6]Regarding assessment of normality, consider also how the qqnorm(), qqline(), and qqplot() functions are typically used when investigating distribution patterns. There remains some degree of inconsistency as to whether the correct usage is either QQ or Q-Q when referencing the term Quantile-Quantile. Both terms (i.e., QQ or Q-Q) may be found in this text.

General Summary of the Dataset

```
head(X_rnorm)                          # First line(s) of data
tail(X_rnorm)                          # Last line(s) of data
summary(X_rnorm)                       # Summary
length(X_rnorm)                        # N
```

R-Based Functions Specific to Distribution Patterns

```
asbio::Mode(X_rnorm)                   # Mode
median(X_rnorm)                        # Median
mean(X_rnorm)                          # Arithmetic Mean
asbio::H.mean(X_rnorm)                 # Harmonic Mean
psych::geometric.mean(X_rnorm)         # Geometric Mean
var(X_rnorm)                           # Variance
sd(X_rnorm)                            # Standard Deviation
range(X_rnorm)                         # Range
asbio::skew(X_rnorm)                   # Skewness
asbio::kurt(X_rnorm)                   # Kurtosis
nortest::ad.test(X_rnorm)              # Anderson-Darling Test
nortest::lillie.test(X_rnorm)          # Lilliefors (KS)
shapiro.test(X_rnorm)                  # Shapiro-Wilk
```

Visual Presentation of Distribution Pattern

```
par(ask=TRUE)                          # Side-by-Side Histogram,
par(mfrow=c(1,3))                      # Density Plot, and QQPlot
hist(X_rnorm,                          # Histogram function
  breaks=25,                           # Adequate bins
  col="red",                           # Color
  font=2,                              # Bold
  font.lab=2,                          # Bold labels
  cex.axis=1.5,                        # Large axis
  main="Histogram of X_rnorm",         # Title
  xlab="X_rnorm Measurement",          # Label text
  xlim=c(50,150))                      # Axis limits
plot(density(X_rnorm), lwd=6, col="red",
  font=2, font.lab=2, cex.axis=1.5,
  main="Density Plot of X_norm",
  xlab="X_rnorm Measurement)",
  xlim=c(50,150))
qqnorm(X_rnorm, col="red", font=2,
  font.lab=2, cex.axis=1.5,
  main="QQPlot of X_rnorm")
qqline(X_rnorm, lwd=3, col="darkblue")
```

Create a Dataset That Fails to Show Normal Distribution

```
X_runif <- round(runif(5000, min=85, max=115))
  # Create an object called X_runif, which consists of 5,000
  # subjects.  The minimum value will be 85 and the maximum
  # value will be 115.  Note how these limits are in general
  # parity of + and - three standard deviations of the above
  # example, where mean was 100 and standard deviation was 5
```

```
# (e.g., 100 - (5 * 3 SDs) = 85 and 100 + (5 * 3 SDs) = 115).
# The object X_runif represents a theoretical representation
# of measurements, but by no means a normal distribution that
# is based on a set mean and a set standard deviation.
# Again, the round() function was used, so that whole numbers
# are generated, only.
#
# When using the rnorm() function and the runif() function,
# be sure to note how the actual values generated will change
# with each use.
```

General Summary of the Dataset

```
head(X_runif)                       # First line(s) of data
tail(X_runif)                       # Last line(s) of data
summary(X_runif)                    # Summary
length(X_runif)                     # N
```

R-Based Functions Specific to Distribution Patterns

```
asbio::Mode(X_runif)                # Mode
median(X_runif)                     # Median
mean(X_runif)                       # Arithmetic Mean
asbio::H.mean(X_runif)              # Harmonic Mean
psych::geometric.mean(X_rnorm)      # Geometric Mean
var(X_runif)                        # Variance
sd(X_runif)                         # Standard Deviation
range(X_runif)                      # Range
asbio::skew(X_runif)                # Skewness
asbio::kurt(X_runif)                # Kurtosis
nortest::ad.test(X_runif)           # Anderson-Darling Test
nortest::lillie.test(X_runif)       # Lilliefors (KS)
shapiro.test(X_runif)               # Shapiro-Wilk
```

These many statistics and associated functions certainly have value and eventually can be used to support decision-making regarding judgment on normal distribution. Yet, it is important to recall that sample size is important when using tests such as the Anderson-Darling Test. With a small sample a large deviation from normality may not be detected. Conversely, with large samples a small deviation from normality may well result in test-based rejection of normality when the opposite is the case. As such, visual presentations have a prime role in the **human decision** to accept or reject whether a dataset exhibits normal distribution (Fig. 1.5).

Visual Presentation of Distribution Pattern

```
par(ask=TRUE)                       # Side-by-Side Histogram,
par(mfrow=c(1,3))                   # Density Plot, and QQPlot
hist(X_runif,                       # Histogram function
  breaks=25,                        # Adequate bins
  col="red",                        # Color
  font=2,                           # Bold
  font.lab=2,                       # Bold labels
```

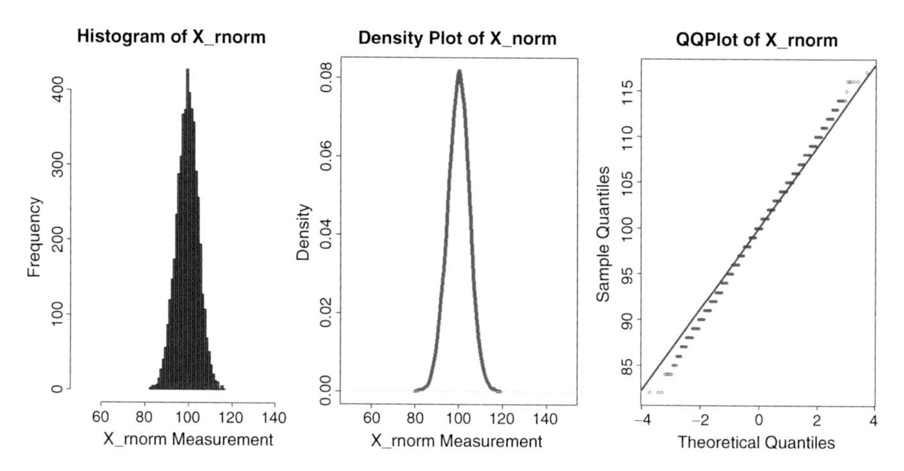

Fig. 1.5 Histogram, density plot, and Quantile-Quantile plot: normal distribution

```
  cex.axis=1.5,                      # Large axis
  main="Histogram of X_runif",       # Title
  xlab="X_runif Measurement",        # Label text
  xlim=c(50,150))                    # Axis limits
plot(density(X_runif), lwd=6, col="red",
  font=2, font.lab=2, cex.axis=1.5,
  main="Density Plot of X_norm",
  xlab="X_runif Measurement)",
  xlim=c(50,150))
qqnorm(X_runif, col="red", font=2,
  font.lab=2, cex.axis=1.5,
  main="QQPlot of X_runif")
qqline(X_runif, lwd=3, col="darkblue")
```

It is beyond the purpose of this lesson to provide explicit notes on statistics such as skewness (focusing on the tails of a distribution) and kurtosis (focusing on the peakedness of a distribution). Many resources could be reviewed for these statistics, as well as tests such as the Anderson-Darling Test for Normality, the Lilliefors (Kolmogorov-Smirnov) Test for Normality, and the Shapiro-Wilk Normality Test. The major focus in this lesson was to review descriptive statistics, such as median and mean, and to then prepare graphical images of distribution patterns to visually observe how the data for a specific variable appear when put into some type of figure.

Ideally, good judgment supported by extensive review of the data will serve as the basis for judgment on whether data are best used from a nonparametric perspective, or if the data meet the conditions needed for use from a parametric perspective.

As a final reminder about this introduction, the many R-based functions and arguments shown in this lesson will be viewed multiple times throughout this set of lessons. These functions and arguments will be detailed in general narrative as well as in R-based syntax comments.

1.8 Addendum: Data Distribution and Sampling

The concept of data distribution patterns and the importance of normal distribution on inferential test selection should not be overlooked. Look again at the reminder about how nonparametric statistics provide a useful purpose for inferential analyses when data: (1) do not meet the purported precision of an interval scale, (2) there are serious concerns about extreme deviation from normal distribution, and (3) there is considerable difference in the number of subjects for each breakout group.

This addendum focuses on different ways that R can be used to visually present data distribution patterns. This visualization provides a perspective of the data that goes beyond review of static numerical statistics. Quite simply, how far can a sample deviate from normal distribution before there are concerns that normal distribution has been violated beyond what can be reasonably accepted? What are the best, or at least most common, tools used to visually represent data distribution? Perhaps the best way to start discussion on this issue is to graphically demonstrate a large dataset that exhibits normal distribution and to then compare this large dataset to a sample from the dataset that is smaller and may, or may not, violate accepted normal distribution.

For this addendum consider Intelligence Quotient (IQ) scores for 100,000 adult subjects. Although IQ is a construct more appropriately associated with psychology, education, and the social sciences (and not biostatistics) it was selected for this demonstration since most adults have some general awareness of IQ scores, IQ testing, the meaning of IQ scores, and the impact of IQ scores throughout society.

A series of R-based functions will be used to create a numeric object variable called IQ (i.e., Intelligence Quotient). In this lesson, the object variable IQ will be populated with 100,000 subjects. The mean will be 100 and the standard deviation will be 15. This Mean and Standard Deviation parallels expected norms for IQ among adult subjects. The object variable IQ, with 100,000 subjects, will then be subjected to a few R functions to eventually generate a sample consisting of 1000 IQ scores. Throughout this addendum, the focus will be on visualization and R-based graphical imagery.

Observe the syntax below to see how the rnorm() function was used to create the object IQ for this demonstration. As the theoretical dataset for this demonstration is constructed, the R function set.seed() will be used to encourage some degree of consistency for data and later outcomes.[7]

```
set.seed(10)                            # Promote consistency
IQ <- rnorm(100000, mean=100, sd=15)    # Create the object
is.vector(IQ)                           # Quality assurance
class(IQ)                               # Quality assurance
```

[7]IQ scores in this demonstration are generated using the rnorm() function. The individual datapoints in the object variable IQ will likely change each time the rnorm() function is used to generate a new set of IQ scores, even though the overall dataset maintains Mean = 100 and SD = 15.

```
head(IQ)                                # Review data
tail(IQ)                                # Review data
length(IQ)                              # Descriptive statistics
summary(IQ)                             # Descriptive statistics
```

```
> set.seed(10)                          # Promote consistency
> IQ <- rnorm(100000, mean=100, sd=15)  # Create the object
> is.vector(IQ)                         # Quality assurance
[1] TRUE
> class(IQ)                             # Quality assurance
[1] "numeric"
> head(IQ)                              # Review data
[1] 100.28119  97.23621  79.43004  91.01248 104.41818 105.84691
> tail(IQ)                              # Review data
[1]  86.33463  88.31597  96.82652  83.29804  75.13473 122.73481
> length(IQ)                            # Descriptive statistics
[1] 100000
> summary(IQ)                           # Descriptive statistics
   Min. 1st Qu.  Median    Mean 3rd Qu.    Max.
  36.05   89.76   99.94   99.91  110.00  167.00
```

Note above how IQ scores show in decimal format. However, IQ scores are expressed as whole numbers, so use the round() function to accommodate the values in this otherwise theoretical dataset.

```
IQ <- round(IQ)                         # Adjust dataset
is.vector(IQ)                           # Quality assurance
class(IQ)                               # Quality assurance
head(IQ)                                # Review data
tail(IQ)                                # Review data
length(IQ)                              # Descriptive statistics
summary(IQ)                             # Descriptive statistics
```

```
> IQ <- round(IQ)                       # Adjust dataset
> is.vector(IQ)                         # Quality assurance
[1] TRUE
> class(IQ)                             # Quality assurance
[1] "numeric"
> head(IQ)                              # Review data
[1] 100  97  79  91 104 106
> tail(IQ)                              # Review data
[1]  86  88  97  83  75 123
> length(IQ)                            # Descriptive statistics
[1] 100000
> summary(IQ)                           # Descriptive statistics
   Min. 1st Qu.  Median    Mean 3rd Qu.    Max.
  36.00   90.00  100.00   99.91  110.00  167.00
```

Note: Remember that R is case sensitive (i.e., iq, Iq, iQ, etc., are not the same as uppercase IQ).

Using no arguments or embellishments, prepare a simple histogram of the vector IQ.

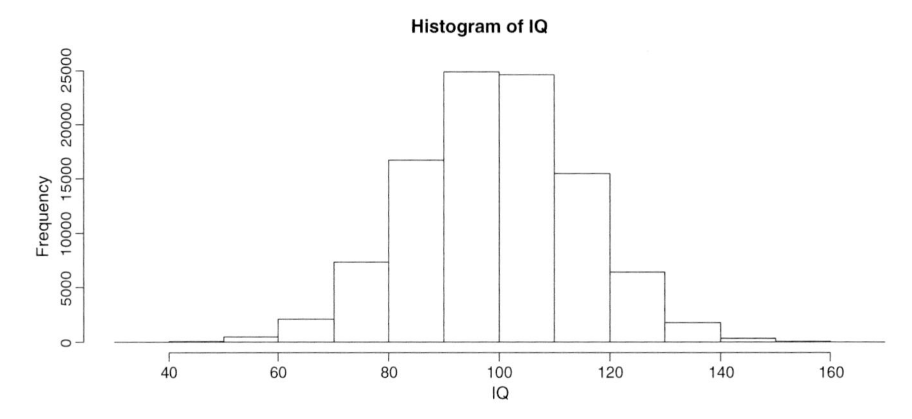

Fig. 1.6 Throwaway histogram

```
par(ask=TRUE); hist(IQ) # ; allows all syntax on one line.
```

From this initial presentation, prepare a slightly more detailed histogram of object variable IQ and then alter the number of intervals (i.e., often called *bins* with other software programs) included in the histogram using the nclass argument. Consolidate the different histograms into one common figure by using the par(mfrow=c(2,3)) function and argument.[8] This action is used to create a graphic with two rows, three columns, and a graphical image placed in each cell (Fig. 1.6).

Be sure to notice how results in the histogram appear as the number of intervals increases, by using the nclass argument. To highlight and contrast data distribution and the number of histogram intervals (i.e., bars), use multiple colors for histogram intervals. The use of multiple colors for histogram intervals is for demonstration purposes only. Usually this would be an undesirable practice in any formal publication or group presentation.

```
par(mfrow=c(2,3))     # 2 by 3 (Row by Column)
par(ask=TRUE)
############################################
hist(IQ, col="red", font=2, cex.lab=1.25,
  main="IQ Scores - Default nclass")
  # font=2 ......... Bold print
  # cex.lab=125 .... Large label(s)
############################################
par(ask=TRUE)
hist(IQ, col=c("red", "green"),
  font=2, cex.lab=1.25, nclass=005,
  main="IQ Scores - nclass = 005")
```

[8]There are six cells in this figure; 2 rows * 3 columns = 6 cells. The individual cells are populated from left to right.

```
###########################################
par(ask=TRUE)
hist(IQ, col=c("red", "green", "blue"),
  font=2, cex.lab=1.25, nclass=010,
  main="IQ Scores - nclass = 010")
###########################################
par(ask=TRUE)
hist(IQ, col=c("red", "green", "blue",
  "magenta"),
  font=2, cex.lab=1.25, nclass=050,
  main="IQ Scores - nclass = 050")
###########################################
par(ask=TRUE)
hist(IQ, col=c("red", "green", "blue",
  "magenta", "black"),
  font=2, cex.lab=1.25, nclass=100,
  main="IQ Scores - nclass = 100")
###########################################
par(ask=TRUE)
hist(IQ, col=c("red", "green", "blue",
  "magenta", "black", "violet"),
  font=2, cex.lab=1.25, nclass=125,
  main="IQ Scores - nclass = 125")
###########################################
```

Going back to a simple histogram, add a title over the top of the histogram and a label under the X axis. Embellish the axis with bold font and larger font, to make it easier to read. Use the rug() function to add a rug below the X axis to provide a sense of N for each place along the continuum of the histogram (Fig. 1.7).

```
par(ask=TRUE)
hist(IQ, nclass=150, col=c("red"),
  main="Histogram of IQ Scores:  N = 100,000,
```

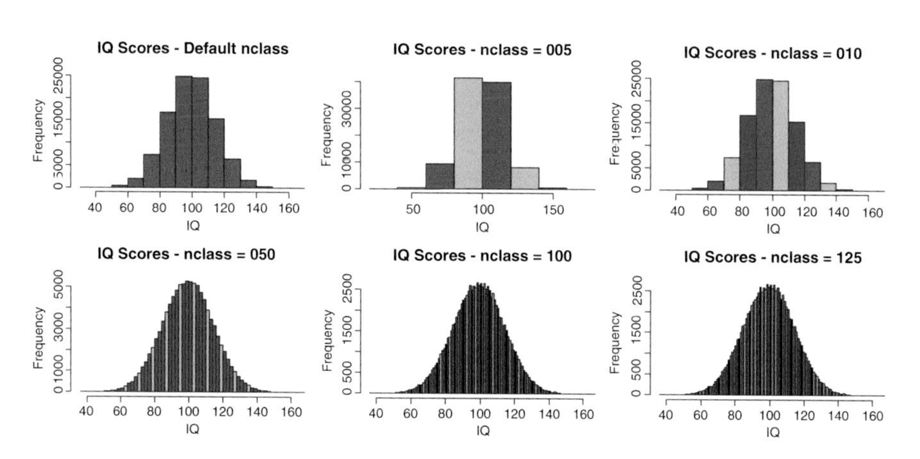

Fig. 1.7 Throwaway histograms showing multiple nclass declarations

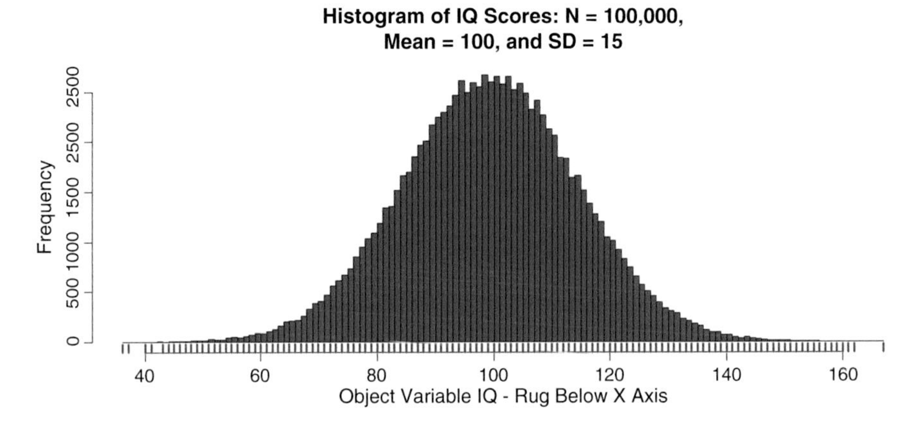

Fig. 1.8 Histogram showing a rug along the X axis

```
  Mean = 100, and SD = 15",
  xlab="Object Variable IQ - Rug Below X Axis",
  cex.lab=1.25, font=2)
rug(IQ, col=c("darkblue"), lwd=3) # Moderate line
```

Show a density curve instead of a histogram for object variable IQ. Use the lwd argument to make the density curve show as a large, dark line (Fig. 1.8).

```
par(ask=TRUE)
plot(density(IQ), col=c("red"),
  main="Density Plot of IQ Scores:  N = 100,000,
  Mean = 100, and SD = 15",
  xlab="Object Variable IQ", cex.lab=1.25, font=2,
  lwd=6)                               # Heavy dark line
```

As useful as these initial views may be, use the descr::histkdnc() function to gain yet another view of how the data in IQ are distributed. Observe how there is multiple visualization of a density curve, histogram, and normal curve in the same figure. A rug (i.e., a graphic device added to a plot and composed of multiple vertical lines) will also be displayed under the histogram, again, to give a sense of the N for each datapoint along the histogram (Fig. 1.9).

```
install.packages("descr")
library(descr)                  # Load the descr package.
help(package=descr)             # Show the information page.
sessionInfo()                   # Confirm all attached packages.
# Select the most local mirror site using Set CRAN mirror.

savelwd      <- par(lwd=6)         # Heavy line
savefont     <- par(font=2)        # Bold
savecex.lab  <- par(cex.lab=1.25)  # Label
```

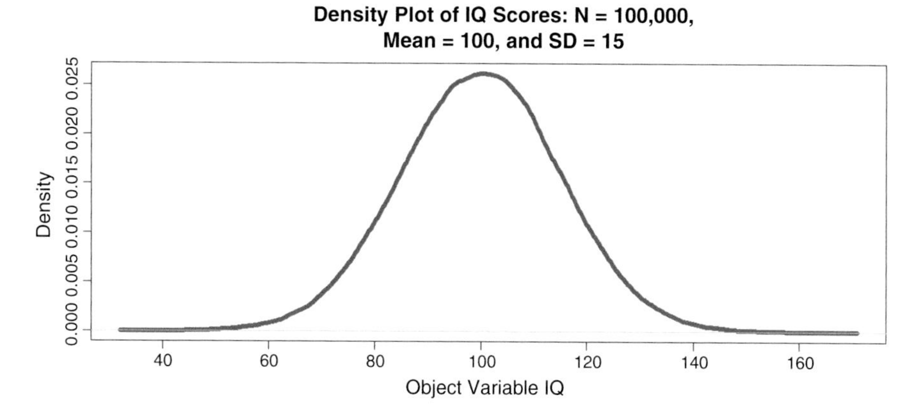

Fig. 1.9 Density plot

```
savecex.axis <- par(cex.axis=1.25) # Axis
par(ask=TRUE)
descr::histkdnc(IQ,
  main="Density Curve, Histogram, and Normal Curve of IQ
  Scores:  N = 100,000, Mean = 100, and SD = 15",
  xlab="Object Variable IQ - Rug Below X Axis",
  col=grey(0.95))          # Allow color contrast with lines
rug(IQ, col=c("deeppink"), lwd=3)
  # The rug is below the histogram.
par(savelwd); par(savefont); par(savecex.lab);
par(savecex.axis)              # Use ; to move to next line
```

To gain another view of distribution patterns, prepare a boxplot (i.e., box-and-whiskers) of IQ and look for the small circles (e.g., bubbles) beyond the whiskers, which show the presence of outliers. Next, embellish the boxplot to improve presentation, whether for later publication or group presentation. As an additional way to view data distribution, prepare a violin plot of the object variable IQ (Figs. 1.10 and 1.11).

```
install.packages("vioplot")
library(vioplot)               # Load the vioplot package.
help(package=vioplot)          # Show the information page.
sessionInfo()                  # Confirm all attached packages.
# Select the most local mirror site using Set CRAN mirror.

par(mfrow=c(1,3))    # 1 by 3 (Row by Column)
par(ask=TRUE)
##################################################
boxplot(IQ, ylim=c(0,200))
##################################################
boxplot(IQ,
  main="Boxplot of IQ Scores:  N = 100,000,
  Mean = 100, and SD = 15",
```

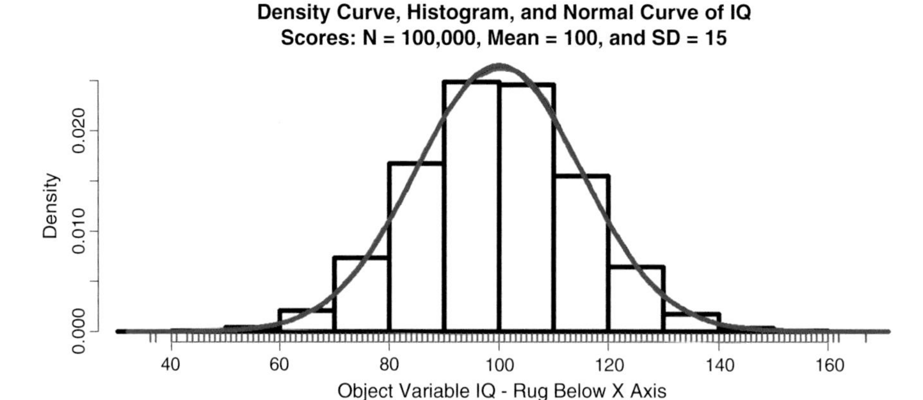

Fig. 1.10 Multiple graphing curves in one figure

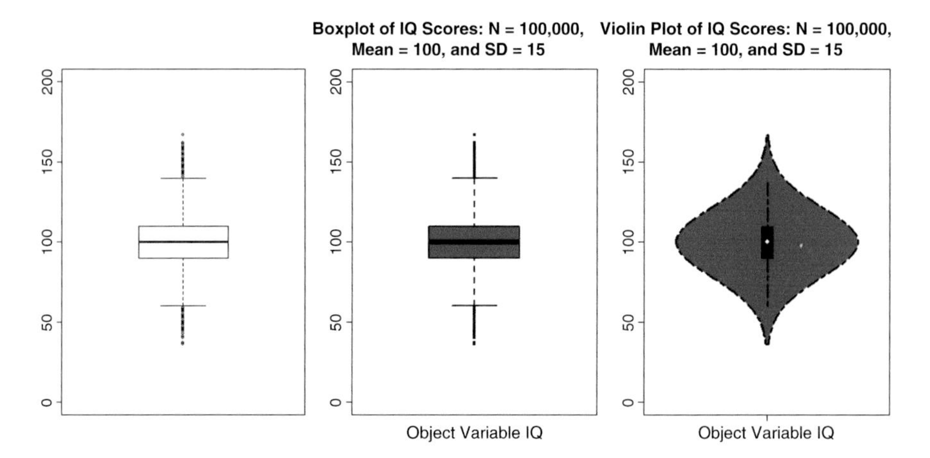

Fig. 1.11 Boxplot and violin plot in one figure

```
  xlab="Object Variable IQ", col=c("red"),
  font.lab=2, font.axis=2, font.main=2,
  cex.lab=1.15, cex.axis=1.15, lwd=2,
  ylim=c(0,200))                 # Scale for Y axis
  # Generate large labels with bold fonts that
  # are slightly enhanced
###############################################
vioplot::vioplot(IQ, col="red", horizontal=FALSE,
  names=c("Object Variable IQ"), lwd=3, lty=6,
  ylim=c(0,200))
  # Double Dash (lty=6) and Moderate (lwd=3) line
  title("Violin Plot of IQ Scores:  N = 100,000,
  Mean = 100, and SD = 15")
###############################################
```

Although these many graphical figures are useful, a fairly complex (but easily prepared) figure may best show distribution of IQ scores and how the data follow normal distribution in this initial theoretical demonstration.

Prepare an object variable representing the Mean of IQ and another object variable representing the Standard Deviation of IQ.

```
IQMean <- mean(IQ)
IQMean

IQStdv <- sd(IQ)
IQStdv
```

```
> IQMean <- mean(IQ)
> IQMean
[1] 99.91027
>
> IQStdv <- sd(IQ)
> IQStdv
[1] 15.05846
```

Next, use these two new objects, along with the syntax that follows, to place a normal curve over the histogram of object variable IQ.

```
par(ask=TRUE)
hist(IQ,
  main="Histogram and Normal Curve Overlay of IQ Scores:
  N = 100,000, Mean = 100, and SD = 15",
  xlab="Object Variable IQ", col=c("red"), breaks=100,
  prob=TRUE, lwd=4, lty=6, cex.lab=1.25, font=2,
  ylim=c(0, 0.045))                          # Define Y axis
curve(dnorm(x, mean=IQMean, sd=IQStdv), col="darkblue",
  lwd=6, lty=3, add=TRUE)  # Heavy dotted line to the curve
# Add a descriptive legend where there is open white space.
savefamily <- par(family="mono") # Courier font
savefont   <- par(font=2)        # Bold text
legend("topleft",
legend = c(
"========================================",
"The normal curve placed over the histogram",
"has the following properties:           ",
"  N ....................... 100,000     ",
"  Mean .....................    100     ",
"  Standard Deviation (SD) ..     15     ",
"========================================"),
ncol=1, locator(1), xjust=1,
text.col="darkblue",
cex=1.05, inset=0.01, bty="n")
par(savefamily)
par(savefont)
```

The normal curve overlay certainly adds to an understanding of how the data are distributed, especially when data deviate from normal distribution. However,

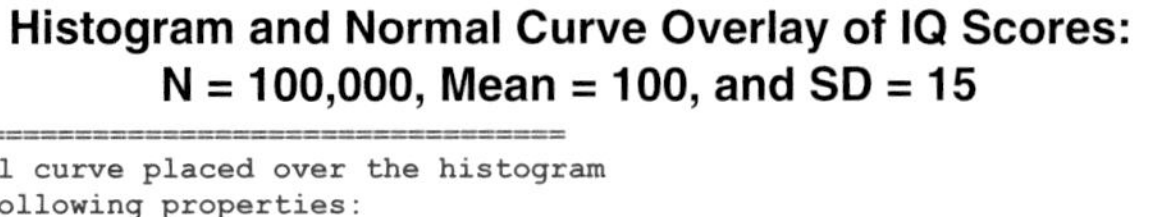

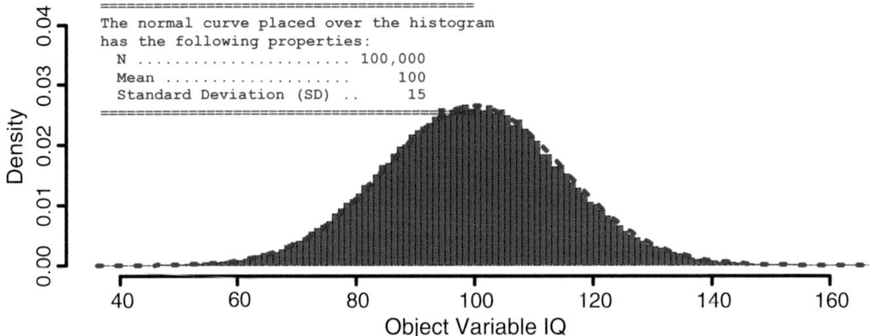

Fig. 1.12 Histogram and normal curve overlay

some type of marker for the standard deviations would also contribute to a better understanding of the data. Follow along with the syntax below to see how more detail can be added to further reinforce how the data for IQ exhibit normal distribution. Notice how additional detail was added using legends (Fig. 1.12).

```
par(ask=TRUE)
hist(IQ,
  main="Histogram and Normal Curve Overlay of IQ Scores:
  N = 100,000, Mean = 100, and SD = 15",
  xlab="Object Variable IQ", col=c("red"), breaks=100,
  prob=TRUE, lwd=4, lty=6, cex.lab=1.25, font=2,
  ylim=c(0, 0.045))                          # Define Y axis
curve(dnorm(x, mean=IQ_Mean, sd=IQ_Stdv),
  col="darkgreen", lwd=4, lty=6, add=TRUE)
abline(v=100, lwd=5)       # Value(s) (v) for vertical line
abline(v=c(055,070,085,115,130,145), # Values - and + 3 SDs
lwd=2, lty=3)
# Add a descriptive legend where there is open white space.
savefamily <- par(family="mono") # Courier font
savefont   <- par(font=2)        # Bold text
legend("topright",
legend = c(
"N ...... 100,000        ",
"Mean ...     100        ",
"SD .....      15        ",
"                        ",
"Mean +1 SD = 115        ",
"Mean +2 SD = 130        ",
"Mean +3 SD = 145        ",
"Mean -1 SD = 085        ",
"Mean -2 SD = 070        ",
"Mean -3 SD = 055        "),
ncol=1, locator(1), xjust=1,
text.col="darkblue",
```

```
cex=1.05, inset=0.01, bty="n")
par(savefamily)
par(savefont)
###############################################################
savefamily <- par(family="mono") # Courier font
savefont   <- par(font=2)        # Bold text
legend("topleft",
legend = c(
"Solid vertical line ...  Mean",
"Dotted vertical line ..    SD",
"Dashed line ........... Curve"),
ncol=1, locator(1), xjust=1,
text.col="darkblue",
cex=1.05, inset=0.005, bty="n")
par(savefamily)
par(savefont)
```

As another visual check, use the qqnorm() function and the qqline() function to examine distribution of IQ data and any possible deviation away from normal distribution. Ideally, if the data exhibit normal distribution, the datapoints in a Quantile-Quantile plot should follow along or at least follow very closely to the line which passes through the quartiles (Fig. 1.13).

```
qqnorm(IQ, main="QQ Plot of IQ",
  ylim=c(40,160), font=2, cex.lab=1.15,
  cex.axis=1.25, lwd=6, col="cyan")
qqline(IQ, lwd=4, col=c("darkblue"))
```

The qqnorm() function and qqline() function in this lesson clearly demonstrate that IQ follows along with normal distribution, even though there are a few noticeable outliers. Outliers are important, and an experienced researcher will check

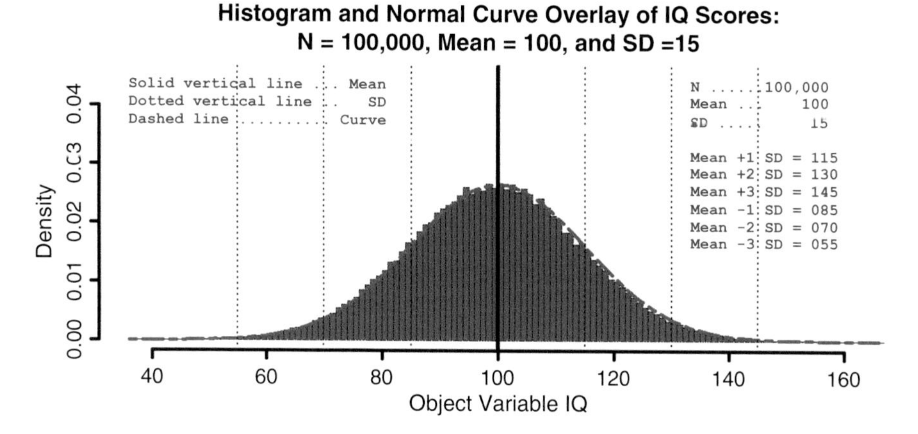

Fig. 1.13 Embellished histogram and normal curve overlay

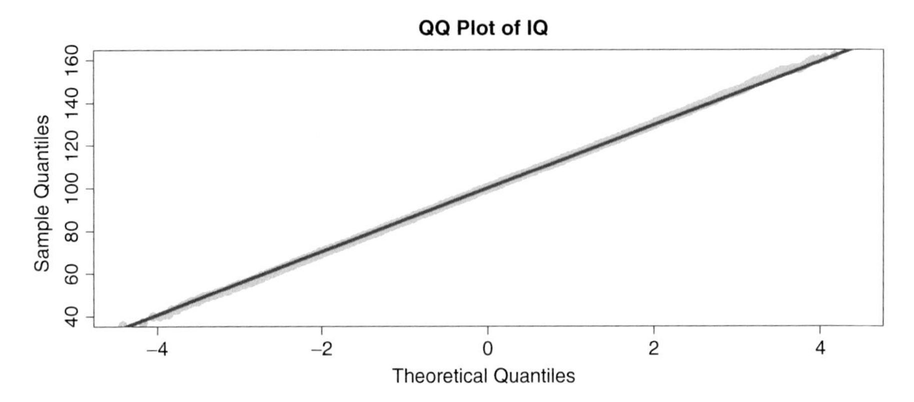

Fig. 1.14 Quantile-Quantile (i.e., QQ or Q-Q) plot

on these values to see if they represent an error or if they represent a true, but extreme, value. However, for this lesson the outliers are so minimal in number that they cause no great concern and are reasonably expected in a population of 100,000 subjects (Fig. 1.14).

Up to this point, the presentation in this addendum has been for IQ, an object created using the rnorm() function with 100,000 datapoints, and with Mean = 100 and SD = 15. The preliminary figures provide visual evidence that IQ exhibits normal distribution.

As desirable as it may be to have a normally distributed object variable consisting of 100,000 datapoints, imagine the command-and-control actions that would be needed to obtain these data. Then, imagine the budget needed to obtain IQ scores from 100,000 adult subjects. It is largely unthinkable to suggest that a proactive study of this magnitude would ever be proposed and funded. Time-on-task, coordination of activities, Institutional Review Board (IRB) permissions, and project budgets are only a few of the many issues that contribute to the need for sampling and the avoidance of queries against entire populations.

- Given concern about the many management actions needed to obtain data from 100,000 subjects, consider a more manageable sample of 1000 subjects.
- Would results (i.e., adherence to normal distribution, expected Mean and SD, etc.) appear the same if a sample of 1000 subjects were used instead of the far larger population of 100,000 subjects?

There are many ways to prepare a sample of 1000 subjects from the overall set of 100,000 IQ scores. Conceivably, it is possible to select the first 1000 datapoints and to discard the remaining 99,000. Although this action might be convenient, the aim should be on random selection and not convenience.

In an effort to eventually select a representative sample of 1000 subjects for the 100,000 subjects found in the object variable IQ, assume that of the 100,000 IQ datapoints, half (i.e., 50,000) are even numbers and half (i.e., 50,000) are odd numbers. Test this assumption using the gtools::odd() function.

```
install.packages("gtools")
library(gtools)                # Load the gtools package.
help(package=gtools)           # Show the information page.
sessionInfo()                  # Confirm all attached packages.
# Select the most local mirror site using Set CRAN mirror.

IQoddeven <- gtools::odd(IQ)
  # Apply the gtools::odd() function against the object
  # variable IQ and direct the output to the new object
  # variable called IQoddeven.  It is expected that the
  # result will consist of a series of TRUE or FALSE
  # listings, where TRUE represents a value that is odd.

head(IQoddeven)          # Quality assurance
tail(IQoddeven)          # Quality assurance

summary(IQoddeven)       # Determine if odd-even is 50/50
```

```
> IQoddeven <- gtools::odd(IQ)
>   # Apply the gtools::odd() function against the object
>   # variable IQ and direct the output to the new object
>   # variable called IQoddeven.  It is expected that the
>   # result will consist of a series of TRUE or FALSE
>   # listings, where TRUE represents a value that is odd.
>
> head(IQoddeven)          # Quality assurance
[1] FALSE  TRUE  TRUE  TRUE FALSE FALSE
> tail(IQoddeven)          # Quality assurance
[1] FALSE FALSE  TRUE  TRUE  TRUE  TRUE
>
> summary(IQoddeven)       # Determine if odd-even is 50/50
   Mode   FALSE    TRUE    NA's
logical   49713   50287       0
```

Reviewing output from the summary() function, it is evident that approximately half of all IQ scores are odd and half are even. Merely to demonstrate Boolean selection and build on needed skills, review the syntax below to see how IQ scores are selected and put into a new object variable, in an effort to eventually achieve a sample of 1000 IQ scores that represent the original population. From among the many possibilities on how R can be used to obtain even numbers only, in this lesson note how the subset() function was wrapped around use of the trunc() function. Note also how two equal signs (i.e., ==) are used to indicate equivalency.

```
IQEven <- subset(IQ, IQ/2==trunc(IQ/2))
is.vector(IQEven)                    # Quality assurance
class(IQEven)                        # Quality assurance
head(IQEven)                         # Review data
tail(IQEven)                         # Review data
length(IQEven)                       # Descriptive statistics
summary(IQEven)                      # Descriptive statistics
```

```
> IQEven <- subset(IQ, IQ/2==trunc(IQ/2))
> is.vector(IQEven)                        # Quality assurance
[1] TRUE
> class(IQEven)                            # Quality assurance
[1] "numeric"
> head(IQEven)                             # Review data
[1] 100 104 106  82  76  96
> tail(IQEven)                             # Review data
[1] 120 108 106 102  86  88
> length(IQEven)                           # Descriptive statistics
[1] 49713
> summary(IQEven)                          # Descriptive statistics
   Min. 1st Qu.  Median    Mean 3rd Qu.    Max.
  36.00   90.00  100.00   99.88  110.00  162.00
```

Already there is a general sense that the sample (IQEven) consists of approximately 50,000 datapoints and that the data in IQEven are all even numbers. Perhaps more importantly for the purpose of this addendum, it is necessary to question whether the data in IQEven follow the normal distribution patterns exhibited in the original vector, IQ. As a data check, prepare a simple histogram of IQEven to gain an overall sense of the data beyond the descriptive information gained from the R functions immediately above. To supplement this visual check, use the qqnorm() function and qqline() function to examine distribution of IQEven data and any possible deviation from normal distribution.

```
par(mfrow=c(1,2))    # 1 by 2 (Row by Column)
par(ask=TRUE)
#################################################
hist(IQEven, col="red", font=2, cex.lab=1.25)
#################################################
qqnorm(IQEven, main="QQ Plot of IQEven",
  ylim=c(40,160), font=2, cex.lab=1.15,
  cex.axis=1.25, lwd=6, col="cyan")
qqline(IQEven, lwd=4, col=c("darkblue"))
#################################################
```

Both the histogram and the qqnorm() function provide some degree of assurance that the distribution of data in IQEven approximates normal distribution, which was the case previously for the distribution of data in IQ. It is appropriate to continue with further sampling in an effort to obtain a sample of 1000 representative subjects.

As another adjustment in preparation of the final sample of representative IQ scores, use the Boolean selection processes supported in R to obtain IQEven scores that range from 55 to 145 to keep within (− or +) three standard deviations in view of Mean = 100 and SD = 15. Use the length() function and summary() function to confirm length, minimum, and maximum values. Then, apply the subset() function to trim extreme values (e.g., the few values below 55 and greater than 145) and then look again at output from the length() function and summary function to see how many datapoints were removed from IQEven (Fig. 1.15).

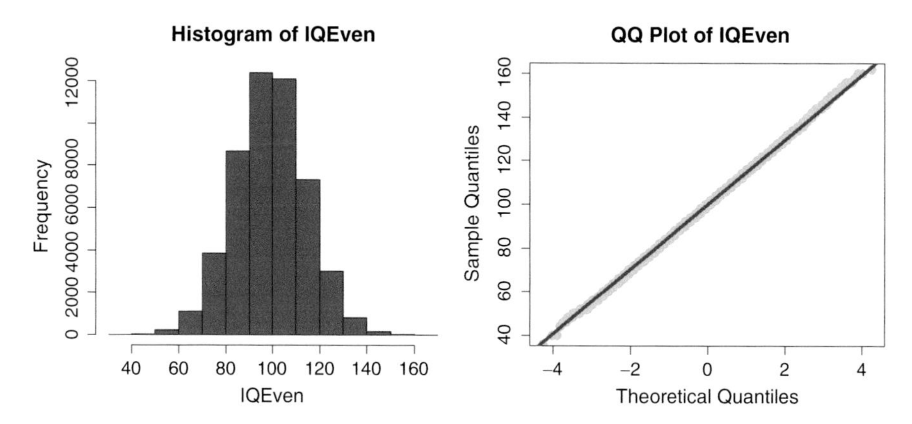

Fig. 1.15 Histogram and Quantile-Quantile plot

```
length(IQEven)
summary(IQEven)

IQEven <- subset(IQEven, (IQEven >= 55) & (IQEven <= 145))
is.vector(IQEven)                          # Quality assurance
class(IQEven)                              # Quality assurance
head(IQEven)                               # Review data
tail(IQEven)                               # Review data
length(IQEven)                             # Descriptive statistics
summary(IQEven)                            # Descriptive statistics
```

```
> length(IQEven)
[1] 49713
> summary(IQEven)
   Min. 1st Qu.  Median    Mean 3rd Qu.    Max.
  36.00   90.00  100.00   99.88  110.00  162.00
>
> IQEven <- subset(IQEven, (IQEven >= 55) & (IQEven <= 145))
> is.vector(IQEven)                          # Quality assurance
[1] TRUE
> class(IQEven)                              # Quality assurance
[1] "numeric"
> head(IQEven)                               # Review data
[1] 100 104 106  82  76  96
> tail(IQEven)                               # Review data
[1] 120 108 106 102  86  88
> length(IQEven)                             # Descriptive statistics
[1] 49565
> summary(IQEven)                            # Descriptive statistics
   Min. 1st Qu.  Median    Mean 3rd Qu.    Max.
  56.00   90.00  100.00   99.87  110.00  144.00
```

With this action and as confirmed using the length() function and summary() function, the few values less than 55 and greater than 145 have been removed from the object IQEven. Most importantly, notice how Median = 100 was the case before and after the extreme values were trimmed.

Given the desire to have a more manageable sample of adult subjects in this presentation on data distribution and sampling, select a sample of 1000 subjects using the sample() function. Use the replace=TRUE argument. Place the output of the sampling process into a new object, called IQEven1000.

```
length(IQEven)     # Confirm length (N) prior to sampling
summary(IQEven)    # Confirm mean and median

IQEven1000 <- sample(IQEven, size=1000, replace=TRUE)
is.vector(IQEven1000)                  # Quality assurance
class(IQEven1000)                      # Quality assurance
head(IQEven1000)                       # Review data
tail(IQEven1000)                       # Review data
length(IQEven1000)                     # Descriptive statistics
summary(IQEven1000)                    # Descriptive statistics
```

```
> length(IQEven)     # Confirm length (N) prior to sampling
[1] 49565
> summary(IQEven)    # Confirm mean and median
   Min. 1st Qu.  Median    Mean 3rd Qu.    Max.
  56.00   90.00  100.00   99.87  110.00  144.00
>
> IQEven1000 <- sample(IQEven, size=1000, replace=TRUE)
> is.vector(IQEven1000)                  # Quality assurance
[1] TRUE
> class(IQEven1000)                      # Quality assurance
[1] "numeric"
> head(IQEven1000)                       # Review data
[1]  86 110  76  94 102 104
> tail(IQEven1000)                       # Review data
[1]  88 110 102 104  88  92
> length(IQEven1000)                     # Descriptive statistics
[1] 1000
> summary(IQEven1000)                    # Descriptive statistics
   Min. 1st Qu.  Median    Mean 3rd Qu.    Max.
   56.0    90.0   100.0   100.2   110.0   144.0
```

As an additional data check, prepare a simple histogram of IQEven1000, which now consists of only 1000 subjects from a dataset that originally represented a population of 100,000 subjects. Then, place the data for IQEven1000 in another histogram, but now include a density curve and normal curve overlay that show in more detail data distribution for the sample IQEven1000.

```
par(mfrow=c(1,2))    # 1 by 2 (Row by Column)
par(ask=TRUE)
###########################################################
hist(IQEven1000, col="red", font=2, cex.lab=1.25,
  xlim=c(50,150), nclass=65,
  main="IQEven Scores Between 55 and 145, Inclusive")
###########################################################
savelwd       <- par(lwd=6)          # Heavy line
savefont      <- par(font=2)         # Bold
savecex.lab   <- par(cex.lab=1.25)   # Label
savecex.axis  <- par(cex.axis=1.25)  # Axis
par(ask=TRUE)
descr::histkdnc(IQEven1000,
  main="Density Curve (Red), Histogram (Grey), and Normal
  Curve (Blue) of IQEven1000 Scores:  N = 1,000,
  Mean = 100, and SD = 15",
  xlab="IQEven1000",
  col=grey(0.95)) # Allow contrast with lines
par(savelwd); par(savefont); par(savecex.lab);
par(savecex.axis)              # Use ; to move to next line
###########################################################
```

As these histograms seem to verify, there is now a more manageable object variable (i.e., IQEven1000) of IQ scores, with length=1000, mean=100, sd=15, min=055, and max=145 (Fig. 1.16).

As a further demonstration of data distribution, use the previously demonstrated syntax to overlay a normal curve over IQEven1000 data and highlight the standard deviations and mean.

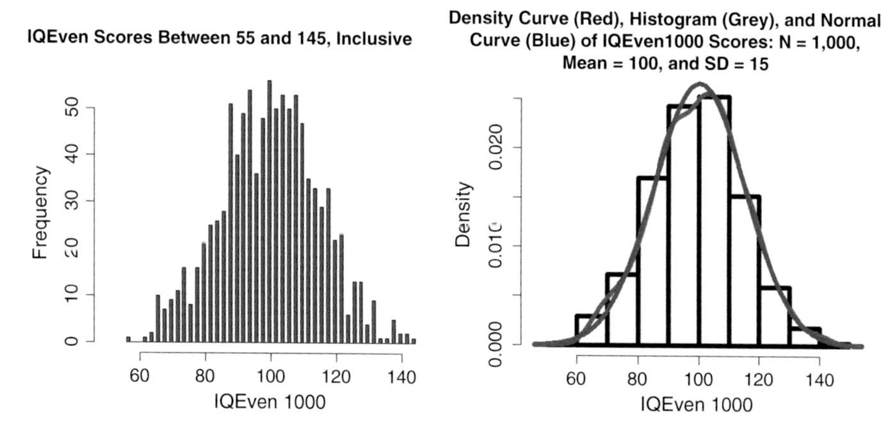

Fig. 1.16 Detailed histograms

```
IQEven1000Mean <- mean(IQEven1000)
IQEven1000Mean

IQEven1000Stdv <- sd(IQEven1000)
IQEven1000Stdv
```

```
> IQEven1000Mean <- mean(IQEven1000)
> IQEven1000Mean
[1] 100.212
>
> IQEven1000Stdv <- sd(IQEven1000)
> IQEven1000Stdv
[1] 14.98972
```

```
par(ask=TRUE)
hist(IQEven1000,
  main="Histogram and Normal Curve Overlay of IQ Scores
  (IQEven1000):  N = 1,000, Mean = 100, and SD = 15",
  xlab="Object Variable IQEven1000", col=c("red"),
  breaks=50, prob=TRUE, xlim=c(45,155), ylim=c(0,0.035),
# Adjust xlim and ylim as needed, to present a full picture
# of data distribution, including all parts of the
# histogram.
  lwd=4, lty=6, cex.lab=1.25, font=2)
curve(dnorm(x, mean=IQEven1000Mean, sd=IQEven1000Stdv),
  col="darkgreen", lwd=4, lty=6, add=TRUE)
abline(v=100, lwd=5)        # Value(s) (v) for vertical line
abline(v=c(055,070,085,115,130,145), # Values - and + 3 SDs
lwd=2, lty=3)    # SD
# Add a descriptive legend where there is open white space.
# As shown below, use spaces to fine-tune placement when
# using a Courier fixed-font presentation.
savefamily <- par(family="mono") # Courier font
savefont   <- par(font=2)        # Bold text
legend("topright",
legend = c(
"N ......   1,000         ",
"Mean ...     100         ",
"SD .....      15         ",
"                         ",
"Mean +1 SD = 115         ",
"Mean +2 SD = 130         ",
"Mean +3 SD = 145         ",
"Mean -1 SD = 085         ",
"Mean -2 SD = 070         ",
"Mean -3 SD = 055         "),
ncol=1, locator(1), xjust=1,
text.col="darkblue",
```

```
cex=1.05, inset=0.01, bty="n")
par(savefamily)
par(savefont)
###############################################################
savefamily <- par(family="mono") # Courier font
savefont   <- par(font=2)        # Bold text
legend("topleft",
legend = c(
"Solid vertical line ...  Mean",
"Dotted vertical line ..    SD",
"Dashed line ........... Curve"),
ncol=1, locator(1), xjust=1,
text.col="darkblue",
cex=1.05, inset=0.005, bty="n")
par(savefamily)
par(savefont)
```

As another visual check, use the qqnorm() function and qqline() function to examine distribution of IQEven1000 data and any possible deviation away from normal distribution (Fig. 1.17).

```
qqnorm(IQEven1000, main="QQ Plot of IQEven1000",
  ylim=c(40,160), font=2, cex.lab=1.15,
  cex.axis=1.25, lwd=6, col="cyan")
qqline(IQEven, lwd=4, col=c("darkblue"))
```

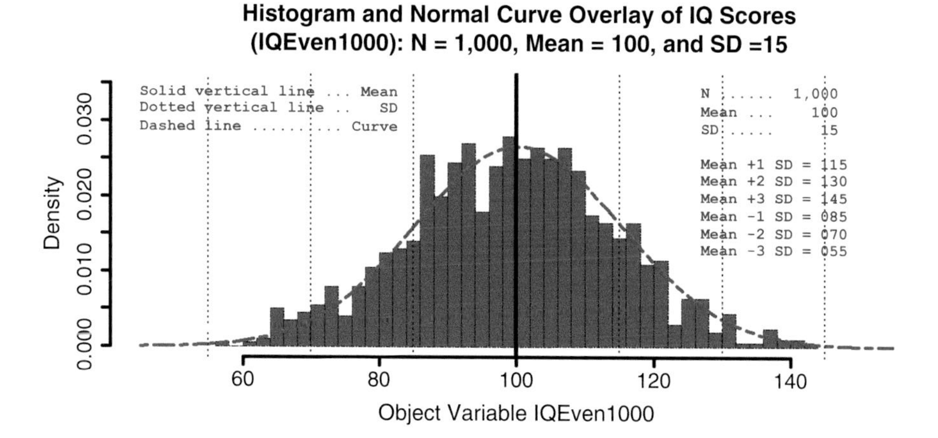

Fig. 1.17 Embellished histogram with multiple legends

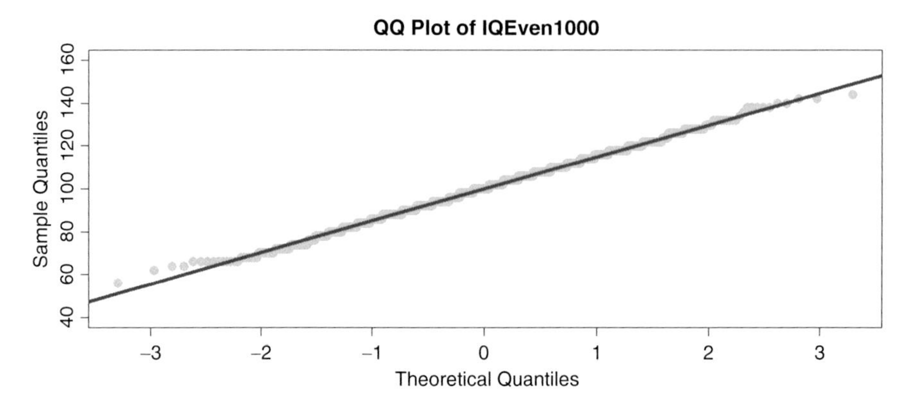

Fig. 1.18 Quantile-Quantile plot with noise showing in the tails

Note especially how there may be some *noise* at the two tails of the QQ plot.[9] It is reasonable to at least question whether data distribution is as ideal as was seen in the QQ plot for the original dataset, IQ, before sampling occurred (Fig. 1.18).

Using these many tools, it is now possible to visually examine and then make some degree of informed judgment on whether the values in the object variable of interest (IQEven1000) follow normal distribution. If normal distribution is not evident, then it is necessary to decide whether the deviation away from normal distribution is so great that a nonparametric inferential test should be considered as an alternate approach over use of a more parametric approach.

A final graphic will help guide decision-making on the visual presentation of data distribution patterns for: IQ, IQEven, and IQEven1000. The function and argument par(mfrow=c(1,3)) is used to create a graphic with one row and three columns with a graphical image placed in each cell.

```
par(mfrow=c(1,3))            # 1 row by 3 column format
par(ask=TRUE)
###############################################################
savelwd        <- par(lwd=6)            # Heavy line
savefont       <- par(font=2)           # Bold font
savecex.lab    <- par(cex.lab=1.25)     # Label size
savefont.lab   <- par(font.lab=2)       # Label bold
savecex.axis   <- par(cex.axis=1.25)    # Axis size
savefont.axis  <- par(font.axis=2)      # Axis font
par(ask=TRUE)
descr::histkdnc(IQ,
  main="Density Curve (Red), Histogram (Grey), and Normal
```

[9]The term *noise* refers to the observation that the small circles used to indicate individual datapoints do not follow along the otherwise straight line of the Quantile-Quantile plot. A few deviations away from the straight line are expected. However, when there are too many deviations it is best to question if the data display normal distribution.

```
  Curve (Blue) of IQ Scores:  N = 100,000,
  Mean = 100, and SD = 15",
  xlab="Object Variable IQ",
  xlim=c(40,160), ylim=c(0,0.03),
  col=grey(0.95))             # Allow contrast with lines
par(savelwd); par(savefont); par(savecex.lab);
par(savefont.lab); par(savecex.axis); par(savefont.axis)
# Use ; to move to next line
################################################################
savelwd       <- par(lwd=6)          # Heavy line
savefont      <- par(font=2)         # Bold font
savecex.lab   <- par(cex.lab=1.25)   # Label size
savefont.lab  <- par(font.lab=2)     # Label bold
savecex.axis  <- par(cex.axis=1.25)  # Axis size
savefont.axis <- par(font.axis=2)    # Axis font
par(ask=TRUE)
descr::histkdnc(IQEven,
  main="Density Curve (Red), Histogram (Grey), and Normal
  Curve (Blue) of IQEven Scores:  N ~ 50,000,
  Mean = 100, and SD = 15",
  xlab="Object Variable IQEven",
  xlim=c(40,160), ylim=c(0,0.03),
  col=grey(0.95))             # Allow contrast with lines
par(savelwd); par(savefont); par(savecex.lab);
par(savefont.lab); par(savecex.axis); par(savefont.axis)
# Use ; to move to next line
################################################################
savelwd       <- par(lwd=6)          # Heavy line
savefont      <- par(font=2)         # Bold font
savecex.lab   <- par(cex.lab=1.25)   # Label size
savefont.lab  <- par(font.lab=2)     # Label bold
savecex.axis  <- par(cex.axis=1.25)  # Axis.size
savefont.axis <- par(font.axis=2)    # Axis font
par(ask=TRUE)
descr::histkdnc(IQEven1000,
  main="Density Curve (Red), Histogram (Grey), and Normal
  Curve (Blue) of IQEven1000 Scores:  N = 1,000,
  Mean = 100, and SD = 15",
  xlab="Object Variable IQEven1000",
  xlim=c(40,160), ylim=c(0,0.03),
  col=grey(0.95))             # Allow contrast with lines
par(savelwd); par(savefont); par(savecex.lab);
par(savefont.lab); par(savecex.axis); par(savefont.axis)
# Use ; to move to next line
################################################################
```

These images, alone, should not be the only guide to determine if a collection of data follows normal distribution. However, graphics are important and they certainly serve as a first consideration to examine distribution patterns. As the lessons in this text progress, other options will be demonstrated and explained. However, never discount the value of graphics and the capability of R to produce graphics that rival all other statistical analysis software—and surpass most (Fig. 1.19).

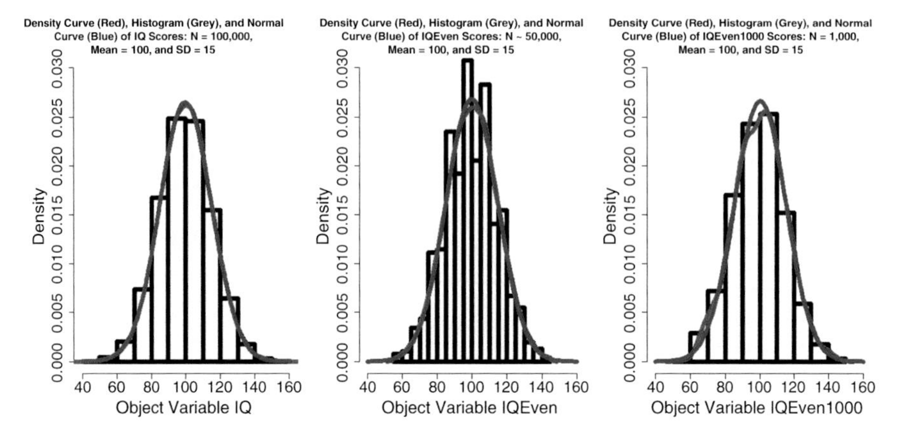

Fig. 1.19 Multiple embellished histograms

1.9 Prepare to Exit, Save, and Later Retrieve This R Session

```
getwd()              # Identify the current working directory.
ls()                 # List all objects in the working
                     # directory.
ls.str()             # List all objects, with finite detail.
list.files()         # List files at the PC directory.

save.image("R_Lesson_Nonparametric_Introduction.rdata")

getwd()              # Identify the current working directory.
ls()                 # List all objects in the working
                     # directory.
ls.str()             # List all objects, with finite detail.
list.files()         # List files at the PC directory.

alarm()              # Alarm, notice of upcoming action.
q()                  # Quit this session.
                     # Prepare for Save workspace image? query.
```

Use the R Graphical User Interface (GUI) to load the saved rdata file: File -> Load Workspace.[10] Otherwise, use the load() function, keying the full pathname, to load the .rdata file and retrieve the session.

Recall, however, that it may be just as useful to simply use the .R script file (typically saved is a .txt ASCII-type file) and recreate the analyses and graphics, provided the data files remain available.

[10]The use of R syntax is stressed in this text. However, this is one case where it may be best to use the R menuing selections (e.g., File - Edit - View - Misc - Packages - Windows - Help), instead of syntax, to ensure that all session activities are placed in the desired location.

Chapter 2
Sign Test

Abstract The Sign Test is typically used to examine differences between two sets of data at the broadest level of comparison. As this lesson is structured, the nonparametric Sign Test is used to examine any possible difference between pretest and posttest measures but with the caution that the Sign Test is by no means as robust as other statistical tests. Even with limited rigor, the Sign Test is an excellent exploratory test and the use of this tool should not be overlooked when working with data that support nonparametric analyses. It is interesting to note that the Sign Test name, itself, is due to signs (i.e., −, +, and o) being derived from measured data. These signs are used to represent direction, as will be shown in this lesson.

Keywords Anderson-Darling test • Bar plot (stacked, side-by-side) • Code book • Continuous scale • Density plot • Descriptive statistics • Distribution-free • Frequency distribution • Histogram • Interval • Mean • Median • Mode • Nominal • Nonparametric • Normal distribution • Null hypothesis • Ordinal • Parametric • Probability (p-value) • Quantile-Quantile (QQ, Q-Q) • Ranking • Ratio • Sign test • Statistical significance

2.1 Background on This Lesson

The Sign Test is an excellent exploratory tool for when it is simply not possible to obtain quantitative measures but it is possible to obtain rank measures between members of a pair, which is demonstrated in this lesson. As suggested in the name for this test, the Sign Test uses the symbols **-** , **+**, and **o** as directional signs.

2.1.1 Description of the Data

This lesson on the Sign Test is based on Pretest v Posttest measures from a study involving 40 individual laboratory rats (*Rattus norvegicus*) and observed change (Pretest and Posttest) after some type of treatment.

T.W. MacFarland, J.M. Yates, *Introduction to Nonparametric Statistics for the Biological Sciences Using R*, DOI 10.1007/978-3-319-30634-6_2

- The subjects are from four different laboratories, and it is assumed that the rats experienced different conditions regarding housing and feeding—at least up to the time the treatment was provided.
- There is equally no assumption that the subjects are of the same strain.
- As the dataset was constructed, the gender and age of each subject are both unidentified.
- The nature of the treatment is currently unknown to the researcher assigned responsibility for statistical analyses:
  - The treatment may have been some type of supplement added to the diet, and Pretest and Posttest measures involve some type of measure for weight or vigor.
  - The treatment may have been some type of behavioral intervention, and the Pretest and Posttest measures involve some type of performance assessment on a structured skills test.
  - The treatment may have been some type of environmental condition, and the Pretest and Posttest measures involve some type of response to light, noise, temperature, etc.
- It is unknown if Pretest measurements were obtained at or near the same time, and equally it is unknown if a consistent amount of time was observed for Posttest measurements after application of the treatment.

The only conditions for this study that are known are that the 40 subjects (i.e., laboratory rats) were measured (Pretest), some type of treatment was applied, and the same subjects were measured (Posttest) some time after application of the treatment. Tracking procedures were used so that each rat was clearly identified when the Pretest measure was taken, when the treatment was applied, and later when the Posttest measure was taken.

This study represents a matched-pair approach, where each subject is measured twice, a Pretest measurement made before application of the treatment and a Posttest measurement made after application of the treatment. However, look at the many previously listed unknown factors associated with this study. Saying all of this, the Sign Test was judged the most appropriate nonparametric test to use given the wide variance in structure for methods and subsequent data, such as the data coming from subjects kept at four different laboratories, with each laboratory possibly using different housing and feeding regimes—all from rats that are genetically similar but that may not be genetically identical.

Regarding the actual Pretest and Posttest measures, for this lesson the only concern is that the Pretest and Posttest measures are viewed as ordinal data and that they lack the assumed precision of interval data. As ordinal data and with the scale used for this lesson, it is known that an 8 is more than a 7 and that a 6 is more than a 5, but there is no assumption that the difference between an 8 and a 7 and the difference between a 6 and a 5 are consistent with each other each time. From this scheme for both methods and measurement, there will be greatest interest in broad comparisons, resulting in the appropriate sign (i.e., or the directional difference between Pretest and Posttest):

- If a Posttest measure is less than a Pretest measure, then the – sign is applied to the comparison.
- If a Posttest measure is greater then a Pretest measure, than the + sign is applied to the comparison.
- If a Posttest measure is equal to a Pretest measure, then the o sign is applied to the comparison.

Given that the data are ordinal and not interval, it is best to focus on the Median when considering measures of central tendency. Statistics such as the Mean and Standard Deviation have value and are used in this lesson for some degree of guidance, but Mean and Standard Deviation should also be viewed with caution in terms of precision when these types of descriptive statistics are gained from ordinal data.

To be brief as to the conditions that support selection of the Sign Test for this design, admittedly a less than rigorous research design but still a design that could yield insight into general trends:

- Although there is a continuous-type scale (01 to 10), there is no assumption of normal distribution of the ordinal data, either for Pretest measures or Posttest measures.
- Although it is known that the rats are all generally similar, different laboratories provided the subjects and there is no assumption that the rats are all drawn from the same population.

Within the reality of these conditions and assumptions about the data, it is judged that the exploratory Sign Test is the best first choice for any attempt at inferential analysis of change in this fairly simple Pretest—Treatment—Posttest study. Other inferential tests may have later value, especially with greater command-and-control over the methods, as future iterations of this study are refined, but the Sign Test is an appropriate first choice—as an exploratory test to discern general trends.

The dataset is fairly simple and as explained later, data for this study were originally entered into a simple text editor, not the a spreadsheet:

- The first line (i.e., row) of data consists of a header, using descriptive variable names: Lab, Subject, Pretest, Posttest, Success, Sign. The header is then followed by 40 lines of data, one line of data for each subject.
- Lab: An alpha code (LA, LB, LC, LD) is used to identify the laboratory that supplied each Subject. Be sure to note later that there is an unequal number of Subjects from each laboratory.
- Subject: There is a coded number (S01 to S40) for each Subject. Adequate tracking protocols were used to correctly identify each Subject when Pretest and Posttest measures were obtained and during application of the Treatment.

- Pretest: The ordinal scale used for Pretest measures ranged from 01 to 10. The exact nature of these numeric values is currently unknown other than that they are viewed as ordinal data.
- Posttest: The ordinal scale used for Posttest measures ranged from 01 to 10. The exact nature of these numeric values is currently unknown other than that they are viewed as ordinal data.
- Success: Given that the dataset is fairly small, with only 40 subjects, the Success variable was hand-calculated, and it is provided to clearly communicate Pretest v Posttest results. Success represents a binary comparison of Pretest and Posttest measures, Y (Yes) if Posttest is greater than Pretest and N (No) if Posttest is not greater than Pretest. Be sure to note how Pretest and Posttest measures that are equivalent (e.g., Pretest = 7 and Posttest = 7) are viewed as N (No) in the coding scheme for Success. Equivalency is not viewed as Success. Use of the term Success is fairly standard for how outcomes are viewed for a Success–Failure, True–False, Go–Stop, Survival–Death, binomial, way of presenting change-type outcomes.
- Sign: The Sign variable was also hand-calculated and equally serves as a comparison of Pretest and Posttest measures. Both use of the term Sign, and the associated − + o symbols are fairly standard for how outcomes of the Sign Test are viewed:
  - The symbol − is used if Posttest is less than Pretest.
  - The symbol + is used if Posttest is greater than Pretest.
  - The symbol o is used if Posttest equals Pretest (i.e., there is a tie between Pretest and Posttest).

Again, very few assumptions are placed on the data and subsequently the Sign Test is viewed as a test that is less robust than other tests in terms of support for later decision-making. Even so, the Sign Test is an excellent tool for initial exploratory analyses and its use should not be overlooked.

2.1.2 *Null Hypothesis (Ho)*

The median of differences between Pretest and Posttest measures of laboratory rats, after application of an otherwise unidentified treatment, equals 0 (`p <= 0.05`).

2.2 Data Entry by Copying Directly into a R Session

The dataset for this lesson originally consisted of Pretest and Posttest measures from 40 laboratory rats, with the rats supplied by four different laboratories. Adequate protocols were used so that the Subjects (i.e., laboratory rats) were identified by a control number (S01 to S40). There are no missing data, with Pretest and Posttest measures obtained for each of the 40 Subjects. Data for the Success and Sign variables were hand-calculated, based on comparisons of Posttest–Pretest measures.

It is common for data to be entered into a spreadsheet, such as the freely-available Gnumeric spreadsheet program or any of the many proprietary spreadsheet programs. It is equally common for the spreadsheet to then be saved in .csv (i.e., comma-separated values) file format so that data in the .csv file can be easily shared with others.

However, for this lesson there are only 40 Subjects and the variables Success and Sign are hand-calculated. The data were instead prepared using a simple text editor (e.g., Crimson Editor, Tinn-R, or vim are all possible selections), copied, and then pasted into the R session, in concert with wrapping the read.table() function around the textConnection() function, as shown below. In later lessons, data will be organized in a spreadsheet, saved in .csv file format, and then as an external .csv file imported directly into R using the R read.table() function. For this lesson, however, consider this example of data entry—data import as another way from among the many possible ways data can be brought into R.

Start a new R session and then attend to beginning actions such as removing unwanted files from prior work, declaring the working directory, etc.

```
###############################################################
# Housekeeping                        Use for All Analyses    #
###############################################################
date()              # Current system time and date.
R.version.string    # R version and version release date.
ls()                # List all objects in the working
                    # directory.
rm(list = ls())     # CAUTION: Remove all files in the working
                    # directory. If this action is not desired,
                    # use the rm() function one-by-one to remove
                    # the objects that are not needed.
ls.str()            # List all objects, with finite detail.
getwd()             # Identify the current working directory.
setwd("F:/R_Nonparametric")
                    # Set to a new working directory.
                    # Note the single forward slash and double
                    # quotes.
                    # This new directory should be the directory
                    # where the data file is located, otherwise
                    # the data file will not be found.
getwd()             # Confirm the working directory.
list.files()        # List files at the PC directory.
###############################################################
```

Create an object called PrePostRats.df. The object PrePostRats.df will be a dataframe, as indicated by the enumerated .df extension to the object name. This object will represent the output of applying the read.table() function wrapped around the textConnection() function against the data that immediately follow, which for this lesson are in an easy-to-read fixed column format. Be sure to note the header=TRUE argument (associated with the read.table() function), that indicates how the first row is a header representing descriptive variable names.

```
PrePostRats.df <- read.table(textConnection("
Lab  Subject  Pretest  Posttest  Success  Sign
LA   S01      05       08        Y        +
LA   S02      04       06        Y        +
LA   S03      03       03        N        o
LA   S04      06       05        N        -
LA   S05      08       09        Y        +
LB   S06      10       09        N        -
LB   S07      08       07        N        -
LB   S08      08       08        N        o
LB   S09      04       08        Y        +
LB   S10      05       05        N        o
LB   S11      08       09        Y        +
LB   S12      03       05        Y        +
LB   S13      05       04        N        -
LB   S14      06       05        N        -
LB   S15      04       04        N        o
LB   S16      07       08        Y        +
LB   S17      07       09        Y        +
LB   S18      09       09        N        o
LB   S19      08       07        N        -
LB   S20      05       08        Y        +
LC   S21      05       06        Y        +
LC   S22      08       08        N        o
LC   S23      03       04        Y        +
LC   S24      05       06        Y        +
LC   S25      06       07        Y        +
LC   S26      04       08        Y        +
LC   S27      07       08        Y        +
LC   S28      09       10        Y        +
LD   S29      10       10        N        o
LD   S30      08       09        Y        +
LD   S31      08       08        N        o
LD   S32      04       06        Y        +
LD   S33      04       05        Y        +
LD   S34      07       08        Y        +
LD   S35      05       07        Y        +
LD   S36      07       09        Y        +
LD   S37      08       10        Y        +
LD   S38      03       06        Y        +
LD   S39      05       06        Y        +
LD   S40      07       08        Y        +    "), header=TRUE)

getwd()                      # Identify the working directory
ls()                         # List objects
attach(PrePostRats.df)       # Attach the data, for later use
str(PrePostRats.df)          # Identify structure
nrow(PrePostRats.df)         # List the number of rows
ncol(PrePostRats.df)         # List the number of columns
```

```
dim(PrePostRats.df)           # Dimensions of the dataframe
names(PrePostRats.df)         # Identify names
colnames(PrePostRats.df)      # Show column names
rownames(PrePostRats.df)      # Show row names
head(PrePostRats.df, n=10)    # Show the head (10 rows)
tail(PrePostRats.df, n=10)    # Show the tail (10 rows)
PrePostRats.df                # Show the entire dataframe
summary(PrePostRats.df)       # Summary statistics
```

2.3 Organize the Data and Display the Code Book

Now that the data have been brought into R, it is usually necessary to check the data for format and then make any changes that may be needed to organize the data (and later coerce the data into desired class). As a typical example, consider the common practice of either numeric, letter, or symbolic codes, as factors, which is the case in this lesson for the object variables Success and Sign:

- The letters Y and N (in CAPS, remember that R is case sensitive) are used with the object variable Success to indicate Yes and No.
- For the object variable Sign, the – + o symbols are used to indicate how Posttest measures compare to prior Pretest measures, or the outcome of Posttest - Pretest.

However data are viewed and whatever symbols are used for factor-type objects, routine data-checking processes should always be used before graphics are prepared and analyses are attempted. These initial actions should be seen as a standard quality assurance practice.

For this simple lesson, the class() function, str() function, and duplicated() function will be sufficient first steps to be sure that data are organized as desired.

```
class(PrePostRats.df)
class(PrePostRats.df$Lab)       # DataFrame$ObjectName notation
class(PrePostRats.df$Subject)   # DataFrame$ObjectName notation
class(PrePostRats.df$Pretest)   # DataFrame$ObjectName notation
class(PrePostRats.df$Posttest)  # DataFrame$ObjectName notation
class(PrePostRats.df$Success)   # DataFrame$ObjectName notation
class(PrePostRats.df$Sign)      # DataFrame$ObjectName notation

str(PrePostRats.df)                        # Structure

duplicated(PrePostRats.df$Subject)         # Duplicates
```

In the dataframe PrePostRats.df, notice how the object variables Pretest and Posttest have no observed decimal values. They show as integers when the class() function is applied. With this caution, the class for each object seems to be currently correct and there are no duplicate subjects in the sample. Saying this, a Code Book will help with future understanding of this dataset, even if the data currently seem simple and obvious.

A Code Book is useful tool for anyone involved in the day-to-day activities of the research and statistics process. The Code Book is typically brief and only serves as a brief reminder for what can be easily forgotten months (or even weeks) later, to make it easy to decipher what may otherwise be seen as arcane numeric codes. Coding schemes that are intuitively obvious today can easily become forgotten tomorrow. Now that the class(), str(), and duplicated() functions have been used for basic diagnostics, consult the Code Book and then coerce each object, as needed, into its correct class.

```
#######################################################
# Code Book for PrePostRats.df                        #
#######################################################
#                                                     #
# Lab ........................ Factor (i.e., nominal) #
#                     A unique ID ranging from LA to LD #
#                                                     #
# Subject .................... Factor (i.e. nominal) #
#                   A unique ID ranging from S01 to S40 #
#                                                     #
# Pretest ................... Numeric (i.e., ordinal) #
#                Pretest measure, ranging from 01 to 10 #
#                                                     #
# Posttest .................. Numeric (i.e., ordinal) #
#               Posttest measure, ranging from 01 to 10 #
#                                                     #
# Success ...................  Factor (i.e., nominal) #
#                      Comparison of Posttest to Pretest #
#                                      N Not Successful #
#                                      S Successful     #
#                                                     #
# Sign ....................... Factor (i.e., nominal) #
#                      Comparison of Posttest to Pretest #
#                                  - Posttest < Pretest #
#                                  + Posttest > Pretest #
#                                  o Posttest = Pretest #
#######################################################
```

Descriptive names for object variables are certainly a good programming practice, as a demonstration of self-documentation. Even with attention to this practice, variable labels are usually needed, as another measure of documentation that supports recall when analyses are reviewed in the future. The epicalc::label.var() function, part of the external epicalc package, is one tool used to provide descriptive labels.[1]

[1]The use of descriptive labels promotes quality analyses. The labels may not be required, but their use will certainly be helpful when the analyses are revisited weeks and months later, which is often the case.

```
install.packages("epicalc")
library(epicalc)              # Load the epicalc package.
help(package=epicalc)         # Show the information page.
sessionInfo()                 # Confirm all attached packages.
# Select the most local mirror site using Set CRAN mirror.

epicalc::des(PrePostRats.df) # Description of the dataset

epicalc::label.var(Lab,       "Laboratory",
  dataFrame=PrePostRats.df)
epicalc::label.var(Subject,   "Subject ID",
  dataFrame=PrePostRats.df)
epicalc::label.var(Pretest,   "Pretest Measures",
  dataFrame=PrePostRats.df)
epicalc::label.var(Posttest, "Posttest Measures",
  dataFrame=PrePostRats.df)
epicalc::label.var(Success,   "Binomial Comparison of Change",
  dataFrame=PrePostRats.df)
epicalc::label.var(Sign,      "- + o Comparison of Change",
  dataFrame=PrePostRats.df)
```

```
epicalc::des(PrePostRats.df) # Description of the dataset
```

```
 No. of observations =  40
  Variable      Class           Description
1 Lab           factor          Laboratory
2 Subject       factor          Subject ID
3 Pretest       integer         Pretest Measures
4 Posttest      integer         Posttest Measures
5 Success       factor          Binomial Comparison of Change
6 Sign          factor          - + o Comparison of Change
```

With assurance that the dataframe is currently in correct format, coerce each object variable into desired format, as a factor object variable, numeric object variable, etc.

```
class(PrePostRats.df)    # Confirm nature of the dataset
str(PrePostRats.df)      # Confirm nature of the dataset

PrePostRats.df$Lab          <- factor(PrePostRats.df$Lab,
  labels=c("Lab A", "Lab B", "Lab C", "Lab D"))
PrePostRats.df$Subject      <- as.factor(PrePostRats.df$Subject)
PrePostRats.df$Pretest      <- as.numeric(PrePostRats.df$Pretest)
PrePostRats.df$Posttest     <- as.numeric(PrePostRats.df$Posttest)
PrePostRats.df$Success      <- factor(PrePostRats.df$Success,
  labels=c("N Not Successful", # Note the ordering of labels, or
           "Y Successful"))    # N and then Y
PrePostRats.df$Sign         <- factor(PrePostRats.df$Sign,
  labels=c("- Posttest < Pretest", # Note the ordering of
           "+ Posttest > Pretest", # labels, or - and then + and
           "o Posttest = Pretest"))# then o
  # Labels were added and from this note use of the factor()
  # function and not as.factor() for PrePostRats.df$Lab,
  # PrePostRats.df$Success, and PrePostRats.df$Sign.
```

As a sidebar comment, at the R prompt, key `help(factor)` and `help(numeric)` to learn more about how data can be coerced into different formats.

Comment: The object variables PrePostRats.df$Pretest and PrePostRats.df$Posttest were coerced from integer to numeric types. In turn, math operations will be used against these two object variables (e.g., calculation of Mean and Standard Deviation). Remember the prior caution that these Pretest and Posttest measures are based on ordinal data, not interval data. Accordingly, use good judgment and perhaps a degree of skepticism when later viewing math-specific statistics gained from these ordinal object variables coerced from integer to numeric class. Measures of central tendency, such as Mean and Standard Deviation, when based on ordinal data, have a role in guidance and decision-making, but, again, only with caution.

```
attach(PrePostRats.df)  # Confirm data are attached correctly

class(PrePostRats.df)           # Confirm nature of the dataset
class(PrePostRats.df$Lab)       # DataFrame$ObjectName notation
class(PrePostRats.df$Subject)   # DataFrame$ObjectName notation
class(PrePostRats.df$Pretest)   # DataFrame$ObjectName notation
class(PrePostRats.df$Posttest)  # DataFrame$ObjectName notation
class(PrePostRats.df$Success)   # DataFrame$ObjectName notation
class(PrePostRats.df$Sign)      # DataFrame$ObjectName notation

ls()                    # List all objects
str(PrePostRats.df)     # Confirm nature of the dataset
summary(PrePostRats.df) # Broad view of descriptive statistics
epicalc::des(PrePostRats.df) # Description of the dataset
```

Use of the attach(), class(), ls(), str(), summary(), and epicalc::des() functions may be somewhat redundant, but it is always a good idea to confirm that actions resulted in desired format. To use the common expression, *Trust, but verify*.

2.4 Conduct a Visual Data Check

It is common to immediately consider descriptive statistics and measures of central tendency when inferential analyses are planned and later completed. Certainly, it is important to know the Mode, Median, Mean, Standard Deviation, etc. However, in these lessons the data are first examined visually, using the strong graphical features supported by R. The images can be simple throwaway graphics (designed only to offer a general sense of the data), or the images can be fully embellished (of high quality, and suitable for presentation or publication). Regardless of details in the final view, graphics provide a composite understanding of the data that may be difficult to grasp when only statistics are viewed.

For initial purposes, the graphical functions of primary interest are hist() and plot(). It is also common to use plot(density()) (i.e., the plot() function wrapped around the density() function). Again, many arguments are available to support the functions used for graphics, but for now the figures will be prepared in fairly simple format.

The par(ask=TRUE) function and argument are used to freeze the presentation on the screen, one figure at a time. When par(ask=TRUE) is used, note how the top line of the figure in the R interface, under File -> Save as, provides a variety of graphical formats to save each figure, with selections showing in this order: Metafile, Postscript, PDF, PNG, BMP, TIFF, and JPEG.[2] It is also possible to perform a simple copy-and-paste against each graphical image. R syntax can also be used to save a graphical image.

```
par(ask=TRUE)
plot(PrePostRats.df$Lab, main="Laboratory", col="red",
  ylim=c(0,16)) # Force Y axis scale to show 15

par(ask=TRUE)
plot(PrePostRats.df$Subject, main="Subject",
  col=c(rainbow(40)))

par(ask=TRUE)
hist(PrePostRats.df$Pretest,
  main="Histogram of Lab Rat Pretest Measures",
  font=2,          # Bold text
  cex.lab=1.15,    # Large font
  col="red")       # Vibrant color

par(ask=TRUE)
hist(PrePostRats.df$Posttest,
  main="Histogram of Lab Rat Posttest Measures",
  font=2,          # Bold text
  cex.lab=1.15,    # Large font
  col="red")       # Vibrant color

par(ask=TRUE)
plot(density(PrePostRats.df$Pretest,
  na.rm=TRUE),   # Required for the density() function
  main="Density Plot of Lab Rat Pretest Measures",
  lwd=6, col="red", font.axis=2, font.lab=2)

par(ask=TRUE)
plot(density(PrePostRats.df$Posttest,
  na.rm=TRUE),   # Required for the density() function
  main="Density Plot of Lab Rat Posttest Measures",
  lwd=6, col="red", font.axis=2, font.lab=2)

par(ask=TRUE)
plot(PrePostRats.df$Success,
  main="Frequency Distribution of Success:  Success is
  Defined as Posttest > Pretest",
```

[2]To keep this text to a manageable number of pages, all figures are not shown. However, as a practice activity they can be easily created with the R syntax in this text and the .csv datasets that are available on the publisher's Web page associated with this text.

```
  lwd=6, col="red", font.axis=2, font.lab=2,
  ylim=c(0,31)) # Force Y axis scale to show 30

par(ask=TRUE)
plot(PrePostRats.df$Sign,
  main="Frequency Distribution of Sign and Comparison
  of Posttest to Pretest",
  lwd=6, col="red", font.axis=2, font.lab=2,
  ylim=c(0,31)) # Force Y axis scale to show 30

par(ask=TRUE)       # Bar and Frequencies of Plot of Success
epicalc::tab1(PrePostRats.df$Success,
  decimal=2,                        # Use the tab1() function
  sort.group=FALSE,                 # from the epicalc
  cum.percent=TRUE,                 # package to see details
  graph=TRUE,                       # about the selected
  missing=TRUE,                     # object variable. (The
  bar.values=c("frequency"),        # 1 of tab1 is the one
  horiz=FALSE,                      # numeric character and
  cex=1.15,                         # it is not the letter
  cex.names=1.15,                   # l).
  cex.lab=1.15, cex.axis=1.15,
  main="Frequency of Success:  N (Posttest !> Pretest) or
  Y (Posttest > Pretest)",
  ylab="Frequency:  N (Not Successful) and Y (Successful)",
  col= c("black", "red"),
  gen=TRUE)
  # Note how a frequency distribution is provided, too.
```

```
PrePostRats.df$Success :
                    Frequency Percent Cum. percent
N Not Successful           14      35           35
Y Successful               26      65          100
  Total                    40     100          100
```

```
par(ask=TRUE)       # Bar and Frequencies of Plot of Sign
epicalc::tab1(PrePostRats.df$Sign,
  decimal=2,                        # Use the tab1() function
  sort.group=FALSE,                 # from the epicalc
  cum.percent=TRUE,                 # package to see details
  graph=TRUE,                       # about the selected
  missing=TRUE,                     # object variable. (The
  bar.values=c("frequency"),        # 1 of tab1 is the one
  horiz=FALSE,                      # numeric character and
  cex=1.15,                         # it is not the letter
  cex.names=1.15,                   # l).
  cex.lab=1.15, cex.axis=1.15,
  main="Frequency of Sign:  - (Posttest < Pretest),
  + (Posttest > Pretest), or 0 (Posttest = Pretest)",
  ylab="Frequency:  - + 0",
  col= c("black", "red", "blue"),
  gen=TRUE)
  # Note how a frequency distribution is provided, too.
```

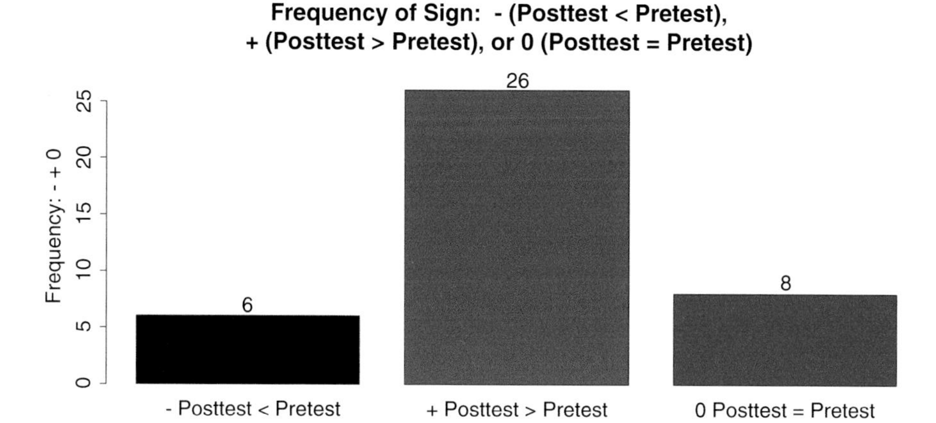

Fig. 2.1 Bar chart using the epicalc::tab1() function

```
PrePostRats.df$Sign :
                         Frequency Percent Cum. percent
- Posttest < Pretest             6      15           15
+ Posttest > Pretest            26      65           80
o Posttest = Pretest             8      20          100
  Total                         40     100          100
```

Because the Pretest data and Posttest data are ordinal, it is best to focus on frequency distributions, at least initially. Although the boxplot() function and different functions for the violin plot could have been used, the above graphic provides sufficient context for this simple dataset where the focus is on ordinal data (Fig. 2.1).[3]

2.5 Descriptive Analysis of the Data

Special accommodations are often needed for missing data. Knowing that missing data can be a concern, it is often helpful to first check for missing data by using the is.na() function and the complete.cases() function against the entire dataset. Both functions return a TRUE or FALSE response, depending on the function and the outcome of whether or not data are missing.

```
is.na(PrePostRats.df)            # Check for missing data
complete.cases(PrePostRats.df)   # Check for complete cases
```

[3]There remains some degree of inconsistency on correct usage for either Boxplot or Box Plot when referencing a Box-and-Whiskers Plot. Both terms may be found in this text.

For the dataset PrePostRats.df, there are no missing data and all cases are complete. That may not be the situation for later lessons, where there will be challenges to accommodation of the dataset.

This dataset consists of only 40 subjects, with the dataset complete for all six object variables. Again, the summary() function is applied, to reinforce an understanding of the data. Note how the summary() function is applied against the entire dataset, thus yielding information about all object variables.

```
summary(PrePostRats.df)
```

The summary() function is very useful and it should always be considered as a first selection when preparing descriptive analyses.

Frequency Distributions of the Factor-Type Object Variables

It is fairly common to provide a general tally of the breakouts for factor-type object variables, such as the number or percentage of individuals who were classified as Not Successful and those who were classified as Successful (the Success object variable) or the number and percentage of individuals who were classified as— (Posttest < Pretest), + (Posttest > Pretest), or o(Posttest = Pretest) (the Sign object variable).

Showing another option available with R, the table() function, by itself or with the cbind() function serving as a wrapper around the table() function may be all that it needed for a fairly simple output of frequency distributions of factor-type object variables:

```
table(PrePostRats.df$Success, useNA = "always")
```

```
cbind(table(PrePostRats.df$Success, PrePostRats.df$Pretest,
  useNA = "always")) # Finite breakouts by specific values
```

```
                 3 4 5 6 7 8 9 10 <NA>
N Not Successful 1 1 2 2 0 5 1  2    0
Y Successful     3 5 6 1 6 4 1  0    0
<NA>             0 0 0 0 0 0 0  0    0
```

```
cbind(table(PrePostRats.df$Success, PrePostRats.df$Posttest,
  useNA = "always"))# Finite breakouts by specific values
```

```
                 3 4 5 6 7 8 9 10 <NA>
N Not Successful 1 2 3 0 2 3 2  1    0
Y Successful     0 1 2 6 2 8 5  2    0
<NA>             0 0 0 0 0 0 0  0    0
```

```
table(PrePostRats.df$Sign, useNA = "always")
```

```
cbind(table(PrePostRats.df$Sign, PrePostRats.df$Pretest,
  useNA = "always")) # Finite breakouts by specific values
```

```
                      3 4 5 6 7 8 9 10 <NA>
- Posttest < Pretest 0 0 1 2 0 2 0  1    0
+ Posttest > Pretest 3 5 6 1 6 4 1  0    0
o Posttest = Pretest 1 1 1 0 0 3 1  1    0
<NA>                 0 0 0 0 0 0 0  0    0
```

```
cbind(table(PrePostRats.df$Sign, PrePostRats.df$Posttest,
  useNA = "always"))# Finite breakouts by specific values
```

```
                      3 4 5 6 7 8 9 10 <NA>
- Posttest < Pretest 0 1 2 0 2 0 1  0    0
+ Posttest > Pretest 0 1 2 6 2 8 5  2    0
o Posttest = Pretest 1 1 1 0 0 3 1  1    0
<NA>                 0 0 0 0 0 0 0  0    0
```

Not surprisingly, there are other functions (many in external packages) that present frequency distributions of factor-type object variables in a somewhat more attractive and concise manner. The xtabs() function and the Epi::stat.table() function, shown immediately below, should both be considered when preparing frequency distributions.

The xtabs() function has value for preparing somewhat more complex summarized frequency distributions of the two factor-type object variables found in this lesson:

```
xtabs(~Sign+Success, data=PrePostRats.df)
```

```
                       Success
Sign                     N Not Successful Y Successful
  - Posttest < Pretest                  6            0
  + Posttest > Pretest                  0           26
  o Posttest = Pretest                  8            0
```

The Epi::stat.table() function is especially helpful for presentation of frequency distributions by percent. Review the following to see the percentage for frequency distributions, overall and by breakouts.

```
install.packages("Epi")
library(Epi)                 # Load the Epi package.
help(package=Epi)            # Show the information page.
sessionInfo()                # Confirm all attached packages.
# Select the most local mirror site using Set CRAN mirror.

Epi::stat.table(index=list("Successful:  Yes or No"=Success,
  "Sign:  - + 0"=Sign), percent(Success,Sign), margin=TRUE,
  data=PrePostRats.df)
  # Table with cell percentages and margin totals
```

```
------------------------------------------------------
                      ------------Sign:  - + o------------
Successful:                    -         +         o    Total
 Yes or No              Posttest Posttest Posttest
                               <         >         =
                         Pretest  Pretest  Pretest
------------------------------------------------------
N Not Successful            15.0       0.0      20.0    35.0
Y Successful                 0.0      65.0       0.0    65.0

Total                       15.0      65.0      20.0   100.0
------------------------------------------------------
>   # Table with cell percentages and margin totals
```

Measures of Central Tendency of the Numeric Object Variables
Even though the summary() function is quite sufficient for a general overview of descriptive statistics, descriptive statistics for individual object variables may be desired. To achieve this aim, review use of the following functions: length(), asbio::Mode(), median(), mean(), sd(), tapply(), and once again summary(). As needed (but not always, depending on specific functions), the na.rm=TRUE argument or some other similar convention will be used to accommodate missing data—which is not a concern for this specific dataset.

Equally, remember that object variables PrePostRats.df$Pretest and PrePostRats.df$Posttest represent ordinal data, and the main focus should be on Median, not Mean and SD (even though these other measures of central tendency have value for understanding the data and are presented in this lesson).

```
length(PrePostRats.df$Pretest)          # N of Pretest
length(PrePostRats.df$Posttest)         # N of Posttest

install.packages("asbio")
library(asbio)                    # Load the asbio package.
help(package=asbio)               # Show the information page.
sessionInfo()                     # Confirm all attached packages.
# Select the most local mirror site using Set CRAN mirror.

asbio::Mode(PrePostRats.df$Pretest) # Mode as average
asbio::Mode(PrePostRats.df$Posttest)# Mode as average
```

```
median(PrePostRats.df$Pretest, na.rm=TRUE)        # Median
```

```
[1] 6
```

```
median(PrePostRats.df$Posttest, na.rm=TRUE)       # Median
```

```
[1] 8
```

```
mean(PrePostRats.df$Pretest, na.rm=TRUE)          # Mean
sd(PrePostRats.df$Pretest, na.rm=TRUE )           # SD

mean(PrePostRats.df$Posttest, na.rm=TRUE)         # Mean
sd(PrePostRats.df$Posttest, na.rm=TRUE )          # SD
```

Descriptive statistics at the summary level are always useful, but breakout statistics are also needed to gain a more complete understanding of the data. There are many ways to obtain breakout statistics, but the tapply() function, epicalc::summ() function, prettyR::brkdn() function, psych::describe.by() function, Hmisc::bystats() function, and the lessR::SummaryStats() function are among the most detailed and easiest to use, to discern differences between breakout groups. For this lesson, given the simple nature of the dataset, only the tapply() function and the epicalc::summ() function are demonstrated. A useful feature for the epicalc::summ() function is that a graphic is prepared, as well as the descriptive statistics.

Comment: Be sure to recall the prior caution that the Pretest and Posttest measures associated with this lesson are viewed as ordinal data. Descriptive statistics (i.e., Mean, SD, etc.) can be easily calculated against ordinal data if the ordinal data are coerced into numeric class, but, as shown below, the meaning of these descriptive statistics should always be viewed with care given the nature of ordinal data as compared to interval data.

```
tapply(Pretest, Success, summary, na.rm=TRUE,
  data=PrePostRats.df) # Pretest by Success, using tapply()

tapply(Posttest, Success, summary, na.rm=TRUE,
  data=PrePostRats.df) # Posttest by Success, using tapply()

tapply(Pretest, Sign, summary, na.rm=TRUE,
  data=PrePostRats.df) # Pretest by Sign using tapply()

tapply(Posttest, Sign, summary, na.rm=TRUE,
  data=PrePostRats.df) # Posttest by Sign using tapply()
```

```
$`- Posttest < Pretest`
   Min. 1st Qu.  Median    Mean 3rd Qu.    Max.
  4.000   5.000   6.000   6.167   7.000   9.000

$`+ Posttest > Pretest`
   Min. 1st Qu.  Median    Mean 3rd Qu.    Max.
  4.000   6.000   8.000   7.423   8.750  10.000

$`o Posttest = Pretest`
   Min. 1st Qu.  Median    Mean 3rd Qu.    Max.
  3.000   4.750   8.000   6.875   8.250  10.000
```

```
par(ask=TRUE) # Use the epicalc package for breakout analyses
epicalc::summ(PrePostRats.df$Pretest,
  by=PrePostRats.df$Success,
  graph=TRUE, pch=18, ylab="auto",
  main="Sorted Dotplot of Pretest by Success",
  cex.X.axis=1.15, cex.Y.axis=1.15, font.lab=2, dot.col="auto")
  # Note the descriptive statistics and not only the graphic
  # that go along with the epicalc::summ() function.

par(ask=TRUE) # Use the epicalc package for breakout analyses
epicalc::summ(PrePostRats.df$Posttest,
  by=PrePostRats.df$Success,
  graph=TRUE, pch=18, ylab="auto",
  main="Sorted Dotplot of Posttest by Success",
  cex.X.axis=1.15, cex.Y.axis=1.15, font.lab=2, dot.col="auto")
  # Note the descriptive statistics and not only the graphic
  # that go along with the epicalc::summ() function.

par(ask=TRUE) # Use the epicalc package for breakout analyses
epicalc::summ(PrePostRats.df$Pretest,
  by=PrePostRats.df$Sign,
  graph=TRUE, pch=18, ylab="auto",
  main="Sorted Dotplot of Pretest by Sign",
  cex.X.axis=1.15, cex.Y.axis=1.15, font.lab=2, dot.col="auto")
  # Note the descriptive statistics and not only the graphic
  # that go along with the epicalc::summ() function.

par(ask=TRUE) # Use the epicalc package for breakout analyses
epicalc::summ(PrePostRats.df$Posttest,
  by=PrePostRats.df$Sign,
  graph=TRUE, pch=18, ylab="auto",
  main="Sorted Dotplot of Posttest by Sign",
  cex.X.axis=1.15, cex.Y.axis=1.15, font.lab=2, dot.col="auto")
  # Note the descriptive statistics and not only the graphic
  # that go along with the epicalc::summ() function.
```

```
For PrePostRats.df$Sign = - Posttest < Pretest
 obs. mean   median  s.d.   min.   max.
 6    6.167  6       1.835  4      9

For PrePostRats.df$Sign = + Posttest > Pretest
 obs. mean   median  s.d.   min.   max.
 26   7.423  8       1.604  4      10

For PrePostRats.df$Sign = o Posttest = Pretest
 obs. mean   median  s.d.   min.   max.
 8    6.875  8       2.532  3      10
```

The Epi::stat.table() function, shown previously for frequency distributions and percentages, can also be used for a limited set of descriptive statistics. Look below at the use of this function for breakout statistics by median (Fig. 2.2).

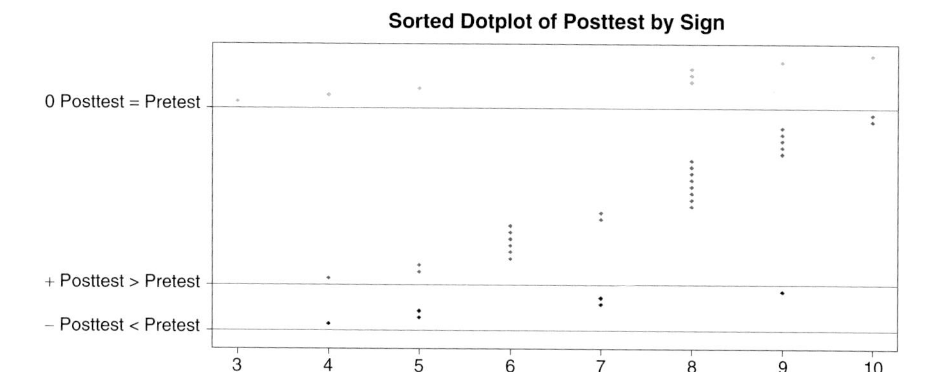

Fig. 2.2 Sorted dotplot using the epicalc::summ() function

```
Epi::stat.table(index=list("Success Y or N"=Success),
  list(N=count(), "Median of Pretest"=median(Pretest)),
  data=PrePostRats.df)
  # Success:  Median of breakouts for Pretest

Epi::stat.table(index=list("Success Y or N"=Success),
  list(N=count(), "Median of Posttest"=median(Posttest)),
  data=PrePostRats.df)
  # Success:  Median of breakouts for Posttest

Epi::stat.table(index=list("Sign   - + o"=Sign),
  list(N=count(), "Median of Pretest"=median(Pretest)),
  data=PrePostRats.df)
  # Sign:  Median of breakouts for Pretest

Epi::stat.table(index=list("Sign   - + o"=Sign),
  list(N=count(), "Median of Posttest"=median(Posttest)),
  data=PrePostRats.df)
  # Sign:  Median of breakouts for Posttest
```

```
 ---------------------------------------
 Sign                         N   Median
 - + o                                of
                                Posttest
 ---------------------------------------
 - Posttest < Pretest         6     6.00
 + Posttest > Pretest        26     8.00
 o Posttest = Pretest         8     8.00
 ---------------------------------------
```

The tables::tabular() function can be used to provide even more detail. Output from the tables::tabular() function is fairly attractive and this output can be easily copied or used in some other fashion in a summary report. Again, the emphasis for this lesson will be on the Median, not the Mean and SD.

```
install.packages("tables")
library(tables)                 # Load the tables package.
help(package=tables)            # Show the information page.
sessionInfo()                   # Confirm all attached packages.
# Select the most local mirror site using Set CRAN mirror.

tables::tabular((Success + 1) ~ (n=1) + Format(digits=2)*
  (Pretest + Posttest)*(min + max + median),
  data=PrePostRats.df)
  # Success (row) by Pretest and Posttest (columns)
  # Focus on the Median, not Mean or SD

tables::tabular((Sign + 1) ~ (n=1) + Format(digits=2)*
  (Pretest + Posttest)*(min + max + median),
  data=PrePostRats.df)
  # Sign (row) by Pretest and Posttest (columns)
  # Focus on the Median, not Mean or SD
```

```
                            Pretest           Posttest
 Sign                     n  min    max median min       max median
 - Posttest < Pretest   6  5      10   7        4         9   6
 + Posttest > Pretest  26  3       9   5        4        10   8
 o Posttest = Pretest   8  3      10   8        3        10   8
 All                   40  3      10   6        3        10   8
```

The output from the tables::tabular() function can also be put into LaTeXformat by using the Hmisc::latex() function as a wrapper. Look below at the professional quality of a table put into LaTeXformat to see why LaTeXis used so frequently for typesetting scientific papers, journal articles, texts, etc.

```
install.packages("Hmisc")
library(Hmisc)                  # Load the Hmisc package.
help(package=Hmisc)             # Show the information page.
sessionInfo()                   # Confirm all attached packages.
# Select the most local mirror site using Set CRAN mirror.

Hmisc::latex(
tables::tabular((Success + 1) ~ (n=1) + Format(digits=2)*
  (Pretest + Posttest)*(min + max + median),
  data=PrePostRats.df)
  # Success (row) by Pretest and Posttest (columns)
  # Focus on the Median, not Mean or SD
) # Note placement of ending ) character
```

Success	n	Pretest Min	Pretest Max	Pretest Median	Posttest Min	Posttest Max	Posttest Median
N not successful	14	3	10	8	3	10	7
Y successful	26	3	9	5	4	10	8
All	40	3	10	6	3	10	8

```
Hmisc::latex(
tables::tabular((Sign + 1) ~ (n=1) + Format(digits=2)*
  (Pretest + Posttest)*(min + max + median),
  data=PrePostRats.df)
  # Sign (row) by Pretest and Posttest (columns)
  # Focus on the Median, not Mean or SD
)
```

Sign	n	Pretest Min	Pretest Max	Pretest Median	Posttest Min	Posttest Max	Posttest Median
− Posttest < Pretest	6	5	10	7	4	9	6
+ Posttest > Pretest	26	3	9	5	4	10	8
o Posttest = Pretest	8	3	10	8	3	10	8
All	40	3	10	6	3	10	8

The R-based output from use of the Hmisc::latex() function may seem more than difficult to read, at first. However, when placed into LaTeX, the table is quite attractive and meets most standards for publication in a professional paper. Remember, of course, that the output has to be compiled as a LaTeXdocument. The original output, as text showing on the R screen, will seem quite odd for those who do not use LaTeX.

Application of the Anderson-Darling Test

Although graphical images and descriptive statistics are helpful in understanding the data, it is also useful to apply selected statistical tests to serve as an additional support for decision making on acceptance of nonparametric or parametric views toward the data. To that end, consider application of the Anderson-Darling Test, the Lilliefors (KS) Test, and the Shapiro-Wilk Test. It should be mentioned that these tests may be influenced by sample size and that they provide one view—but not the only view—on the nature of distribution patterns. Experience, needs, and practical judgment, supported by careful review of graphical images, descriptive statistics, and statistical tests should be used when deciding if variables from a dataset are best viewed from a nonparametric or parametric perspective.

```
install.packages("nortest")
library(nortest)              # Load the nortest package.
help(package=nortest)         # Show the information page.
sessionInfo()                 # Confirm all attached packages.
# Select the most local mirror site using Set CRAN mirror.
```

From among a few different possible tests, the Anderson-Darling Test is used for this lesson to examine distribution. The Null Hypothesis for the Anderson-Darling Test is structured to examine if the data follow a specified distribution:

Anderson-Darling Null Hypothesis: The data follow the normal distribution.

```
nortest::ad.test(PrePostRats.df$Pretest)
  # Anderson-Darling Test
```

```
        Anderson-Darling normality test

data:  PrePostRats.df$Pretest
A = 0.9737, p-value = 0.01279
```

```
nortest::ad.test(PrePostRats.df$Posttest)
  # Anderson-Darling Test
```

```
        Anderson-Darling normality test

data:  PrePostRats.df$Posttest
A = 1.0195, p-value = 0.009813
```

The calculated Anderson-Darling Test for normality p-value is fairly small for both object variables, PrePostRats.df$Pretest and PrePostRats.df$Posttest:

- Anderson-Darling Test PrePostRats.df$Pretest p-value = 0.01279
- Anderson-Darling Test PrePostRats.df$Posttest p-value = 0.009813

Given these p-values, reject the Anderson-Darling Null Hypotheses that the data are from a normal distribution. In this lesson, the data for object variables PrePostRats.df$Pretest and PrePostRats.df$Posttest do not display normal distribution.

```
par(ask=TRUE)
par(mfrow=c(1,2))                     # Side-by-Side QQ Plots
qqnorm(PrePostRats.df$Pretest,
  col="black", bg="red", pch=23,  # Points in the plot
  font=2, font.lab=2, cex.axis=1.5,
  main="QQPlot of PrePostRats.df$Pretest")
qqline(PrePostRats.df$Pretest, lwd=4, col="darkblue")
qqnorm(PrePostRats.df$Posttest,
  col="black", bg="red", pch=23,  # Points in the plot
  font=2, font.lab=2, cex.axis=1.5,
  main="QQPlot of PrePostRats.df$Posttest")
qqline(PrePostRats.df$Posttest, lwd=4, col="darkblue")
```

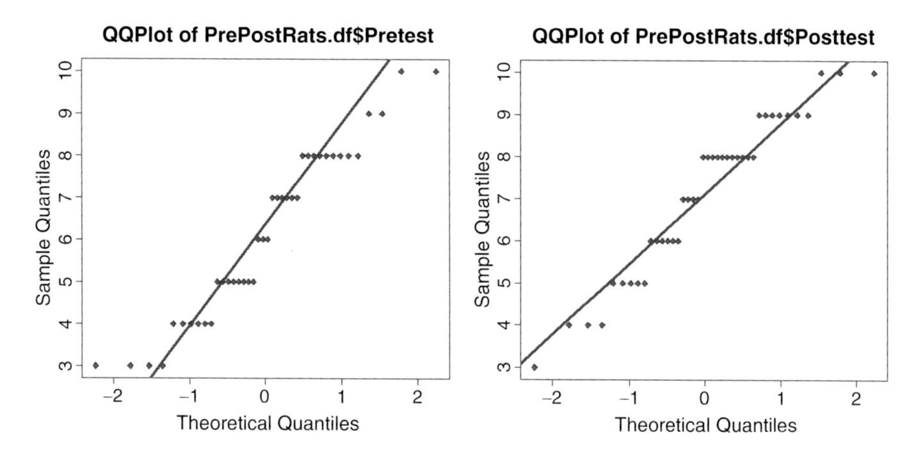

Fig. 2.3 QQ plots comparing two separate object variables

The QQ plot (i.e., normal probability plot) provides additional confirmation that the data are best viewed from a nonparametric perspective.[4] Note the placement of the data along the qqline, especially at the tails (Fig. 2.3).

2.6 Conduct the Statistical Analysis

Use the BSDA::SIGN.test() function to conduct a Dependent Samples Sign Test of differences in Pretest and Posttest measures, at the level of:

- – or Posttest < Pretest
- + or Posttest > Pretest
- o or Posttest = Pretest (scores are tied)

By no means are these three classifications seen as robust measures (i.e., the Pretest = 5 to Posttest = 6 difference yields a + and a Pretest = 5 to Posttest = 9 also yields a +), but it has been judged that design and/or measurement process for this exploratory lesson on the Sign Test does not support more exact measures.

```
install.packages("BSDA", dependencies=TRUE)
library(BSDA)                    # Load the BSDA package.
help(package=BSDA)               # Show the information page.
sessionInfo()                    # Confirm all attached packages.
# Select the most local mirror site using Set CRAN mirror.

BSDA::SIGN.test(PrePostRats.df$Pretest,
  PrePostRats.df$Posttest, md=0)
```

[4]The Quantile-Quantile (Q-Q or QQ) plot is a graphical tool that is used to examine data distribution patterns.

```
        Dependent-samples Sign-Test

data:  PrePostRats.df$Pretest and PrePostRats.df$Posttest
S = 6, p-value = 0.0005351
alternative hypothesis: true median difference is not equal to 0
95 percent confidence interval:
 -1.0000000 -0.2729644
sample estimates:
median of x-y
           -1

                          Conf.Level L.E.pt U.E.pt
Lower Achieved CI             0.9193     -1 -1.000
Interpolated CI               0.9500     -1 -0.273
Upper Achieved CI             0.9615     -1  0.000
```

2.7 Summary

For a dependent samples Sign Test (i.e., a two-sample dependent Sign Test), the Null Hypothesis is focused on the median and the median for the differences of x and y, or Pretest and Posttest in this sample lesson. Consider, again, the Null Hypothesis:

The median of differences between Pretest and Posttest measures of laboratory rats, after application of an otherwise unidentified treatment, equals 0 (p <= 0.05).

Going beyond the use of frequency distributions and measures of central tendency such as the Median, the Sign Test provides evidence that there is a statistically significant difference in outcomes between Pretest and Posttest measures after application of the treatment, given a calculated p-value of 0.0005351, which is certainly less than p <= 0.05.

Accordingly, the Null Hypothesis is rejected and it has been determined that there is a statistically significant difference (p <= 0.05) in Pretest and Posttest measures among laboratory rats after application of the otherwise unknown treatment.

The finding of a statistically significant difference between Pretest and Posttest measures is in parity with the descriptive statistics associated with this lesson. Observe the Median value for both the Pretest and the Posttest, both at a simple level of comparison using the median() function and with greater detail using the tables::tabular() function.

```
median(PrePostRats.df$Pretest)
```

```
[1] 6
```

```
median(PrePostRats.df$Posttest)
```

```
[1] 8
```

```
tables::tabular((Sign + 1) ~ (n=1) + Format(digits=2)*
  (Pretest + Posttest)*(min + max + median),
  data=PrePostRats.df)
  # Sign (row) by Pretest and Posttest (columns)
  # Focus on the Median, not Mean or SD
```

```
                               Pretest            Posttest
Sign                         n min    max median min      max median
- Posttest < Pretest  6  5     10   7      4        9   6
+ Posttest > Pretest 26  3      9   5      4       10   8
o Posttest = Pretest  8  3     10   8      3       10   8
All                  40  3     10   6      3       10   8
```

For the collection of all 40 laboratory rats, Median Pretest = 6 and Median Posttest = 8. Equally, review the Sign Test and how the calculated p-value of 0.0005351 was less than the p-value associated with the Null Hypothesis, `p <= 0.05`. These two outcomes support judgment that the treatment (i.e., intervention) resulted in a difference.

When interpreting the frequency distributions associated with this lesson, it is often best to use the following methodology to interpret the meaning of the calculated p value:

- − changes = 06 (Posttest < Pretest)
- + changes = 26 (Posttest > Pretest)
- o changes = 08 (Posttest = Pretest)

After careful analysis of the data, the Null Hypothesis is rejected and instead it is declared that there is a statistically significant difference (`p <= 0.05`) between Pretest and Posttest measures of laboratory rats after application an unidentified treatment. The outcome (as indicated by difference in Pretest and Posttest measures) was influenced by the treatment (i.e., intervention) activity. To be more exact, the lab rats associated with this lesson showed gain (however gain was viewed) after the treatment:

- 26 rats showed an increase from Pretest to Posttest
- 06 rats showed a decrease from Pretest to Posttest
- 08 rats showed no change from Pretest to Posttest

The treatment, overall, resulted in gain. However, avoid saying that there was a 65 % (26/40) positive change because of the intervention. This type of statement is sometimes observed in publications, but it should be recalled that the Sign Test does not support this level of measurement and subsequent conclusion. Instead, it is only possible to claim that there was an overall difference (viewed as gain, in this lesson—whatever gain means) as evidenced by use of the Sign Test.

Again, view the Sign Test as an exploratory tool and use more robust analyses (based on more controlled research designs) for more finite conclusions. As shown in this lesson, with little known about the laboratories providing the subjects and other command-and-control issues, more precise methodologies and inferential tests would be needed to offer a greater level of judgment on the magnitude of change. Even so, for initial attempts to examine a problem, the Sign Test may be a very appropriate test to gain a sense of general direction in trends.

2.8 Prepare to Exit, Save, and Later Retrieve This R Session

```
getwd()             # Identify the current working directory.
ls()                # List all objects in the working
                    # directory.
ls.str()            # List all objects, with finite detail.
list.files()        # List files at the PC directory.

save.image("R_Lesson_Sign-Test.rdata")

getwd()             # Identify the current working directory.
ls()                # List all objects in the working
                    # directory.
ls.str()            # List all objects, with finite detail.
list.files()        # List files at the PC directory.

alarm()             # Alarm, notice of upcoming action.
q()                 # Quit this session.
                    # Prepare for Save workspace image? query.
```

Use the R Graphical User Interface (GUI) to load the saved rdata file: File -> Load Workspace. Otherwise, use the load() function, keying the full pathname, to load the .rdata file and retrieve the session.

Recall, however, that it may be just as useful to simply use the .R script file (typically saved is a .txt ASCII-type file) and recreate the analyses and graphics, provided the data files remain available.

Chapter 3
Chi-Square

Abstract The Chi-square test is perhaps the most frequently used (or overused) nonparamteric statistical test. The Chi-square test, named for the Greek letter χ (i.e., Chi or the Greek letter for x), is typically used to test for differences in proportions between two or more groups. The Chi-square test is also called a *goodness of fit* test. That is to say, the Chi-square test is used to see if grouped data actually fit into declared groups, or if the data instead do not fit into the group. For this lesson, Chi-square will be demonstrated using data in two formats: (1) Chi-square using R will first be demonstrated where the data are presented as an external file imported into R, with data organized at the level of individual subjects, (i.e., each row represents the data for an individual subject) and (2) Chi-square using R will also be demonstrated where data are not at the level of individual subjects but data are instead presented in summary format, as a collapsed contingency table.

Keywords Bar plot (stacked, side-by-side) • Boolean • Central tendency • Chi-square • Code book • Comma-separated values (.csv) • Contingency table • Crosstabs • Distribution-free • Dotplot • Frequency distribution • Goodness of fit • Histogram • Mosaic plot • Nominal • Nonparametric • Normal distribution • Null hypothesis • Parametric • Probability (p-value) • Proportion • Representation • Statistical significance • Yates correction

3.1 Background on This Lesson

Chi-square is used to test for differences in proportions between two or more groups. The Chi-square test is typically used when the data are represented as frequency counts (i.e., headcounts) grouped into specific categories. It is common to use Chi-square analyses with nominal data presented as counts in assigned cells.

The general approach with Chi-square is to determine if the number of subjects in identified groups differ by relative frequency. The proportion of cases from one group are compared to the proportion of cases from a different group.

Electronic supplementary material The online version of this chapter (doi: 10.1007/978-3-319-30634-6_3) contains supplementary material, which is available to authorized users.

T.W. MacFarland, J.M. Yates, *Introduction to Nonparametric Statistics for the Biological Sciences Using R*, DOI 10.1007/978-3-319-30634-6_3

The compelling advantage of Chi-square is that it supports well-accepted analyses with data that are only nominal (e.g., Gender—Female or Male, Location—Sect. 3.1 or Sect. 3.2, etc.) in terms of measurement. The samples in this lesson will provide more insight into the use of Chi-square.

3.1.1 Description of the Data

This lesson on Chi-square analysis is based on the occurrence of a specific trait between female and male members of a biological organism. In this lesson, assume that 60 subjects of a specific biological organism are examined by a team of trained technicians for two immediate judgments: Gender (i.e., Female or Male) and Trait (i.e., Trait is Absent or Trait is Present). For the purpose of this lesson, it is not necessary to know the type of biological organism (e.g., possible examples could include *Alces alces*, Moose; *Carcharodon carcharias*, Great White Shark; *Homo sapien*, Human), and it is equally not necessary to know the nature of the trait. It is only necessary to know that the technicians have received adequate training for all protocols and it is therefore assumed that the data are correct and are presented as frequency counts:

- Assume that the gender has been identified correctly.
- Assume that the absence or presence of the trait has also been identified correctly. Further, the *degree* of absence or presence of the trait is not measured. Instead, for this lesson the measure is binary. The trait in question is either absent or the trait in question is present.

Although it is beyond the purpose of this lesson, be sure to recall that many measurements in the biological sciences must be made quickly and often with less precision than may be desired.

- In a laboratory setting when working with non-moving organisms or perhaps small docile animals, it may be possible to use protocols that allow for close examination and careful measurement.
- Under field conditions, however, speed and safety may override the desire for precision, either for protection of the technicians taking measurements or for protection of the organism under study, such as when working with large unsedated animals that have sharp teeth and large claws, hooves, or talons.

In this study, a team of field technicians gained data on Gender and Trait from 60 unique subjects, all of the same organism. The lead technician then reviewed individual field notes (i.e., paper-based data sheets) and prepared a dataset at the level of the individual subject. A Gnumeric-based spreadsheet was originally prepared, but to further assure future data compatibility with other professionals the .gnumeric spreadsheet was then also saved in .csv (comma-separated values) format. The data are summarized below, and they are also found in original format (by subject row-by-row) in the file GenderTrait.csv, which is found on the publisher's Web page associated with this text.

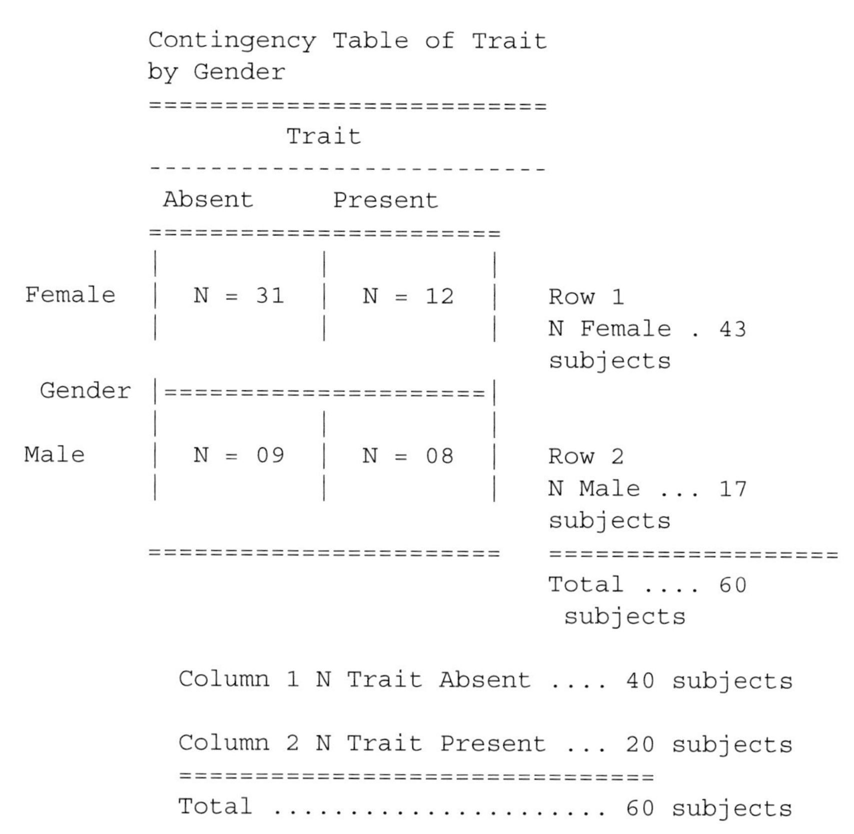

```
          Contingency Table of Trait
          by Gender
          ==========================
                   Trait
          --------------------------
           Absent      Present
          =======================
          |          |          |
Female    |  N = 31  |  N = 12  |   Row 1
          |          |          |   N Female . 43
                                    subjects
 Gender   |=====================|
          |          |          |
Male      |  N = 09  |  N = 08  |   Row 2
          |          |          |   N Male ... 17
                                    subjects
          =======================   ===================
                                    Total .... 60
                                     subjects

            Column 1 N Trait Absent .... 40 subjects

            Column 2 N Trait Present ... 20 subjects
            ===============================
            Total ...................... 60 subjects
```

To summarize this simple, and fairly common, 2 by 2 (i.e., 2 rows by 2 columns) contingency table:

- The trait in question is absent in 31 female subjects and it is absent in 09 male subjects.
- The trait in question is present in 12 female subjects and it is present in 08 male subjects.

Because of distinguishing characteristics, assume that it is fairly easy to determine Gender. However, recall that there is no precise measurement for the object variable Trait. Neither a sphygmomanometer, thermometer, or weighing scale were used to obtain data for Trait. Instead, trained technicians examined subjects, made informed but quick judgment, and then immediately recorded field notes on paper-based worksheets. The data were only later put into electronic format.

When viewing the data found in GenderTrait.csv, be sure to note how numerical codes have been purposely used for the data (Gender and Trait) in this lesson. Numerical codes are quite common, and the creation of a later Code Book is essential so that there is a record of what each code represents.

When using Chi-square, there are a few criteria that must be observed regardless of the field conditions or nature of individual subjects, whether human or otherwise:

- Data must be presented as frequency (i.e., counted) data, such as the number of Yes responses to a specific survey statement or the number of left-handed batters on a baseball team. Recall, however, that ordinal and even interval data can be organized (i.e., collapsed or grouped) into categories such as *The number of human subjects with Systolic Blood Pressure GTE (greater than or equal to) 114* and *The number of human subjects with Systolic Blood Pressure LT (less than) 114.*[1]
- Due to the undesired impact of low cell counts in a contingency table, the number of observed frequencies for each cell should be five or more. Some reference materials suggest that the number of observed frequencies for each cell should be ten or more. Otherwise, it may be necessary to use the Yates correction formula along with Chi-square, to accommodate low cell counts.
- Regardless of the organization scheme, the data must be arranged in a logical manner. All subjects must be considered once and only once.

3.1.2 Null Hypothesis (Ho)

There is no statistically significant difference (`p <= 0.05`) between the two genders (Female or Male) in regard to the presence (Absent or Present) of a specific unnamed trait of an otherwise unidentified biological organism.

Notice how the Null Hypothesis (Ho) uses `p <= 0.05`. The expression `p <= 0.05` is used to identify the declared probability level specific to the Null Hypothesis. Many exploratory inferential analyses in the biological sciences are conducted at `p <= 0.05`. However, it is not uncommon to see some analyses set at the more restrictive level of `p <= 0.01` and even `p <= 0.001`.

Along with the use of p, you will also see the term *alpha* in many discussions about the level of probability, but p will be used in this lesson.

3.2 Data Import of a .csv Spreadsheet-Type Data File into R

The dataset for this lesson represents data from 60 subjects, all of the same but unnamed biological species. Adequate protocols were used so that the organisms (i.e., Subjects) were identified by a control number (S01 to S60). There are no missing data, with data for Gender and Trait obtained for each of the 60 Subjects. As previously mentioned, data were transferred from paper-based field notes to a Gnumeric-based spreadsheet and then to a .csv file.

[1]Although it is beyond the immediate purpose of this text on R, it is still useful to have some background with Boolean terms used for selection. As time permits, become acquainted with the following terms: EQ (equals), NE (not equals), LT (less than), LTE or LE (less than or equal), GT (greater than), and GTE or GE (greater than or equal).

Start a new R session and then attend to beginning actions such as removing unwanted files from prior work, declaring the working directory, etc.

```
###############################################################
# Housekeeping                              Use for All Analyses    #
###############################################################
date()                # Current system time and date.
R.version.string      # R version and version release date.
ls()                  # List all objects in the working
                      # directory.
rm(list = ls())       # CAUTION: Remove all files in the working
                      # directory. If this action is not desired,
                      # use the rm() function one-by-one to remove
                      # the objects that are not needed.
ls.str()              # List all objects, with finite detail.
getwd()               # Identify the current working directory.
setwd("F:/R_Nonparametric")
                      # Set to a new working directory.
                      # Note the single forward slash and double
                      # quotes.
                      # This new directory should be the directory
                      # where the data file is located, otherwise
                      # the data file will not be found.
getwd()               # Confirm the working directory.
list.files()          # List files at the PC directory.
###############################################################

GenderTrait.df <- read.table (file =
  "GenderTrait.csv",
  header = TRUE,
  sep = ",")                    # Import the  csv file

getwd()                         # Identify the working directory
ls()                            # List objects
attach(GenderTrait.df)          # Attach the data, for later use
str(GenderTrait.df)             # Identify structure
nrow(GenderTrait.df)            # List the number of rows
ncol(GenderTrait.df)            # List the number of columns
dim(GenderTrait.df)             # Dimensions of the dataframe
names(GenderTrait.df)           # Identify names
colnames(GenderTrait.df)        # Show column names
rownames(GenderTrait.df)        # Show row names
head(GenderTrait.df)            # Show the head
tail(GenderTrait.df)            # Show the tail
GenderTrait.df                  # Show the entire dataframe
summary(GenderTrait.df)         # Summary statistics
```

By completing these actions, an object called GenderTrait.df has been created. This R-based object is a dataframe, and it consists of the data originally included in the file GenderTrait.csv, a comma-separated values .csv file. To avoid possible conflicts, make sure that there are no prior R-based objects called GenderTrait.df in the current working directory. The prior use of rm(list = ls()) accommodates this concern, removing all prior objects in the current R session.

Observe how it was only necessary to key the filename for the .csv file and not the full pathname since the R working directory is currently set to the directory and/or subdirectory where this .csv file is located. See the Housekeeping section at the beginning of this lesson.

3.3 Organize the Data and Display the Code Book

Now that the data have been imported into R, it is usually necessary to check the data for format and then make any changes that may be needed to organize the data. This dataset consists of 60 subjects and the data are fairly simple, with an identifying code for Subject, a numeric code for Gender, and a numeric code for Trait. Although the data are simple, it will be necessary to accommodate the numeric codes for the factor-type object variables, Gender (i.e., factors Female or Male) and Trait (i.e., factors Absent or Present) and put them into a format that is easier to understand.

This lesson will also use rownames for the dataset, using the rownames() function. Although this action is not required, rownames may be helpful when working with increasingly large datasets. The rownames() function assigns a unique identifier for each row in the dataset. In this lesson, each rowname begins with the term Subject.

```
rownames(GenderTrait.df) <- paste('Subject', 1:60)

tail(GenderTrait.df)   # Show the tail, now to confirm rownames
```

For this lesson, the class() function, str() function, and duplicated() function will be used to confirm that data are organized correctly.

```
class(GenderTrait.df)
class(GenderTrait.df$Subject)
class(GenderTrait.df$Gender)
class(GenderTrait.df$Trait)
# Use DataFrame$ObjectName notation for object variables

str(GenderTrait.df)              # Structure

duplicated(GenderTrait.df)       # Duplicates
```

Based on the above actions, the class for each object seems to be correct, and there are no duplicate rows of data in the dataframe. A Code Book will help with future understanding of this dataset.

For anyone involved in the day-to-day activities of the research and statistics process, a Code Book is an essential aid—especially when data need to be reviewed in the future when object variable names and values are forgotten. The Code Book is typically brief and only serves as a useful reminder for what can be easily forgotten months (or even weeks) later. Coding schemes that are intuitively obvious today can easily become forgotten tomorrow.

Now that the class(), str(), and duplicated() functions have been used for basic diagnostics, consult the Code Book and coerce each object, as needed, into its correct class.

```
#######################################################
# Code Book for GenderTrait.df                        #
#######################################################
# Subject .................. S01 (Low) to S60 (High) #
#                                                     #
# Gender ................... Female = 1 and Male = 2 #
#                                                     #
# Trait ................ Absent = 1 and Present = 2 #
#######################################################
```

After data are brought into the current R session and there is agreement that the data are in correct format, it is usually necessary to organize the data to some degree. In this lesson, note how numeric codes have been used to identify Gender and Trait. Note also how these numeric codes are currently viewed as integers, as communicated by output from the str() function.

With assurance that the dataframe is in correct format and that labels are correct, coerce objects into correct format. A set of simple R-based actions can easily:

- Transform (i.e., recode) GenderTrait.df$Gender and GenderTrait.df$Trait into new object variables.
- Change the recoded object variables from original integer format to factor format.
- Apply narrative text labels for the otherwise cryptic numeric codes.

This transformation (again, typically called a recode action) is needed and the process, using R-based syntax, follows:

```
GenderTrait.df$Gender.recode <- factor(GenderTrait.df$Gender,
  labels=c("Female", "Male"))

GenderTrait.df$Trait.recode  <- factor(GenderTrait.df$Trait,
  labels=c("Absent", "Present"))
```

As a reminder, in this lesson, Gender has been recoded from 1s and 2s into two separate groups (i.e., Female and Male). Equally, Trait has been recoded from 1s and 2s into two separate groups (e.g., Absent and Present):

- The object variable GenderTrait.df$Gender.recode was created by putting the object variable GenderTrait.df$Gender into factor format. Labels were then applied in sequential order for this new object, with Female used to represent every occurrence of the numeric value 1 and Male used to represent every occurrence of the numeric value 2.
- The object variable GenderTrait.df$Trait was created by putting the object variable GenderTrait.df$Trait into factor format. Labels were applied in sequential

order for this new object, with Absent used to represent every occurrence of the numeric value 1 and Present used to represent every occurrence of the numeric value 2.

Note the formal nomenclature for this recode action and use of DataframeName$ObjectName when working with object variable names. Note also how the $ symbol is used to separate the name of the dataframe from the name of the object: DataframeName$ObjectName.

A confirming set of functions may not be necessary, but a redundant data check is always helpful to provide assurance that data in the current R session are correct prior to use of the data. Trust that the data are correct, but verify—as a continuous quality assurance process, as shown below in the following R syntax:

```
getwd()                         # Identify the working directory
ls()                            # List objects
attach(GenderTrait.df)          # Attach the data, for later use
str(GenderTrait.df)             # Identify structure
nrow(GenderTrait.df)            # List the number of rows
ncol(GenderTrait.df)            # List the number of columns
dim(GenderTrait.df)             # Dimensions of the dataframe
names(GenderTrait.df)           # Identify names
colnames(GenderTrait.df)        # Show column names
rownames(GenderTrait.df)        # Show row names
head(GenderTrait.df)            # Show the head
tail(GenderTrait.df)            # Show the tail
GenderTrait.df                  # Show the entire dataframe
summary(GenderTrait.df)         # Summary statistics
```

```
summary(GenderTrait.df[, 2:5])              # Variables 2 to 5
     Gender          Trait          Gender.recode   Trait.recode
 Min.   :1.000   Min.   :1.000   Female:43       Absent :40
 1st Qu.:1.000   1st Qu.:1.000   Male  :17       Present:20
 Median :1.000   Median :1.000
 Mean   :1.283   Mean   :1.333
 3rd Qu.:2.000   3rd Qu.:2.000
 Max.   :2.000   Max.   :2.000
```

3.4 Conduct a Visual Data Check

Graphics are important for multiple reasons. Throwaway graphics serve as a useful quality assurance tool, identifying data that may be either out-of-range or illogical. Graphics also provide a general sense of outcomes and comparisons between and among variables. Although the precise statistics presented in tables are important to those who regularly work with data, publishable quality graphics are perhaps the most common medium for communication with the general public on research findings.

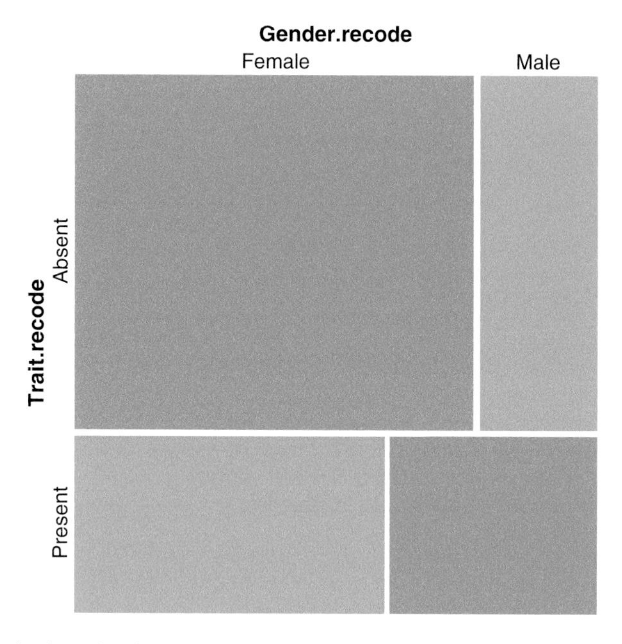

Fig. 3.1 Mosaic plot using the vcd::mosaic() function

First, prepare a throwaway graphic of each main variable simply to see general trends and to also serve as a review of the data. Avoid making any attempt to overly embellish these initial figures.

```
par(ask=TRUE)       # Barchart of Subject
plot(GenderTrait.df$Subject,
  main="Barplot of Subject")

par(ask=TRUE)       # Dotchart of Gender
dotchart(GenderTrait.df$Gender,
  main="Dotchart of Gender Before Recode")

par(ask=TRUE)       # Dotchart of Trait
dotchart(GenderTrait.df$Trait,
  main="Dotchart of Trait Before Recode")
```

A conditional mosaic-type plot may help explain the relationship between and among data of interest, or Gender.recode and Trait.recode for this lesson. The vcd::mosaic() function is a good first choice for this simple graphic (Fig. 3.1).

```
install.packages("vcd")
library(vcd)                  # Load the vcd package.
help(package=vcd)             # Show the information page.
sessionInfo()                 # Confirm all attached packages.
```

```
# Select the most local mirror site using Set CRAN mirror.

par(ask=TRUE)
vcd::mosaic(~ Gender.recode + Trait.recode,
  data = GenderTrait.df, legend=FALSE,
  gp = shading_diagonal)

par(ask=TRUE)
vcd::mosaic(~ Trait.recode + Gender.recode,
  data = GenderTrait.df, legend=FALSE,
  gp = shading_diagonal)
```

In the figures that follow, notice how the barplot() function wraps around the table() function.

```
par(ask=TRUE)       # Barplot of Gender.recode
barplot(table(GenderTrait.df$Gender.recode),
  main="Barplot of Gender After Recode")

par(ask=TRUE)       # Barplot of Trait.recode
barplot(table(GenderTrait.df$Trait.recode),
  main="Barplot of Trait After Recode")

par(ask=TRUE)       # Stacked barplot
barplot(table(GenderTrait.df$Gender.recode,
  GenderTrait.df$Trait.recode),
  beside=FALSE,     # Stacked barplot
  main="Stacked Barplot")

par(ask=TRUE)       # Side-by-side barplot
barplot(table(GenderTrait.df$Gender.recode,
  GenderTrait.df$Trait.recode),
  beside=TRUE,      # Side-by-side barplot
  main="Side-by-Side Barplot")
```

Then, when there is agreement that data are correct and the general approach for the graphic is acceptable, prepare a more embellished figure if desired. Remember to make colors vibrant and use print that is large and dark, whenever possible, to support future public display of the figure.

There are many R-based functions to select from when preparing graphics. The tools that come with initial download of R typically meet immediate needs for the production of graphics. However, with practice and more experience, be sure to explore the many additional R-based functions available in the thousands of external packages currently available to the R community.

Along with producing graphical figures, many functions also produce statistics of some type, usually measures of central tendency or frequency distributions. Again, explore the many possibilities available here and recall that when using R, rarely if ever is there a one-and-only-one function available to support production of a graphic.

```
par(ask=TRUE)
barplot(table(GenderTrait.df$Gender.recode),
  main="Barplot of Gender",         # Title
  xlab="Gender",                    # X axis label
  ylab="Frequency",                 # Y axis label
  cex.axis=1.25,                    # Axis size
  cex.names=1.25,                   # Names size
  cex.lab=1.25,                     # Label size
  col=c("pink", "blue"),            # Color of bar
  font.lab=2)                       # Bold font

par(ask=TRUE)
barplot(table(GenderTrait.df$Trait.recode),
  main="Barplot of Trait",          # Title
  xlab="Trait",                     # X axis label
  ylab="Frequency",                 # Y axis label
  cex.axis=1.25,                    # Axis size
  cex.names=1.25,                   # Names size
  cex.lab=1.25,                     # Label size
  col=c("red", "green"),            # Color of bar
  font.lab=2)                       # Bold font
```

A legend may help better identify groups and group membership, while still keeping the figures simple. To achieve this aim, use the table() function to create a new object variable that represents a crosstab table of GenderTrait.df$Gender.recode by GenderTrait.df$Trait.recode. Then, see how this newly created object variable (GenderTrait.crosstab) is used in concert with the barplot() function and the legend argument.

```
GenderTrait.crosstab <- table(     # Organize the data
  GenderTrait.df$Gender.recode,    # into a table, to
  GenderTrait.df$Trait.recode)     # ease later actions.
rownames(GenderTrait.crosstab) <- c("Female", "Male")
colnames(GenderTrait.crosstab) <- c("Absent", "Present")
GenderTrait.crosstab               # Print the table.
str(GenderTrait.crosstab)          # Object structure
attributes(GenderTrait.crosstab)   # Object attributes

par(ask=TRUE)     # Barplot of Gender.recode by Trait.recode
barplot(GenderTrait.crosstab,
  main="Gender by Trait (Stacked)",          # Title
  xlab="Trait",                              # X axis label
  ylab="Frequency",                          # Y axis label
  cex.axis=1.25,                             # Axis size
  cex.names=1.25,                            # Names size
  cex.lab=1.25,                              # Label size
  font.lab=2,                                # Bold font
```

```
  col=c("pink", "blue"),                     # Factor colors
  legend=rownames(GenderTrait.crosstab),     # Legend
  beside=FALSE)                              # Stacked

par(ask=TRUE)    # Barplot of Gender.recode by Trait.recode
barplot(GenderTrait.crosstab,
  main="Gender by Trait (Side-by-Side)",     # Title
  xlab="Trait",                              # X axis label
  ylab="Frequency",                          # Y axis label
  cex.axis=1.25,                             # Axis size
  cex.names=1.25,                            # Names size
  cex.lab=1.25,                              # Label size
  font.lab=2,                                # Bold font
  col=c("pink", "blue"),                     # Factor colors
  legend=rownames(GenderTrait.crosstab),     # Legend
  beside=TRUE)                               # Side-by-side

TraitGender.crosstab <- table(     # Organize the data
  GenderTrait.df$Trait.recode,     # into a table, to
  GenderTrait.df$Gender.recode)    # ease later actions.
rownames(TraitGender.crosstab) <- c("Absent", "Present")
colnames(TraitGender.crosstab) <- c("Female", "Male")
TraitGender.crosstab               # Print the table.
str(TraitGender.crosstab)          # Object structure
attributes(TraitGender.crosstab)   # Object attributes

par(ask=TRUE)    # Barplot of Trait.recode by Gender.recode
barplot(TraitGender.crosstab,
  main="Trait by Gender (Stacked)",          # Title
  xlab="Gender",                             # X axis label
  ylab="Frequency",                          # Y axis label
  cex.axis=1.25,                             # Axis size
  cex.names=1.25,                            # Names size
  cex.lab=1.25,                              # Label size
  font.lab=2,                                # Bold font
  col=c("red", "green"),                     # Factor colors
  legend=rownames(TraitGender.crosstab),     # Legend
  beside=FALSE)                              # Stacked

par(ask=TRUE)    # Barplot of Trait.recode by Gender.recode
barplot(TraitGender.crosstab,
  main="Trait by Gender (Side-by-Side)",     # Title
  xlab="Gender",                             # X axis label
  ylab="Frequency",                          # Y axis label
  cex.axis=1.25,                             # Axis size
  cex.names=1.25,                            # Names size
  cex.lab=1.25,                              # Label size
  font.lab=2,                                # Bold font
  col=c("red", "green"),                     # Factor colors
  legend=rownames(TraitGender.crosstab),     # Legend
  beside=TRUE)                               # Side-by-side
```

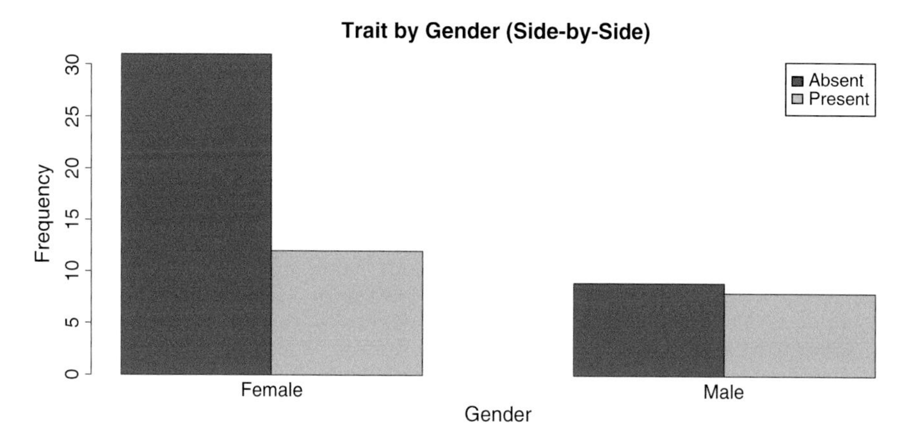

Fig. 3.2 Side-by-side bar plot of two separate object variables

Although these figures prepared by using the barplot() function are both useful and visually appealing, use the epicalc package to produce additional information (i.e., frequency distributions and percentage representation) about the factor object variables in question, Gender.recode and Trait.recode for this sample (Fig. 3.2).

```
install.packages("epicalc")
library(epicalc)              # Load the epicalc package.
help(package=epicalc)         # Show the information page.
sessionInfo()                 # Confirm all attached packages.
# Select the most local mirror site using Set CRAN mirror.

epicalc::tableStack(Gender.recode,
  dataFrame=GenderTrait.df,
  by="none", count=TRUE, decimal=2,
  percent=c("column", "row"),
  frequency=TRUE, name.test=TRUE,
  total.column=TRUE, test=TRUE)

par(ask=TRUE)      # Bar Plot of Gender.recode
epicalc::tab1(GenderTrait.df$Gender.recode,
  decimal=2,                      # Use the tab1() function
  sort.group=FALSE,               # from the epicalc
  cum.percent=TRUE,               # package to see details
  graph=TRUE,                     # about the selected
  missing=TRUE,                   # object variable. (The
  bar.values=c("frequency"),      # 1 of tab1 is the one
  horiz=FALSE,                    # numeric character and
  cex=1.15,                       # it is not the letter
  cex.names=1.15,                 # l).
  cex.lab=1.15, cex.axis=1.15,
  main="Gender",
  ylab="Frequency of Gender, Includings NAs if Any",
  col= c("pink", "blue"),
```

```
  gen=TRUE)

epicalc::tableStack(Trait.recode,
  dataFrame=GenderTrait.df,
  by="none", count=TRUE, decimal=2,
  percent=c("column", "row"),
  frequency=TRUE, name.test=TRUE,
  total.column=TRUE, test=TRUE)

par(ask=TRUE)       # Bar Plot of Trait.recode
epicalc::tab1(GenderTrait.df$Trait.recode,
  decimal=2,                       # Use the tab1() function
  sort.group=FALSE,                # from the epicalc
  cum.percent=TRUE,                # package to see details
  graph=TRUE,                      # about the selected
  missing=TRUE,                    # object variable. (The
  bar.values=c("frequency"),       # 1 of tab1 is the one
  horiz=FALSE,                     # numeric character and
  cex=1.15,                        # it is not the letter
  cex.names=1.15,                  # l).
  cex.lab=1.15, cex.axis=1.15,
  main="Trait",
  ylab="Frequency of Trait, Includings NAs if Any",
  col= c("red", "green"),
  gen=TRUE)
```

3.5 Descriptive Analysis of the Data

Measures of central tendency (e.g., Mode, Median, Mean, SD, etc.) are not needed for this lesson since there are no data of interest that have measured, as opposed to counted, numerical values. Instead, the focus of this lesson is on frequency counts, percentages, and breakouts of frequency counts.

For this simple dataset, the summary() function may be all that is necessary to gain a sense of the data. Note how the summary() function is applied against the entire dataset, thus yielding information about all object variables including those that are not directly used in this lesson, including ostensibly unnecessary information about Subject, Gender (prior to recode), and Trait (prior to recode).

```
summary(GenderTrait.df)            # Entire dataframe

summary(GenderTrait.df[, 4:5])     # Variables 4 to 5
```

However, there are many other R-based functions that support analysis of frequency-type data. A few of these functions are demonstrated below.

Two way frequency tables are easily achieved in different presentations by using the table() function, the margin.table() function, and the prop.table() function. As always, use the interactive help(function_name) at the R prompt to learn more about the specific use of these many functions.

```
table(GenderTrait.df$Gender.recode,
  GenderTrait.df$Trait.recode)
  # Breakouts, row by column

margin.table(table(GenderTrait.df$Gender.recode,
  GenderTrait.df$Trait.recode))
  # Total

margin.table(table(GenderTrait.df$Gender.recode,
  GenderTrait.df$Trait.recode), 1)
  # Breakouts for Gender.recode

margin.table(table(GenderTrait.df$Gender.recode,
  GenderTrait.df$Trait.recode), 2)
  # Breakouts for Trait.recode

prop.table(table(GenderTrait.df$Gender.recode,
  GenderTrait.df$Trait.recode))
  # Total
```

```
             Absent   Present
  Female 0.5166667 0.2000000
  Male   0.1500000 0.1333333
```

```
prop.table(table(GenderTrait.df$Gender.recode,
  GenderTrait.df$Trait.recode), 1)
  # Breakouts for Gender.recode to total 100 percent
  # for Trait.recode

prop.table(table(GenderTrait.df$Gender.recode,
  GenderTrait.df$Trait.recode), 2)
  # Breakouts for Trait.recode to total 100 percent
  # for Gender.recode
```

The xtabs() function should also be considered for presentation of a frequency distribution table. The xtabs() function produces attractive output and label headers make a useful addition.

```
xtabs(~Gender.recode+Trait.recode,
  data=GenderTrait.df, sparse=FALSE)
```

```
             Trait.recode
Gender.recode Absent Present
       Female     31      12
       Male        9       8
```

A few more specialized functions will be demonstrated later in this lesson, since these functions not only present frequency distributions, but they also provide statistical analyses, such as the Chi-square statistic.

3.6 Conduct the Statistical Analysis

chisq.test() Function

The chisq.test() function is used to conduct this Chi-square analysis of Gender.recode by Trait.recode. Specifically, the Pearson's Chi-square Test for Count Data is used to determine if there is a statistically significant difference in the relative frequency of occurrence of Gender (Female and Male) by a specific trait (Absent and Present). At the R prompt, key `help(chisq.test)` to learn more about this function. This interactive approach for obtaining immediate help with R applies to all R functions available in the active R session.

Perspective of Gender (row) by Trait (column)

```
table(GenderTrait.df$Gender.recode,
  GenderTrait.df$Trait.recode)
  # Gender (row) by Trait (column)
```

```
         Absent Present
  Female     31      12
  Male        9       8
```

```
chisq.test(GenderTrait.df$Gender.recode,
  GenderTrait.df$Trait.recode, correct=TRUE)
  # Use continuity correction, (e.g., Yates) which is a
  # concern whenever N <= 10 for any individual cell in
  # a 2 by 2 table.
```

```
  Pearson's Chi-squared test with Yates' continuity correction

data:  GenderTrait.df$Gender.recode and
       GenderTrait.df$Trait.recode
X-squared = 1.2415, df = 1, p-value = 0.2652
```

```
chisq.test(GenderTrait.df$Gender.recode,
  GenderTrait.df$Trait.recode, correct=FALSE)
  # Do not use continuity correction.
```

```
        Pearson's Chi-squared test

data:  GenderTrait.df$Gender.recode and
       GenderTrait.df$Trait.recode
X-squared = 2.0109, df = 1, p-value = 0.1562
```

```
chisq.test(GenderTrait.crosstab, correct=TRUE)
  # Use continuity correction, (e.g., Yates) which is a
  # concern whenever N <= 10 for any individual cell in
  # a 2 by 2 table.

chisq.test(GenderTrait.crosstab, correct=FALSE)
  # Do not use continuity correction.

summary(GenderTrait.crosstab)
```

Perspective of Trait (row) by Gender (column)

```
table(GenderTrait.df$Trait.recode,
  GenderTrait.df$Gender.recode)
  # Trait (row) by Gender (column)
```

```
          Female Male
  Absent      31    9
  Present     12    8
```

```
chisq.test(GenderTrait.df$Trait.recode,
  GenderTrait.df$Gender.recode, correct=TRUE)
  # Use continuity correction, (e.g., Yates) which is a
  # concern whenever N <= 10 for any individual cell in
  # a 2 by 2 table.
```

```
  Pearson's Chi-squared test with Yates' continuity correction

data:  GenderTrait.df$Trait.recode and
       GenderTrait.df$Gender.recode
X-squared = 1.2415, df = 1, p-value = 0.2652
```

```
chisq.test(GenderTrait.df$Trait.recode,
  GenderTrait.df$Gender.recode, correct=FALSE)
  # Do not use continuity correction.
```

```
        Pearson's Chi-squared test

data:  GenderTrait.df$Trait.recode and
       GenderTrait.df$Gender.recode
X-squared = 2.0109, df = 1, p-value = 0.1562
```

```
chisq.test(TraitGender.crosstab, correct=TRUE)
  # Use continuity correction, (e.g., Yates) which is a
  # concern whenever N <= 10 for any individual cell in
  # a 2 by 2 table.

chisq.test(TraitGender.crosstab, correct=FALSE)
  # Do not use continuity correction.

summary(TraitGender.crosstab)
```

When using the chisq.test() function and more specifically by using the argument correct=TRUE and later changing the argument to correct=FALSE, note how the Chi-square statistic was calculated using Yates correction (correct=TRUE) and how it was calculated without Yates correction (correct=FALSE). Yates correction is often used when any individual cell has an observed N of five or fewer datapoints, whereas others suggest that Yates correction should be used when any individual cell has an observed N of ten or fewer datapoints. In this sample:

- With Yates Correction, p-value = 0.2652
- Without Yates Correction, p-value = 0.1562

It was a simple task to use both approaches toward the use of Yates correction and later it will be decided which of the two approaches (e.g., use Yates or not use Yates) is the better choice. Recall that there are two cells (Gender = Male and Trait = Absent, where N = 9; Gender = Male and Trait = Present, where N = 8) in the two by two contingency table where observed N is less than ten. Accordingly, it is possible that Yates correction may be appropriate for this problem.

gmodels::CrossTable() Function

Along with use of the chisq.test() function, the gmodels::CrossTable() function should also be considered as a perhaps redundant, but still useful, check of all calculations. Note the way data are summarized in the crosstabs table gained from the gmodels::CrossTable() function. Equally, notice how the statistics are provided for both calculations, with Yates correction (for this sample, Chi-square = 1.24145, d.f. = 1, and p = 0.2651918) and also without Yates correction (for this sample, Chi-square = 2.010944, d.f. = 1, and p = 0.1561681).

```
install.packages("gmodels")
library(gmodels)                # Load the gmodels package.
help(package=gmodels)           # Show the information page.
sessionInfo()                   # Confirm all attached packages.
# Select the most local mirror site using Set CRAN mirror.

gmodels::CrossTable(GenderTrait.df$Gender.recode,
  GenderTrait.df$Trait.recode,
  expected=TRUE,          # Include expected cell counts.
  prop.r=TRUE,            # Include row proportions.
  prop.c=TRUE,            # Include column proportions.
  prop.t=TRUE,            # Include table proportions.
  chisq = TRUE,           # Include Chi-square test results,
  format=c("SPSS"))       # Model SPSS output format.
```

```
Pearson's Chi-squared test
-------------------------------------------------------------
Chi^2 =  2.010944     d.f. =  1     p =  0.1561681

Pearson's Chi-squared test with Yates' continuity correction
-------------------------------------------------------------
Chi^2 =  1.24145     d.f. =  1     p =  0.2651918
```

Along with Chi-square statistics, note in the complete gmodels::CrossTable() function output how this function also provides a set of percentages for all cells in the contingency table: row percentages, column percentages, and total percentages. Even if it were not necessary to calculate the Chi-Square statistic, the way these percentages are presented support use of the gmodels::CrossTable() function.

summary(xtabs()) Functions
Another useful function is the xtabs() function, with the summary() function wrapped around it. Consider below how the combined use of these two functions generates the Chi-square statistic.

```
summary(xtabs(~Gender.recode+Trait.recode,
  data=GenderTrait.df, sparse=FALSE))
```

```
Number of cases in table: 60
Number of factors: 2
Test for independence of all factors:
        Chisq = 2.0109, df = 1, p-value = 0.1562
```

The output gained from use of the summary(xtabs()) functions is certainly not verbose and there is no accompanying graphic, but all relevant statistics are provided in support of later decision-making.

vcd::table2d_summary() Function
Consider the vcd::table2d_summary() function as an another tool to calculate the Chi-square statistic. The output provides an attractive frequency distribution table and all relevant statistics for a Chi-square analysis: Chi-square statistic, Degrees of Freedom (df), and p-value. Below, note how the vcd::table2d_summary() function is applied against the previously created table, GenderTrait.crosstab and then again against TraitGender.crosstab.

```
vcd::table2d_summary(GenderTrait.crosstab)

vcd::table2d_summary(TraitGender.crosstab)
```

However, consider the use of selected arguments with the vcd::table2d_summary() function to provide margin totals, enhancing understanding of relationships between and among data in one simple presentation.

```
vcd::table2d_summary(GenderTrait.crosstab,
  margins=TRUE, percentages=TRUE)
  # Use arguments for more information.
```

```
             Absent Present  TOTAL

Female freq   31.00   12.00  43.00
       %      51.67   20.00  71.67
Male   freq    9.00    8.00  17.00
       %      15.00   13.33  28.33
TOTAL  freq   40.00   20.00  60.00
       %      66.67   33.33 100.00

Number of cases in table: 60
Number of factors: 2
Test for independence of all factors:
        Chisq = 2.0109, df = 1, p-value = 0.1562
```

```
vcd::table2d_summary(TraitGender.crosstab,
  margins=TRUE, percentages=TRUE)
  # Use arguments for more information.
```

```
                 Female   Male  TOTAL

Absent  freq     31.00    9.00  40.00
        %        51.67   15.00  66.67
Present freq     12.00    8.00  20.00
        %        20.00   13.33  33.33
TOTAL   freq     43.00   17.00  60.00
        %        71.67   28.33 100.00

Number of cases in table: 60
Number of factors: 2
Test for independence of all factors:
        Chisq = 2.0109, df = 1, p-value = 0.1562
```

Note especially how the vcd::table2d_summary() function produces an easy-to-read frequency distribution table of cell counts and percentages.

lessR::BarChart() Function

Although these many (and other) functions are sufficient for Chi-square analyses, there are many cases where functions in external packages have been developed that combine both graphic output and statistical analysis. Below, look at the way the barplot() function will be improved upon by using the lessR::BarChart() function. The lessR::BarChart() function will not only produce a barplot, but by using the quiet=FALSE argument the lessR::BarChart() function will also generate useful tables and an output of the Chi-square statistic, which can easily serve as another quality assurance check against the chisq.test() function.

```
install.packages("lessR")
library(lessR)                  # Load the lessR package.
help(package=lessR)             # Show the information page.
sessionInfo()                   # Confirm all attached packages.
# Select the most local mirror site using Set CRAN mirror.
```

Prepare an initial graphic of Gender by Trait, with supporting Chi-square analysis in the Gender by Trait crosstabs.

```
par(ask=TRUE)       # Barplot of Gender.recode by Trait.recode
lessR::BarChart(Gender.recode, # Gender.recode
  by=Trait.recode,             # Trait.recode
  data=GenderTrait.df,         # Data source
  beside=TRUE,                 # Side-by-Side barchart
  col.fill=c("red", "green"),  # Legend colors
  col.bg=c("white"),           # Background color
  col.grid=c("grey"),          # Grid color
  xlab="Gender",               # X axis label
  ylab="Frequency",            # Y axis label
  main="Frequency of Gender and Trait",
```

```
  cex.axis=1.25,                 # Adjust axis
  col.axis="black",              # Color axis
  font.lab=2,                    # Bold font
  legend.title="Trait Legend",   # Legend title
  legend.loc="topright",         # Legend location
  quiet=FALSE)                   # Produce statistics
```

```
--------------------------------
Joint and Marginal Frequencies
--------------------------------
    Gender.recode
Trait.recode   Female Male  Sum
  Absent           31    9   40
  Present          12    8   20
  Sum              43   17   60

-------------------
Chi-square Analysis
-------------------
Number of cases (observations) in analysis: 60
Number of variables: 2
Test of independence:   Chisq = 2.010944, df = 1,
  p-value = 0.1562
```

Be sure to view the full set of statistics generated along with the barchart figure. Again, note how the accompanying statistics produced by the lessR::BarChart() function (Chisq = 2.010944, df = 1, p-value = 0.1562) are consistent with what has been generated by using the chisq.test() function, the gmodels::CrossTable() function, and the other previously demonstrated functions. Redundancy is often useful as a quality assurance check.

3.7 Summary

In this lesson, the graphical and text output provided a great deal of information. Of immediate importance, however, focus on the 2 by 2 (2 rows by 2 columns) contingency table of Gender.recode by Trait.recode or Trait.recode by Gender.recode and, most importantly, give attention to the calculated p value both with Yates correction and without Yates correction:

```
chisq.test(table(
GenderTrait.df$Gender.recode, GenderTrait.df$Trait.recode),
  correct=TRUE) # Yates correction, for low N cells
```

```
  Pearson's Chi-squared test with Yates' continuity correction

data:  table(GenderTrait.df$Gender.recode,
             GenderTrait.df$Trait.recode)
X-squared = 1.2415, df = 1, p-value = 0.2652
```

```
chisq.test(table(
GenderTrait.df$Gender.recode, GenderTrait.df$Trait.recode),
  correct=FALSE) # Not Yates correction, for low N cells
```

```
        Pearson's Chi-squared test

data:  table(GenderTrait.df$Gender.recode,
             GenderTrait.df$Trait.recode)
X-squared = 2.0109, df = 1, p-value = 0.1562
```

```
chisq.test(table(
GenderTrait.df$Trait.recode, GenderTrait.df$Gender.recode),
  correct=TRUE) # Yates correction, for low N cells
```

```
  Pearson's Chi-squared test with Yates' continuity correction

data:  table(GenderTrait.df$Trait.recode,
             GenderTrait.df$Gender.recode)
X-squared = 1.2415, df = 1, p-value = 0.2652
```

```
chisq.test(table(
GenderTrait.df$Trait.recode, GenderTrait.df$Gender.recode),
  correct=FALSE) # Not Yates correction, for low N cells
```

```
        Pearson's Chi-squared test

data:  table(GenderTrait.df$Trait.recode,
             GenderTrait.df$Gender.recode)
X-squared = 2.0109, df = 1, p-value = 0.1562
```

```
chisq.test(GenderTrait.crosstab, correct=TRUE)
  # Yates correction
```

```
  Pearson's Chi-squared test with Yates' continuity correction

data:  GenderTrait.crosstab
X-squared = 1.2415, df = 1, p-value = 0.2652
```

```
chisq.test(GenderTrait.crosstab, correct=FALSE)
  # Not Yates correction
```

```
        Pearson's Chi-squared test

data:  GenderTrait.crosstab
X-squared = 2.0109, df = 1, p-value = 0.1562
```

```
chisq.test(TraitGender.crosstab, correct=TRUE)
  # Yates correction
```

```
    Pearson's Chi-squared test with Yates' continuity correction

data:  TraitGender.crosstab
X-squared = 1.2415, df = 1, p-value = 0.2652
```

```
chisq.test(TraitGender.crosstab, correct=FALSE)
  # Not Yates correction
```

```
        Pearson's Chi-squared test

data:  TraitGender.crosstab
X-squared = 2.0109, df = 1, p-value = 0.1562
```

With Yates correction, the calculated p value is 0.2652 (which rounds to 0.27). Without Yates correction, the calculated p value is 0.1562 (which rounds to 0.16).

Both p values (0.2652 with Yates correction and 0.1562 without Yates correction) exceed the previously declared value of `p <= 0.05`, associated with the Null Hypothesis. In this case, the calculated p value of 0.16 (or 0.27, depending on use of Yates correction) exceeds `p <= 0.05`, providing another measure to confirm that for the sample in question, there is no difference (`p <= 0.05`) in the occurrence of a specific trait for the two genders.

Null Hypothesis (Ho) There is no statistically significant difference (`p <= 0.05`) between the two genders (Female or Male) in regard to the presence (Absent or Present) of a specific unnamed trait of an otherwise unidentified biological organism.

Although the nature of the study was masked in this sample, it can be stated with a fair degree of confidence that there is no difference between the two genders in terms of the absence or presence of the trait relevant to this lesson.

Of course, more precise measures may have been desirable, along with a larger sample. Recall that in this sample an individual technician determined both gender and presence or absence of the trait. It is assumed that gender is fairly easily identified, but that is not always the case. More problematic, however, is declaration of the nature of the trait and how it may have benefited from some type of empirical measure, such as a reading on a scaled or calibrated instrument, but that was not the case in this lesson. Perhaps the sample consisted of a biological organism that was captured in the wild and needed to be released quickly to avoid harm to either the organism or field staff. Under these conditions, a quick call may be the only choice for data collection. Of course, there may be other equally compelling reasons for the way data were obtained, but that is not evident in what was provided to the researcher charged with analysis. For this sample, it is only sufficient to know that there was no statistically significant difference (`p <= 0.05`) between the two genders regarding presence or absence of the trait in question.

3.8 Addendum: Calculate the Chi-Square Statistic from Contingency Tables

This lesson demonstrated calculation of the Chi-square statistic for data that were eventually organized into a 2 by 2 contingency table. A 2 by 2 table with four cells is perhaps the most common approach to use of Chi-square analyses, but other configurations are possible.

Consider another typical scenario for a Chi-square test where data have been organized into discrete categories where there are six cells. In this sample, data are organized by gender (rows) in regard to responses to a survey-based health-related question that allowed Yes, No, or Undecided as possible responses (columns), allowing for three possible selections to the question.

As opposed to the 2 (rows) by 2 (columns) table presented previously, in this sample the data are organized into a 2 (rows) by 3 (columns) table, consisting of $2 \star 3 = 6$ cells. Again, totals are provided to the right and bottom:

Response to a Health-Related Survey Question by Gender

Gender	Response			
	Yes	No	Undecided	Total
Female	N = 09	N = 11	N = 14	34
Male	N = 12	N = 07	N = 08	27
Total	N = 21	N = 18	N = 22	61

The original data file is not available, which is often quite common, but notice how a contingency table can be built using R if totals for each cell are known. For this sample, observe how the cbind() function is used to construct a dataframe called GenderSurveyQ.cross:

```
GenderSurveyQ.cross <- cbind(c(09, 12), c(11, 07), c(14, 08))
rownames(GenderSurveyQ.cross) <- c("Female", "Male")
colnames(GenderSurveyQ.cross) <- c("Yes", "No", "Undecided")
str(GenderSurveyQ.cross)          # Object structure
attributes(GenderSurveyQ.cross)   # Object attributes
GenderSurveyQ.cross               # Print the table.

GenderSurveyQ.cross <- data.frame(GenderSurveyQ.cross)
```

```
str(GenderSurveyQ.cross)          # Object structure
attributes(GenderSurveyQ.cross)   # Object attributes
GenderSurveyQ.cross               # Print the table.
```

First, calculate the Chi-square statistic using the fairly terse chisq.test() function.

```
chisq.test(GenderSurveyQ.cross)
```

```
        Pearson's Chi-squared test

data:  GenderSurveyQ.cross
X-squared = 2.1792, df = 2, p-value = 0.3363
```

Then, in an effort to obtain a better cell-by-cell understanding of outcomes, calculate the Chi-square statistic using the far more verbose mosaic::xchisq.test() function.

```
install.packages("mosaic")
library(mosaic)                 # Load the mosaic package.
help(package=mosaic)            # Show the information page.
sessionInfo()                   # Confirm all attached packages.
# Select the most local mirror site using Set CRAN mirror.

mosaic::xchisq.test(GenderSurveyQ.cross)
```

```
        Pearson's Chi-squared test

data:  x
X-squared = 2.1792, df = 2, p-value = 0.3363

   9.00     11.00     14.00
(11.70)   (10.03)   (12.26)
[0.625]   [0.093]   [0.246]
<-0.79>   < 0.31>   < 0.50>

  12.00      7.00      8.00
( 9.30)   ( 7.97)   ( 9.74)
[0.787]   [0.117]   [0.310]
< 0.89>   <-0.34>   <-0.56>

key:
        observed
        (expected)
        [contribution to X-squared]
        <residual>
```

From this organization of data, the p-value was calculated (`p-value <= 0.3363`) and subsequent decision-making can used to determine if overall differences between observed and expected counts in each cell are due to chance, or if the differences are instead due to true differences between the two genders and responses to the survey question, at `p <= 0.05`.

Using the appropriate statistical analysis, it was determined in this example of Gender (Female or Male) by Survey Question Response (Yes, No, or Undecided) that Chi-square = 2.179, degrees of freedom = 2, and `p <= 0.3363`. Given that calculated p (0.34) is greater than the typically declared p value of `p <= 0.05`, it can be declared there is no statistically significant difference (`p <= 0.05`) in survey question response by gender from among subjects in this sample. Again, this sample presented a 2 by 3 contingency table (2 rows by 3 columns) instead of the more common 2 by 2 contingency table. Yet, R-based functions are easily used for this expanded contingency table, where data were not available at the level of the individual subject but were instead only available in collapsed (i.e., grouped) format for each cell in the contingency table.

3.9 Prepare to Exit, Save, and Later Retrieve This R Session

```
getwd()                  # Identify the current working directory.
ls()                     # List all objects in the working
                         # directory.
ls.str()                 # List all objects, with finite detail.
list.files()             # List files at the PC directory.

save.image("R_Lesson_Chi-square.rdata")

getwd()                  # Identify the current working directory.
ls()                     # List all objects in the working
                         # directory.
ls.str()                 # List all objects, with finite detail.
list.files()             # List files at the PC directory.

alarm()                  # Alarm, notice of upcoming action.
q()                      # Quit this session.
                         # Prepare for Save workspace image? query.
```

Use the R Graphical User Interface (GUI) to load the saved rdata file: File -> Load Workspace. Otherwise, use the load() function, keying the full pathname, to load the .rdata file and retrieve the session.

Recall, however, that it may be just as useful to simply use the .R script file (typically saved is a .txt ASCII-type file) and recreate the analyses and graphics, provided the data files remain available.

Chapter 4
Mann–Whitney U Test

Abstract The Mann–Whitney U test is often viewed as the nonparametric equivalent of Student's t-Test for Independent Samples, but this comparison may be somewhat too convenient. The two tests (the nonparametric Mann–Whitney U-Test and the parametric Student's t-Test for Independent Samples) may have similar purposes in that they are both used to determine if there are statistically significant differences between two groups. However, the Mann–Whitney U-Test is used with nonparametric data (typically, ordinal data) whereas the Student's t-Test for Independent Samples is used with data that meet the assumptions associated with parametric distributions (typically interval data that approximate an acceptable level of normal distribution). Even so, the Mann–Whitney U-Test has many appropriate uses and it should be considered when using ranked data, data that deviate from acceptable distribution patterns, or for when there are noticeable differences in the number of subjects in the two comparative groups.

Keywords Anderson-Darling Test • Bar plot (stacked, side-by-side) • Box plot • Code Book • Comma-separated values (.csv) • Continuous scale • Density plot • Descriptive statistics • Distribution-free • Frequency distribution • Histogram • Interval • Mann–Whitney U Test • Mean • Median • Mode • Nominal • Nonparametric • Normal distribution • Null hypothesis • Ordinal • Parametric • Probability (p-value) • Quantile-Quantile (QQ, Q-Q) • Ranking • Stacked data • Statistical significance • Student's t-Test for Independent Samples • Unstacked data

4.1 Background on this Lesson

Typically using ordinal data, the Mann–Whitney U Test is used to determine if two independent groups are from the same population. The Mann–Whitney Test is quite powerful and by no means should it be considered anything but equivalent to Student's t-Test for Independent Samples in terms of utility. However, the data

---

Electronic supplementary material The online version of this chapter (doi: 10.1007/978-3-319-30634-6_4) contains supplementary material, which is available to authorized users.

T.W. MacFarland, J.M. Yates, *Introduction to Nonparametric Statistics for the Biological Sciences Using R*, DOI 10.1007/978-3-319-30634-6_4

for Mann–Whitney are usually ordinal, whereas the data for Student's t-Test are interval. Of course, there are those who suggest that far too many studies use data that are declared interval, and, subsequently, Student's t-Test is used to examine differences. Yet, in reality, the data are ordinal and the Mann–Whitney Test would be the more appropriate choice.

4.1.1 Description of the Data

This lesson on the Mann–Whitney U-Test is based on a study about goats (*Capra aegagrus hircus*) and more specifically judgments about two groups of goats after a mineral supplement was introduced into the diet of one group of goats (i.e., experimental group) but not the other group of goats (i.e., control group). To be more specific about the conditions associated with the data:

- A herd (i.e., tribe) of 30 goats was divided into two separate groups. From among the 30 goats available for placement into the two groups, assignment into either Group 1 or Group 2 was based on random selection.
  - Group 1 served as a control group and these goats received regular feed during the treatment period.
  - Group 2 served as the experimental group and these goats received a mineral supplement during the treatment period, in addition to the regular feeding program. Application of the mineral supplement treatment was consistent for the 15 goats receiving the treatment. However, the nature of the mineral supplement, amount, means of introduction into the feeding program (e.g, powder, liquid, granules, etc.), regularity of treatment, etc., remain unknown to the researcher responsible for data analysis.
- At the end-of-treatment, each goat was judged against a measure that potentially ranged from 40 to 100. The nature of the judgment remains unknown to the researcher responsible for data analysis.

It should be emphasized that the exact nature of the treatment (i.e., object variable Treatment) used for the two groups of goats is currently unidentified. The treatment consisted of some type of mineral supplement to the diet, but there is no other usable information about the treatment.

It is also necessary to recognize that the measure used to determine outcomes at the end-of-treatment (i.e., object variable Judgment) is equally unidentified. The data for Judgment may refer to some measure about hair color, some measure about overall vigor, some measure of milk production (such as protein content or butterfat content), etc.

- A key point here regarding the object variable Judgment is that based on prior experience with the treatment process and later measures obtained at time-of-judgment, there is no expectation that outcomes are normally distributed and follow along some semblance of the bell-shaped curve. This view toward normal distribution of data may occur, but normal distribution is not expected.

- Another issue involving the object variable Judgment is that there are concerns about the nature of the data and whether the data are ordinal or if they rise to meet conditions necessary to consider the data interval. For the purpose of this lesson, the data associated with object variable Judgment are viewed as ordinal data.

Given the nature of the data associated with this study and, specifically, the data associated with the object variable Judgment, Student's t-Test for Independent Samples is not the appropriate test to use to critically examine if there are statistically significant differences between the two groups.

Instead, this lesson will be based on use of the Mann–Whitney U-Test, with no expectation for Judgment measures other than that the data are assumed to be ordered and distribution-free. Accordingly, the data for Judgment are therefore viewed from a nonparametric perspective.

The dataset is fairly simple, and the entire dataset is found as stacked data in the file Goats.csv:

- The first line consists of a header that uses descriptive variable names: Goat, Treatment, and Judgment.
- The header is then followed by 30 lines of data, one line of data for each goat (i.e., subject).
- Goat: There is a coded identifier (G01 to G30) for each goat. Adequate tags and tracking protocols were used to correctly identify each goat throughout the study.
- Treatment: Binary values of 1 and 2 are used to differentiate between the two groups of goats associated with this study:
  - Group 1 (i.e., control group): Regular Feed
  - Group 2 (i.e., experimental group): Regular Feed and Added Mineral Supplement
- Judgment: At the end-of-treatment, each goat was individually judged by a qualified technician for an otherwise unidentified characteristic, measure, trait, etc. The scale for Judgment ranged from 40 (low) to 100 (high). Based on prior experience it is assumed that:
  - The data do not follow along any consistent pattern of normal distribution.
  - The data do not have a consistent scale and they should be viewed as ordinal data and not interval data. That is to say, the difference between a measure of 89 and 90 may not be consistently equal to the difference between a 90 and 91, 93 and 94, 98 and 99, etc.

Given these conditions and the view that Judgment measures are ordinal data that do not follow normal distribution, the nonparametric Mann–Whitney U-Test is viewed as the most appropriate inferential test to determine if there is a statistically significant difference (`p <= 0.05`) between the two groups, goats who experienced Treatment 1 (i.e., control group) and their counterparts who experienced Treatment 2 (i.e., experimental group).

It is beyond the purpose of this lesson to offer a detailed lecture on experimental designs for the biological sciences. By no means is the design for this lesson offered as an ideal, but this design is an accurate portrayal of the realities of exploratory biological research, especially when faced with field conditions, as opposed to research with greater control under laboratory conditions.

- There is no attempt to select subjects beyond this one herd of 30 goats.
- No background information about the herd of 30 goats is known and from this limited information there is no differentiation in selected subjects by breed, age, gender, etc.
- There is no pretest measure of Judgment for either Group 1 (i.e., control group) or Group 2 (i.e., experimental group). As such, it is not possible to assess change over time, and instead it is only possible to assess differences between the two groups on a posttest measure only.

Given the nature of the data, the nonparametric Mann–Whitney U-Test is judged the most appropriate inferential test for this analysis of differences between goats in Group 1 (i.e., the control group) and goats in Group 2 (i.e., the experimental group).

4.1.2 Null Hypothesis (Ho)

There is no statistically significant difference (`p <= 0.05`) between goats that received regular feed during a treatment period (i.e., the control group) and their counterparts that received regular feed and an otherwise unidentified mineral supplement added to the feeding program during the same treatment period (i.e., the experimental group).

The Null Hypothesis (Ho) uses `p <= 0.05`, which is quite common for exploratory research. Saying that, it is equally common to see more restrictive probability levels (i.e., the term *alpha* is sometimes seen) used in research that benefits from a more rigorous design, with `p <= 0.01` frequently used.

4.2 Data Import of a .csv Spreadsheet-Type Data File into R

The data for this lesson were originally entered into a Gnumeric-based spreadsheet. The data were then also saved in .csv (i.e., comma-separated values) file format as Goats.csv. The data in the .csv file are separated by commas, not tabs and not spaces. As a .csv file the data can be easily sent to, and opened by, other researchers without the need for specialized software or proprietary software that may be cost prohibitive for many.

Start a new R session and then attend to beginning actions such as removing unwanted files from prior work, declaring the working directory, etc.

```
###############################################################
# Housekeeping                              Use for All Analyses    #
###############################################################
date()              # Current system time and date.
R.version.string    # R version and version release date.
ls()                # List all objects in the working
                    # directory.
rm(list = ls())     # CAUTION: Remove all files in the working
                    # directory. If this action is not desired,
                    # use the rm() function one-by-one to remove
                    # the objects that are not needed.
ls.str()            # List all objects, with finite detail.
getwd()             # Identify the current working directory.
setwd("F:/R_Nonparametric")
                    # Set to a new working directory.
                    # Note the single forward slash and double
                    # quotes.
                    # This new directory should be the directory
                    # where the data file is located, otherwise
                    # the data file will not be found.
getwd()             # Confirm the working directory.
list.files()        # List files at the PC directory.
###############################################################
```

With R set to work in the desired directory, create an object called Goats.df. The object Goats.df will be a dataframe, as indicated by the enumerated .df extension to the object name. This object will represent the output of applying the read.table() function against the comma-separated values file called Goats.csv. The arguments used with the read.table() function show that there is a header with descriptive variable names (header = TRUE) and that the separator between fields is a comma (sep = ",").

```
Goats.df <- read.table (file =
  "Goats.csv",
  header = TRUE,
  sep = ",")                  # Import the .csv file

getwd()                       # Identify the working directory
ls()                          # List objects
attach(Goats.df)              # Attach the data, for later use
str(Goats.df)                 # Identify structure
nrow(Goats.df)                # List the number of rows
ncol(Goats.df)                # List the number of columns
dim(Goats.df)                 # Dimensions of the dataframe
names(Goats.df)               # Identify names
colnames(Goats.df)            # Show column names
rownames(Goats.df)            # Show row names
head(Goats.df, n=10)          # Show the head
tail(Goats.df, n=10)          # Show the tail
Goats.df                      # Show the entire dataframe
summary(Goats.df)             # Summary statistics
```

These actions result in the creation of an object called Goats.df. This R-based object is a dataframe and it consists of the data originally included in the file Goats.csv, a comma-separated values .csv file. To avoid possible conflicts, make sure that there are no prior R-based objects called Goats.df. The prior use of rm(list = ls()) accommodates this concern, removing all prior objects in the current R session.

Observe how it was only necessary to key the filename for the .csv file and not the full pathname since the R working directory is currently set to the directory and/or subdirectory where this .csv file is located. See the Housekeeping section at the beginning of this lesson.

4.3 Organize the Data and Display the Code Book

After the data are imported into R, it is always best to organize the data by checking format and then making any changes that may be needed. The dataset for this lesson is fairly small (N = 30 subjects), and there are no missing data.

To support tracking purposes, a rowname will be used with this dataset, using the rownames() function. Although the dataset for this lesson is small and this action is not required, the addition of rownames is helpful—especially when working with large datasets. The rownames() function assigns a unique identifier for each row in the dataset, each beginning with the term Goat in this example.

```
rownames(Goats.df) <- paste('Goat', 1:30)

head(Goats.df)     # Show the first few lines of the dataset
tail(Goats.df)     # Show the last few lines of the dataset
Goats.df           # Show the entire dataset since it is small
```

For this lesson, the class() function, str() function, and duplicated() function will be used to be sure that data are organized as desired.

```
class(Goats.df)
class(Goats.df$Goat)        # DataFrame$ObjectName notation
class(Goats.df$Treatment) # DataFrame$ObjectName notation
class(Goats.df$Judgment)   # DataFrame$ObjectName notation

str(Goats.df)               # Structure

duplicated(Goats.df)        # Duplicates
```

The class for each object is currently correct and there are no duplicate rows of data in the dataframe. With the data in correct format, a Code Book will help with future understanding of the data in this dataset.

The Code Book is typically brief and only serves as a useful reminder for what can be easily forgotten months (or even weeks) later, and to also make it easy to decipher what may otherwise be seen as arcane numeric codes (e.g., For Gender, does 1 = Female and 2 = Male or does 1 = Male and 2 = Female? Without a Code

Book it is only too easy to make mistakes with the way codes are organized.). Coding schemes that are intuitively obvious today can easily become forgotten tomorrow.

The Code Book below represents how data are desired before analyses begin. Recoding may be needed to put data into new formats.

```
########################################################
# Code Book for Goats.df                               #
########################################################
#                                                      #
# Goat ...................... Factor (i.e., nominal) #
#                   A unique ID ranging from G01 to G30 #
#                                                      #
# Treatment ...................Factor (i.e., nominal) #
#                                     Regular Feed = 1 #
#      Regular Feed and Added Mineral Supplement = 2 #
#                                                      #
# Judgment ............... .. Numeric (i.e., ordinal) #
#                           A numeric measure that ranges #
#                                      from 40 to 100 #
########################################################
```

The str() function is then again applied against the dataframe to show the nature of each object variable as well as to confirm that the data are collectively viewed as a dataframe.

```
str(Goats.df)       # Structure, before recoding
```

```
'data.frame':   30 obs. of  3 variables:
 $ Goat      : Factor w/ 30 levels "G01","G02","G03",..: 1 2 ...
 $ Treatment: int  1 1 1 1 1 1 1 1 1 1 ...
 $ Judgment : int  80 82 91 100 76 65 85 88 97 55
```

Recall that the Code Book shows data in their desired formats, which often requires some degree of recoding, which has not yet occurred.

Once there is agreement that the data were brought into R in correct format, it is usually necessary to organize the data to some degree:

- The object variable Goat is only used to identify specific subjects. Each datum for Goat begins with the letter G, and this object variable is currently recognized as a factor object variable.
- In this lesson, note how whole numbers (e.g., 1 and 2, as integer-type codes) have been used in the original file to identify groups for the factor object variable named Treatment. A set of simple R-based actions can easily:
  - Transform (i.e., recode) the object variable Goats.df$Treatment into a new object variable.

  – Change the recoded object variable from original integer format to enumerated factor format.[1]
  – Apply narrative labels for the otherwise cryptic numeric codes (e.g., 1 and 2).

- Values for Judgment are currently whole numbers, and as such they are first treated in R as integers. A simple recode action will instead be used to put these values into numeric format.

```
Goats.df$Goat              <- as.factor(Goats.df$Goat)

Goats.df$Treatment.recode <- factor(Goats.df$Treatment,
  labels=c("Regular Feed", "Added Mineral Supplement"))
  # Use factor() and not as.factor().

Goats.df$Judgment          <- as.numeric(Goats.df$Judgment)

str(Goats.df)      # Structure, after recoding
```

```
'data.frame':   30 obs. of  4 variables:
 $ Goat             : Factor w/ 30 levels "G01","G02","G03",..:
                      1 2 ...
 $ Treatment        : int  1 1 1 1 1 1 1 1 1 1 ...
 $ Judgment         : num  80 82 91 100 76 65 85 88 97 55 ...
 $ Treatment.recode: Factor w/ 2 levels "Regular Feed",..: 1 1 1
                      1 ...
```

Before continuing, a few redundant actions will help confirm that the data are in correct and desired format.

```
getwd()                       # Identify the working directory
ls()                          # List objects
attach(Goats.df)              # Attach the data, for later use
str(Goats.df)                 # Identify structure
nrow(Goats.df)                # List the number of rows
ncol(Goats.df)                # List the number of columns
dim(Goats.df)                 # Dimensions of the dataframe
names(Goats.df)               # Identify names
colnames(Goats.df)            # Show column names
rownames(Goats.df)            # Show row names
head(Goats.df)                # Show the head
tail(Goats.df)                # Show the tail
Goats.df                      # Show the entire dataframe
summary(Goats.df)             # Summary statistics

summary(Goats.df[, 2:4])      # Variables 2 to 4
```

[1] Review the factor() function and the as.factor() function to see appropriate applications of each, specifically for when object variables are recoded from one class to another class.

```
  Treatment       Judgment                              Treatment.recode
 Min.   :1.0   Min.    : 47.00   Regular Feed                :15
 1st Qu.:1.0   1st Qu.: 76.75   Added Mineral Supplement:15
 Median :1.5   Median : 84.50
 Mean   :1.5   Mean    : 82.87
 3rd Qu.:2.0   3rd Qu.: 90.50
 Max.   :2.0   Max.    :100.00
```

The object variable Goats.df$Treatment.recode was created by putting the object variable Goats.df$Treatment into factor format. Labels were then applied in sequential order for this new object, with Regular Feed used to represent every occurrence of the numeric value 1 and Added Mineral Supplement used to represent every occurrence of the numeric value 2.

The object variable Goats.df$Judgment was recoded from integer format to numeric format by applying the as.numeric() function.

Note the formal nomenclature used in this recode action and DataframeName$ObjectName notation when working with object variables that are part of a dataframe. Note also how the $ symbol is used to separate the name of the dataframe from the name of the object: DataframeName$ObjectName.

4.4 Conduct a Visual Data Check

It is common to immediately consider descriptive statistics and measures of central tendency when inferential analyses are planned and later completed. When working with numeric data viewed from a parametric perspective it is critical to know the Mode, Median, Mean, Standard Deviation, etc. However, in these lessons the data are first examined visually, using the strong graphical features supported by R. The images can be simple throwaway graphics, designed only to offer a general sense of the data. Or, the images can be fully embellished, high quality, and suitable for presentation or publication. Regardless of details in the final view, graphics provide a composite understanding of the data that may be difficult to grasp when statistics, only, are viewed.

For initial purposes, the graphical functions of primary interest are plot() and epicalc::tab1() for factor-type object variables and boxplot(), hist(), and plot(density()) for numeric-type object variables. More specialized functions from the lattice package will then be demonstrated to provide a brief demonstration of how R supports a wide range of graphical functions—functions that often go far beyond what is available when R is first downloaded.

The par(ask=TRUE) function and argument are used to freeze the presentation on the screen, one figure at a time. Note how the top line of the figure, under the selection *File—Save as*, provides a variety of graphical formats to save each figure, listed in the following order: Metafile, Postscript, PDF, PNG, BMP, TIFF, and

JPEG.[2] It is also possible to perform a simple copy-and-paste against each graphical image. R syntax can also be used to save a graphical image.

Visual Presentation of Factor-Type Object Variables

```
par(ask=TRUE)
plot(Goats.df$Goat, main="Goat - Subject")

par(ask=TRUE)
plot(Goats.df$Treatment.recode,
  main="Frequency Distribution of Treatment:  Regular Feed v
  Regular Feed and Added Mineral Supplement",
  lwd=6, col="red", font.axis=2, font.lab=2)
```

As a general comment about this figure and other figures, titles should be adequately descriptive, often at the point of being somewhat lengthy. However, labels need to be somewhat brief, or even terse, if they are to fit on the graph in the allowed space.

```
install.packages("epicalc")
library(epicalc)              # Load the epicalc package.
help(package=epicalc)         # Show the information page.
sessionInfo()                 # Confirm all attached packages.
# Select the most local mirror site using Set CRAN mirror.

par(ask=TRUE)      # Bar and Frequencies Treatment.recode
epicalc::tab1(Goats.df$Treatment.recode,
  decimal=2,                     # Use the tab1() function
  sort.group=FALSE,              # from the epicalc
  cum.percent=TRUE,              # package to see details
  graph=TRUE,                    # about the selected
  missing=TRUE,                  # object variable. (The
  bar.values=c("frequency"),     # 1 of tab1 is the one
  horiz=FALSE,                   # numeric character and
  cex=1.15,                      # it is not the letter
  cex.names=1.15,                # l).
  cex.lab=1.15, cex.axis=1.15,
  main="Regular Feed (Control Group) v Regular Feed and
  Added Mineral Supplement (Experimental Group)",
  ylab="Regular Feed and Added Mineral Supplement",
  col= c("black", "red"),
  gen=TRUE)
  # Note how a frequency distribution is provided, too.
```

Visual Presentation of Numeric-Type Object Variables

As these visual presentations of the numeric-type object variable Goats.df$Judgment are prepared, recall that the data for this object variable are considered ordinal, not

[2]Each format has specific advantages. All figures associated with this text were saved in .PNG (i.e., Portable Network Graphics) format, because .PNG figures are effective and their inclusion eliminates any concerns about free use.

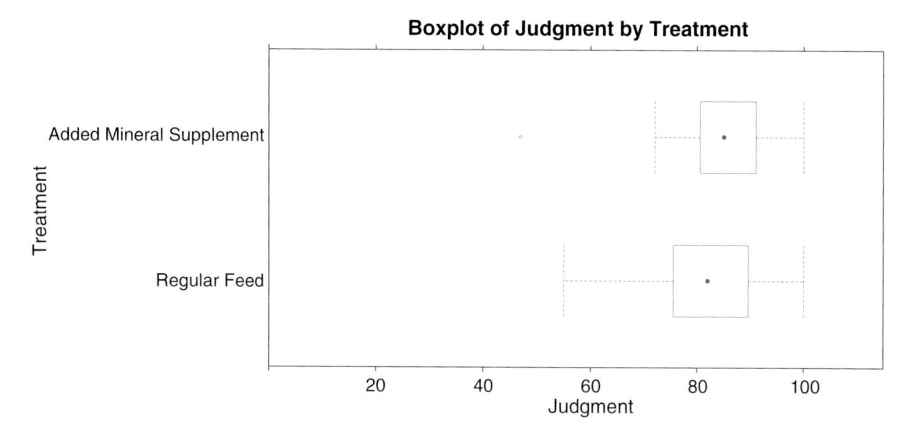

Fig. 4.1 Boxplot using the lattice::bwplot() function

interval. The object variable Goats.df$Judgment has been presented as a numeric variable and indeed it should be viewed this way—the object variable Judgment in this lesson is certainly a number. However, merely keep in mind that the scale is not consistent as would be expected if the data followed along a more parametric perspective associated with interval measurement.

Look carefully, below, as the following R syntax is reviewed. The subtle difference of a named object variable, a | (i.e., pipe) instead of a ~ (i.e., tilde), the selection of one argument over another, etc., can make all the difference in how a figure appears. The comments are helpful, but the best way to approach this syntax is to copy it then use it for individual practice (Fig. 4.1).

```
par(ask=TRUE)
boxplot(Goats.df$Judgment,
  main="Boxplot of Judgment (End-of-Treatment Measure)",
  font=2,          # Bold text
  cex.lab=1.15,    # Large font
  cex.axis=1.25,   # Large axis text
  lwd=2,           # Thick line
  col="red")       # Vibrant color

par(ask=TRUE)
boxplot(Goats.df$Judgment ~ Goats.df$Treatment.recode,
  main="Boxplot of Judgment (End-of-Treatment Measure) by
    Treatment:
  Regular Feed v Regular Feed and Added Mineral Supplement",
  font=2,          # Bold text
  cex.lab=1.15,    # Large font
  cex.axis=1.25,   # Large axis text
  lwd=2,           # Thick line
  col="red")       # Vibrant color
```

```
par(ask=TRUE)
hist(Goats.df$Judgment,
  main="Histogram of Judgment (End-of-Treatment Measure)",
  font=2,          # Bold text
  xlab="Judgment",# X axis label
  cex.lab=1.15,    # Large font
  cex.axis=1.25,   # Large axis text
  lwd=2,           # Thick line
  col="red")       # Vibrant color

par(ask=TRUE)
plot(density(Goats.df$Judgment,
  na.rm=TRUE),     # Required for the density() function
  main="Density Plot of Judgment (End-of-Treatment Measure)",
  font=2,          # Bold text
  cex.lab=1.15,    # Large font
  cex.axis=1.25,   # Large axis text
  lwd=6,           # Thick line
  col="red")       # Vibrant color
```

There are also many other ways to show the numeric variables, individually and by breakout groups. From among the many possible selections, the lattice package and specifically the lattice::histogram() and lattice::bwplot() functions will be used to show valuable displays of Judgment individually and then by Treatment (i.e., Regular Feed v Regular Feed and Added Mineral Supplement).

```
install.packages("lattice")
library(lattice)              # Load the lattice package.
help(package=lattice)         # Show the information page.
sessionInfo()                 # Confirm all attached packages.
# Select the most local mirror site using Set CRAN mirror.

par(ask=TRUE) # 1 Column by 1 Row Histogram
lattice::histogram(~ Goats.df$Judgment,
  type="count", # Note: count
  par.settings=simpleTheme(lwd=2),
  par.strip.text=list(cex=1.15, font=2),
  scales=list(cex=1.15),
  main="Histogram (Count) of Judgment",
  xlab=list("Judgment", cex=1.15, font=2),
  xlim=c(0,115), # Note the range.
  ylab=list("Count", cex=1.15, font=2),
  aspect=1, breaks=10,
  layout = c(1,1), # Note: 1 Column by 1 Row.
  col="red")

par(ask=TRUE) # 1 Column by 2 Rows Histogram
lattice::histogram(~ Goats.df$Judgment |
  Goats.df$Treatment.recode,
  type="count", # Note: count
  par.settings=simpleTheme(lwd=2),
  par.strip.text=list(cex=1.15, font=2),
  scales=list(cex=1.15),
```

```
  main="Histograms (Count) of Judgment by Treatment",
  xlab=list("Judgment", cex=1.15, font=2),
  xlim=c(0,115), # Note the range.
  ylab=list("Count", cex=1.15, font=2),
  aspect=0.25, breaks=10,
  layout = c(1,2), # Note: 1 Column by 2 Rows.
  col="red")

par(ask=TRUE) # Singular boxplot.
lattice::bwplot(Goats.df$Judgment,
  par.settings = simpleTheme(lwd=2),
  par.strip.text=list(cex=1.15, font=2),
  scales=list(cex=1.15),
  main="Boxplot of Judgment",
  xlab=list("Judgment", cex=1.15, font=2),
  xlim=c(0,115), aspect=0.5, layout=c(1,1),
  col="red")

par(ask=TRUE) # Breakout group by measured object
lattice::bwplot(Goats.df$Treatment.recode ~
  Goats.df$Judgment,
  par.settings = simpleTheme(lwd=2),
  par.strip.text=list(cex=1.15, font=2),
  scales=list(cex=1.15),
  main="Boxplot of Judgment by Treatment",
  xlab=list("Judgment", cex=1.15, font=2),
  xlim=c(0,115),
  ylab=list("Treatment", cex=1.15, font=2),
  aspect=0.5, layout=c(1,1), col="red")
```

Although histograms and boxplots are certainly useful graphical tools, the density plot is especially helpful for visualizing how data are distributed individually and by breakout groups, which is why syntax for the density plot was included earlier in this lesson.[3] That demonstration of the density plot was dependent on wrapping the plot() function around the density() function, deployed as plot(density()).

For this lesson, look again at the density plot as a useful tool for visualizing data and, more importantly, the distribution of data. First, prepare a throwaway density plot with the UsingR::DensityPlot() function and then, if the outcomes show promise, use the lattice::densityplot() function for more aesthetic and visually appealing density plot images.

[3]Separate from the use of R or any other software, be sure to study the many possibilities for how data can be graphically displayed. Start with simple tools, such as the histogram and boxplot. Then, with more practice and understanding, move to more sophisticated tools such as density plot, violin plot, etc. An Internet search on *graphical display of data* or some similar term will provide an ample number of quality resources on this topic.

```
install.packages("UsingR")
library(UsingR)              # Load the UsingR package.
help(package=UsingR)         # Show the information page.
sessionInfo()                # Confirm all attached packages.
# Select the most local mirror site using Set CRAN mirror.

par(ask=TRUE)
UsingR::DensityPlot(Judgment ~ Treatment.recode, data=Goats.df)
```

As demonstrated in the R syntax, a density plot is used to visualize how measured data are organized at the singular level and also by breakout groups. Look at the way these density plots have been prepared, only this time with more detail by using the lattice::densityplot() function. Statistical analyses are certainly necessary and should never be neglected, no matter how visual presentations appear. In this lesson, note how the density plot presentation of Judgment by Treatment brings to attention a visual reminder that the distribution of Judgment measures is certainly not equivalent for the two Treatment breakout groups: Regular Feed (Control Group) vs Regular Feed and Added Mineral Supplement (Experimental Group). Of course, this visual difference does not mean that there is a statistically significant difference, but the visual image provides a reminder of trends (Fig. 4.2).

```
par(ask=TRUE) # 1 Column by 1 Row Density Plot
lattice::densityplot(~ Goats.df$Judgment,
  type="count", # Note: count
  par.settings=simpleTheme(lwd=2),
  par.strip.text=list(cex=1.15, font=2),
  scales=list(cex=1.15),
```

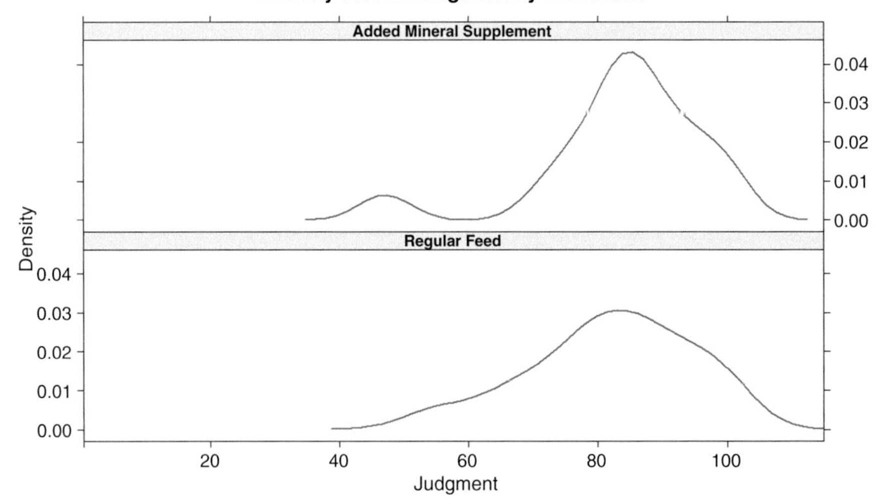

Fig. 4.2 Comparative density plots using the lattice::densityplot() function

```
  main="Density Plot of Judgment",
  xlab=list("Judgment", cex=1.15, font=2),
  xlim=c(0,115), # Note the range.
  ylab=list("Density", cex=1.15, font=2),
  aspect=1,
  layout = c(1,1), # Note: 1 Column by 1 Row.
  col="red")

par(ask=TRUE) # 1 Column by 2 Rows Density Plot
lattice::densityplot(~ Goats.df$Judgment |
  Goats.df$Treatment.recode,
  type="count", # Note: count
  par.settings=simpleTheme(lwd=2),
  par.strip.text=list(cex=1.15, font=2),
  scales=list(cex=1.15),
  main="Density Plot of Judgment by Treatment",
  xlab=list("Judgment", cex=1.15, font=2),
  xlim=c(0,115), # Note the range.
  ylab=list("Density", cex=1.15, font=2),
  aspect=0.25,
  layout = c(1,2), # Note: 1 Column by 2 Rows.
  col="red")
```

Of course, the lattice package is by no means the only package with functions that support breakout group comparisons for density plots. As shown previously, consider the plot(density()) function and the UsingR::DensityPlot() function as initial tools for preparation of throwaway density-type graphical comparisons.

However, the sm::sm.density.compare() function is possibly more useful, in part because it is easier to embellish for bolder presentation. As the syntax has been prepared, a left-click on the mouse is used to place the legend at any desired location, typically at an open area with sufficient white space (Fig. 4.3).

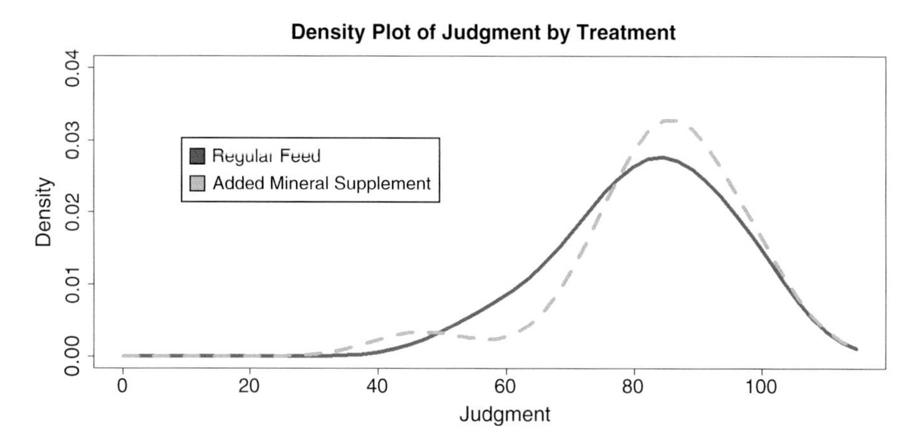

Fig. 4.3 Comparative density plots using the sm::sm.density.compare() function

```
install.packages("sm")
library(sm)                    # Load the sm package.
help(package=sm)               # Show the information page.
sessionInfo()                  # Confirm all attached packages.
# Select the most local mirror site using Set CRAN mirror.

savecexaxis  <- par(cex.axis=1.25)
par(ask=TRUE)
sm::sm.density.compare(Goats.df$Judgment,
  Goats.df$Treatment.recode,
  lwd=6,
  xlab=list("Judgment", cex=1.15, font=2),
  ylab=list("Density", cex=1.15, font=2),
  xlim=c(0,115), ylim=c(0,0.04))    # Adjust as needed
  title(main="Density Plot of Judgment by Treatment")
colorfill <- c(2:(2+length(levels(
  Goats.df$Treatment.recode))))
savefont     <- par(font=2)  # Local to the legend
legend(locator(1), levels(
  Goats.df$Treatment.recode),
  fill=colorfill, bty="n")
  # There is no box around the legend (bty="n") so
  # that bold text does not write lines in the legend
  # box.
par(savefont)                  # Local to the legend
  # Remember to click on an open location to paste the
  # legend into the figure.
par(savecexaxis)
  # Return to the original value.
```

Although descriptive statistics and inferential tests (Mann–Whitney U-Test for this lesson) are needed to make final judgment, graphics provide a sense of general trends and how the data compare to each other, individually and by group breakouts. Remember that the syntax used in this lesson can, of course, be used with future analyses. Simply alter the syntax, typically the dataframe name and object names, and adjust margins as needed to account for different scales.

4.5 Descriptive Analysis of the Data

Before the descriptive analyses are attempted for this lesson, it is important to once again mention that data for the object variable Goats.df$Judgment are viewed as ordinal data:

- A Judgment of 95 has a greater value than a Judgment of 94 and a Judgment of 75 has a greater value than a Judgment of 74. The data are certainly numeric, and as such it is possible to calculate descriptive statistics such as Mean and SD.

- However, the difference between 95 and 94 and the difference between 75 and 74, as displayed above, may not be consistently equivalent to the difference between 92 and 91, 88 and 87, etc. Equivalency in scale is essential if the data are classified as interval. Such equivalency is not assumed in this lesson.

Measures of Central Tendency of the Numeric Object Variables

The data for Goats.df$Judgment are ordinal, and because of this declaration there should be a degree of caution when viewing statistics such as Mean and SD for ordinal data. There are those who would argue that statistics such as Mean and SD are more appropriately associated with interval data and these descriptive statistics should be viewed with a degree of skepticism, or possibly avoided, when calculated against ordinal data. It is far beyond the purpose of this lesson, however, to go into this somewhat theoretical discussion. There are certainly many resources that would be of value to an interested reader on the appropriate use of descriptive statistics and measures of central tendency with ordinal data.

For this lesson, descriptive statistics such as Mean and SD are presented to understand better the object variable Goats.df$Judgment, even though the data associated with this object are ordinal.

Given the different ways missing data can impact analyses, it is best to first check for missing data (there are no missing data in Goats.df, the dataset used in this lesson) by using the is.na() function and the complete.cases() function against the entire dataset. Both functions return a TRUE or FALSE response, depending on the function and the outcome of whether data are missing or data are not missing.

```
is.na(Goats.df)                # Check for missing data
complete.cases(Goats.df)       # Check for complete cases
```

For this simple dataset, the summary() function may be all that is necessary to gain a sense of the data. Note how the summary() function is applied against the entire dataset, thus yielding information about all object variables including those that are not directly used in this sample, including ostensibly unnecessary information about Subject and also Treatment, prior to the transformation of Treatment into Treatment.recode.

Although the summary() function is quite sufficient, descriptive statistics for individual object variables may be desired. To achieve this need, review the help pages and other documentation for the following functions: length(), asbio::Mode(), median(), mean(), sd(), table(), and summary(). Additionally, consider function arguments needed to accommodate missing data, such as na.rm=TRUE. Using these available tools, look at the way measures of central tendency are approached:

```
length(Goats.df$Treatment.recode)       # N
length(Goats.df$Judgment)               # N

install.packages("asbio")
library(asbio)                 # Load the asbio package.
help(package=asbio)            # Show the information page.
sessionInfo()                  # Confirm all attached packages.
```

```
# Select the most local mirror site using Set CRAN mirror.

asbio::Mode(Goats.df$Judgment)          # Mode

median(Goats.df$Judgment, na.rm=TRUE)   # Median

mean(Goats.df$Judgment, na.rm=TRUE)      # Mean
sd(Goats.df$Judgment,na.rm=TRUE )        # SD
  # Measures of Central Tendency

table(Goats.df$Treatment.recode)
  # Frequency Distribution of Nominal Variable

summary(Goats.df)           # All variables

summary(Goats.df[, 3:4])    # Variables 3 to 4
```

```
    Judgment                         Treatment.recode
 Min.    : 47.00   Regular Feed               :15
 1st Qu.: 76.75   Added Mineral Supplement:15
 Median : 84.50
 Mean   : 82.87
 3rd Qu.: 90.50
 Max.   :100.00
```

The epicalc::summ() function, below, is also useful in that it can provide descriptive statistics and a representative figure of individual object variables.

```
par(ask=TRUE) # Use the epicalc package.
epicalc::summ(Goats.df$Judgment,
  by=NULL, graph=TRUE, box=TRUE, # Make a boxplot
  pch=18, ylab="auto",
  main="Sorted Dotplot and Boxplot of Judgment",
  cex.X.axis=1.15, cex.Y.axis=1.15, font.lab=2,
  dot.col="auto")
  # Note the descriptive statistics that go
  # along with the epicalc::summ() function.

savefont     <- par(font=2)  # Bold text
par(ask=TRUE) # Use the epicalc package.
epicalc::summ(Goats.df$Judgment,
  by=Goats.df$Treatment.recode,
  graph=TRUE, box=FALSE,              # No boxplot
  pch=18, ylab="auto",
  main="Sorted Dotplot Judgment by Treatment",
  cex.X.axis=1.15, cex.Y.axis=1.05,
  dot.col="auto")
  # Note the descriptive statistics that go
  # along with the epicalc::summ() function.
par(savefont)
```

```
For Goats.df$Treatment.recode = Regular Feed
 obs. mean    median  s.d.    min.    max.
 15   81.93   82      12.572 55      100

For Goats.df$Treatment.recode = Added Mineral
  Supplement
 obs. mean    median  s.d.    min.    max.
 15   83.8    85      12.857 47      100
```

The epicalc::summ() by=NULL argument can be set to either TRUE or FALSE, to either obtain or limit breakout descriptive statistics, as desired.

Although the epicalc::summ() function may be sufficient for production of descriptive statistics by different groups, there are many other functions that serve the same purpose, including the tapply() function and the psych::describeBy() function. As time permits, explore the many other R functions that serve a similar purpose.

```
tapply(Judgment, Treatment.recode, summary, na.rm=TRUE,
  data=Goats.df) # Breakouts of Judgment by Treatment.recode
```

```
$'Regular Feed'
   Min. 1st Qu.  Median    Mean 3rd Qu.    Max.
  55.00   75.50   82.00   81.93   89.50  100.00

$'Added Mineral Sup    plement'
   Min. 1st Qu.  Median    Mean 3rd Qu.    Max.
   47.0    80.5    85.0    83.8    91.0   100.0
```

```
install.packages("psych")
library(psych)                # Load the psych package.
help(package=psych)           # Show the information page.
sessionInfo()                 # Confirm all attached packages.
# Select the most local mirror site using Set CRAN mirror.

psych::describeBy(Goats.df$Judgment,
  Goats.df$Treatment.recode, mat=TRUE) # Matrix output
  # Breakouts of Judgment by Treatment.recode
```

The tables::tabular() function can be used to provide even more detail, in a fairly attractive table format that can be easily copied into a summary report.

```
install.packages("tables")
library(tables)               # Load the tables package.
help(package=tables)          # Show the information page.
sessionInfo()                 # Confirm all attached packages.
# Select the most local mirror site using Set CRAN mirror.

tables::tabular((Treatment.recode + 1) ~ (n=1) +
  Format(digits=4) * (Judgment)*(min + max + median + mean + sd)
  data=Goats.df)
  # Treatment.recode (row) by Judgment (columns)
```

```
                              Judgment
Treatment.recode            n  min      max     median mean   sd
Regular Feed                15  55.00   100.00  82.00  81.93  12.5
Added Mineral Supplement 15  47.00   100.00  85.00  83.80  12.8
All                         30  47.00   100.00  84.50  82.87  12.5
```

Although it may at first seem redundant, another function used to produce descriptive statistics in detailed tables is the etable::tabular.ade() function. The output can be easily copied and pasted into a standard word processing editor and, with minor editing, the output can be formatted into tables that have a great deal of specificity.

```
install.packages("etable")
library(etable)             # Load the etable package.
help(package=etable)        # Show the information page.
sessionInfo()               # Confirm all attached packages.
# Select the most local mirror site using Set CRAN mirror.

etable::tabular.ade(x_vars="Judgment",
  data=Goats.df,
  xname="Judgment",
  rows=c("Treatment.recode", "ALL"),
  rnames="Treatment",
  y_vars=c("N", "MIN", "MAX", "MEDIAN", "MEAN", "SD"),
  allnames=TRUE,
  FUN=stat_cell)
  # Treatment.recode (row) by Judgment (column)
```

```
1 Treatment
2                            N  MIN  MAX MEDIAN MEAN SD
3 Regular Feed               15 55.0 100 82.0   81.9 12.6
4 Added Mineral Supplement 15 47.0 100 85.0   83.8 12.9
5 Total                      30 47.0 100 84.5   82.9 12.5
```

From among the many possible R functions used for descriptive statistics, whether statistics are presented as singular values or table format, consider the prettyR::brkdn() function that provides output that can be copied from R and pasted into a word processing document, often with minimal if any editing for presentation.

```
install.packages("prettyR")
library(prettyR)            # Load the prettyR package.
help(package=prettyR)       # Show the information page.
sessionInfo()               # Confirm all attached packages.
# Select the most local mirror site using Set CRAN mirror.

prettyR::brkdn(Judgment ~ Treatment.recode,
  data=Goats.df, maxlevels=2,
  num.desc=c("valid.n", "median", "mean", "sd"),
  width=10, round.n=2)
  # Treatment.recode (row) by Judgment (column)
```

```
Breakdown of Judgment by Treatment.recode
Level                          valid.n   median   mean    sd
Regular Feed                   15        82       81.93   12.57
Added Mineral Supplement       15        85       83.8    12.86
```

Application of the Anderson-Darling Test

Graphical images and descriptive statistics are helpful in understanding data. It is also useful to apply selected statistical tests to serve as an additional support for decision-making on acceptance of nonparametric or parametric views toward the data. To that end, consider application of the Anderson-Darling Test, the Lilliefors (KS) Test, and the Shapiro-Wilk Test. These tests may be influenced by sample size and they provide one view, but not the only view, on the nature of distribution patterns. Experience, needs, and practical judgment, supported by careful review of graphical images, descriptive statistics, and statistical tests, should be used when deciding if variables from a dataset are best viewed from a nonparametric or parametric perspective.

```
install.packages("nortest")
library(nortest)              # Load the nortest package.
help(package=nortest)         # Show the information page.
sessionInfo()                 # Confirm all attached packages.
# Select the most local mirror site using Set CRAN mirror.
```

For this lesson is will be sufficient to apply the Anderson-Darling Test only. The Null Hypothesis for the Anderson-Darling Test is structured to examine whether data follow a specified distribution:

Anderson-Darling Null Hypothesis: The data follow the normal distribution.

For this lesson there will be three approaches to the Anderson-Darling Test and subsequent examination of p-values for each approach[4]:

- The Anderson-Darling Test will be applied against the values for Goats.df$Judgment, overall.
- The Anderson-Darling Test will be applied against the values for Goats.df$Judgment, where Treatment.recode is Regular Feed (i.e., Treatment is 1).
- The Anderson-Darling Test will be applied against the values for Goats.df$Judgment, where Treatment.recode is Added Mineral Supplement (i.e., Treatment is 2).

```
with(Goats.df, nortest::ad.test(Judgment))
  # All values for Goats.df$Judgment
```

[4]In the R syntax shown immediately below, notice how the with() function was used for selection. In association with this approach, note the use of two equal signs (i.e., ==) and not one equal sign.

```
        Anderson-Darling normality test

data:  Judgment
A = 0.5469, p-value = 0.1462
```

```
with(Goats.df, nortest::ad.test(Judgment[Treatment.recode ==
  "Regular Feed"]))
  # Values for Goats.df$Judgment where there was Regular Feed
```

```
        Anderson-Darling normality test

data:  Judgment[Treatment.recode == "Regular Feed"]
A = 0.1922, p-value = 0.8759
```

```
with(Goats.df, nortest::ad.test(Judgment[Treatment.recode ==
  "Added Mineral Supplement"]))
  # Values for Goats.df$Judgment where there was Regular Feed
  # and Added Mineral Supplement
```

```
        Anderson-Darling normality test

data:  Judgment[Treatment.recode == "Added Mineral Supplement"]
A = 0.6173, p-value = 0.08771
```

The calculated Anderson-Darling Test for normality p-value is fairly large overall (p-value = 0.1462) and for subjects that had regular feed only (p-value = 0.8759). However, for subjects that had a mineral supplement added to the regular feeding program the calculated p-value begins to approach 0.05 (p-value = 0.08771):

- Anderson-Darling Test Goats.df$Judgment p-value = 0.1462 for all subjects.
- Anderson-Darling Test Goats.df$Judgment p-value = 0.8759 for those subjects that had regular feed only.
- Anderson-Darling Test Goats.df$Judgment p-value = 0.08771 for those subjects that had regular feed and an added mineral supplement.

The p-values associated with these three attempts at the Anderson-Darling Test all exceed the p-value of 0.05 and it could be stated that the Null Hypothesis is confirmed and relative to this critical p-value (0.05) the data follow normal distribution. That is to say, for all three iterations of the Anderson-Darling Test, the Null Hypothesis is confirmed and the data follow the normal distribution.

However, for those subjects that had regular feed and an added mineral supplement, the result is not quite clear-cut, because a calculated p-value of 0.08771 begins to approach a critical p-value of 0.05. This type of finding is where personal experience with the research process and a broad view of the data need to be applied.

In an abundance of caution, and equally based on review of the graphical images of distribution patterns, a nonparametric approach will be used in this lesson for Judgment and comparisons of Judgment by Treatment, even though all three Anderson-Darling Test p-values exceed 0.05.

The QQ plot (i.e., normal probability plot) provides additional confirmation that the data are best viewed from a nonparametric perspective. Note placement of the data along the qqline, especially at the tails.

```
par(ask=TRUE)
par(mfrow=c(1,2))                        # Side-by-Side QQ Plots
with(Goats.df, qqnorm(Judgment[Treatment.recode ==
  "Regular Feed"],
  pch=22, col="red", bg="black", font=2, font.lab=2,
  cex.axis=1.5,                 # Adjust points in the QQ Plot
  main="QQPlot:  Judgment with Regular Feed Only"))
with(Goats.df, qqline(Judgment[Treatment.recode ==
  "Regular Feed"],
  lwd=4, col="darkblue"))                    # Adjust the QQ Line
with(Goats.df, qqnorm(Judgment[Treatment.recode ==
  "Added Mineral Supplement"],
  pch=22, col="red", bg="black", font=2, font.lab=2,
  cex.axis=1.5,                 # Adjust points in the QQ Plot
  main="QQPlot:  Judgment with Regular Feed and
  Added Mineral Supplement"))
with(Goats.df, qqline(Judgment[Treatment.recode ==
  "Added Mineral Supplement"],
  lwd=4, col="darkblue"))                    # Adjust the QQ Line
```

4.6 Conduct the Statistical Analysis

The dataset for this lesson was originally prepared as a Gnumeric spreadsheet and saved as Goats.gnumeric. The Gnumeric *File—Save as* feature was then used to save Goats.gnumeric into Goats.csv, a comma-separated values file. Goats.csv was then imported into R and saved as the object Goats.df. Additional changes were made to the dataset, after the data were imported into R, by using a few recoding techniques. As an example, the object variable Goats.df$Treatment.recode was created to understand the data more fully, given the stark numeric values used for the object variable Goats.df$Treatment.

```
class(Goats.df)    # Confirm the data
names(Goats.df)    # Confirm the data
str(Goats.df)      # Confirm the data
```

This lesson is focused on determining if there is a statistically significant difference in Judgment between those goats that received Treatment 1 (the control group that received regular feed) and goats that received Treatment 2 (the experimental group that received a mineral supplement added to the regular feeding program). To be more precise, consider the exact wording of the Null Hypothesis:

Null Hypothesis (Ho) There is no statistically significant difference (`p <= 0.05`) between goats that received regular feed during a treatment period (i.e., the control group) and their counterparts that received regular feed and an otherwise unidentified mineral supplement added to the feeding program during the same treatment period (i.e., the experimental group).

Again, the data associated with Judgment are viewed as ordinal data, not interval data. The data are numerical, and there is certainly an ordering to Judgment data (i.e., Judgment = 88 is greater than Judgment = 87 and Judgment = 77 is less than Judgment = 78).

Yet, data distribution and precision in scale are such that it is only prudent to view the data as ordinal data. Because of this view toward the data, the Mann–Whitney U-Test is viewed as the most appropriate test to determine if there is a statistically significant difference in Judgment between the two groups (i.e., control vs experimental). If the data were viewed as interval data, then Student's t-Test for Independent Samples would receive consideration, but that is not the case in this lesson.

Note: Use the transformed object variable Treatment.recode, to have output show as narrative text instead of output showing as a cryptic numeric code, which would be the case if the object variable Treatment, alone, were used.

As is often the situation with R, there are more than a few functions available for the Mann–Whitney U Test and three will be demonstrated below. Notice how the primary information is consistent for each function, but the visual presentation and supplementary information are different for each of the three functions: wilcox.test() function, coin::wilcox_test() function, and exactRankTests::wilcox.exact() function. As time permits, review reputable resources on the Internet as to why the Mann–Whitney U-Test is associated with the Wilcox Test, but that discussion is beyond the purpose of this lesson.

wilcox.test() Function

```
wilcox.test(Goats.df$Judgment ~ Goats.df$Treatment.recode,
  alternative = c("two.sided"),
  paired=FALSE, exact=TRUE, correct=TRUE)
  # Note the use of ~ between the two object variables
```

```
        Wilcoxon rank sum test with continuity correction

data:  Goats.df$Judgment by Goats.df$Treatment.recode
W = 98, p-value = 0.5611
alternative hypothesis: true location shift is not equal to 0

Warning message:
In wilcox.test.default(x = c(80, 82, 91, 100, 76, 65, 85, 88,:
  cannot compute exact p-value with ties
```

The statistic of greatest importance in this application of the wilcox.test() function is the calculated p-value of 0.5611, which more than exceeds the criterion p-value of 0.05.

coin::wilcox_test() Function

```
install.packages("coin")
library(coin)                      # Load the coin package.
help(package=coin)                 # Show the information page.
sessionInfo()                      # Confirm all attached packages.
# Select the most local mirror site using Set CRAN mirror.

coin::wilcox_test(Judgment ~ Treatment.recode,
  data = Goats.df,
  distribution = "exact", conf.int = TRUE)
  # Note the use of ~ between the two object variables
```

```
        Exact Wilcoxon Mann-Whitney Rank Sum Test

data:  Judgment by Treatment.recode
  (Regular Feed, Added Mineral Supplement)
Z = -0.602, p-value = 0.5595
alternative hypothesis: true mu is not equal to 0
95 percent confidence interval:
 -11   6
sample estimates:
difference in location
                    -2
```

The statistic of greatest importance in this application of the coin::wilcox_test() function is the calculated p-value of 0.5595, which more than exceeds the criterion p-value of 0.05.

exactRankTests::wilcox.exact() Function

```
install.packages("exactRankTests")
library(exactRankTests)        # Load the exactRankTests package.
help(package=exactRankTests)   # Show the information page.
sessionInfo()                  # Confirm all attached packages.
# Select the most local mirror site using Set CRAN mirror.

exactRankTests::wilcox.exact(Judgment ~ Treatment.recode,
  data=Goats.df,
  paired=FALSE, conf.int=TRUE, alternative="two.sided")
  # Note the use of ~ between the two object variables
```

```
        Exact Wilcoxon rank sum test

data:  Judgment by Treatment.recode
W = 98, p-value = 0.5595
alternative hypothesis: true mu is not equal to 0
95 percent confidence interval:
 -12   7
sample estimates:
difference in location
                  -2.5
```

The statistic of greatest importance in this application of the exactRankTests::wilcox.exact() function is the calculated p-value of 0.5595, which more than exceeds the criterion p-value of 0.05.

4.7 Summary

In this lesson, the graphics and descriptive statistics provided a great deal of information about the object variable Judgment and Judgment by Treatment breakouts. Of immediate importance, however, are the Null Hypothesis and the subsequent p-value associated with each of the three attempts at the Mann–Whitney U-Test. Compare the calculated p-value from each of the three tests (using wilcox.test(), coin::wilcox_test(), and exactRankTests::wilcox.exact() functions) to the criterion p-value of 0.05 associated with the Null Hypothesis.

Although more detail about the nature of the object variable Judgment and exactly what it represents would have been useful, for the immediate purpose of this lesson this detail is not needed and may only cause confusion, which is why the analyst knew very little about the biological experiment associated with this lesson. What is important to know is that one group of goats received regular feed throughout the experiment and another group received an added mineral supplement to go along with their regular feeding program. Judgment represents some type of measurement at the end-of-treatment.

Saying this, the analyses supported the observation that there is no statistically significant difference (`p <= 0.05`) in Judgment by Treatment. That is to say, for this one-time, non-replicated, posttest-only experiment, there was no difference in Judgment by the two Treatment breakouts (i.e., control group vs experimental group). Goats that received the added mineral supplement did not have a significantly different (`p <= 0.05`) Judgment measure than their counterparts that did not receive the added mineral supplement.

Although the Mann–Whitney U Test provided the information needed to make this assessment about Judgment and more specifically, Judgment by the two Treatment groups, it is helpful to once again review the descriptive statistics associated with this lesson. Because the data are ordinal, give special attention to the Median. Review prior comments for why it is appropriate to review other descriptive statistics such as Mean and SD even though the data are not interval.

```
prettyR::brkdn(Judgment ~ Treatment.recode,
  data=Goats.df, maxlevels=2,
  num.desc=c("valid.n", "median", "mean", "sd"),
  width=10, round.n=2)
  # Treatment.recode (row) by Judgment (column)
```

```
Breakdown of Judgment by Treatment.recode
Level                        valid.n   median  mean   sd
Regular Feed                 15        82      81.93  12.57
Added Mineral Supplement     15        85      83.8   12.86
```

As confirmed by using three different R-based functions associated with the Mann–Whitney U Test, there is no statistically significant difference (`p <= 0.05`) in Judgment between goats who had regular feed and goats who had an added mineral supplement.

4.8 Addendum: Stacked Data vs Unstacked Data

It was previously mentioned that the data in Goats.gnumeric, Goats.csv, and Goats.df were presented in stacked format as opposed to the use of unstacked data. A brief visual display of the two ways data can be organized (stacked data and unstacked data) follows. Using data totally separate from this lesson on goats, the example shown below is simple and shows data for six dogs: Breed (Labrador vs Beagle) and Weight (measured in pounds).

```
Stacked Data

Breed (Grouping Variable)  Weight (Measured Variable)
Labrador L1                53
Labrador L2                58
Labrador L3                49
Beagle   B1                33
Beagle   B2                25
Beagle   B3                28

Unstacked Data

Labrador_Weight            Beagle_Weight
53                         33
58                         25
49                         28
```

Experienced researchers typically work with data in multiple formats. Because of the need for exposure to a variety of formats, the stacked data previously found in the object Goats.df are presented below as unstacked data. Because the dataset for 30 goats is fairly small, the data will be entered directly into this R session. The data could have easily been saved in a separate file and then imported into R, but for this small collection of data it was deemed useful to demonstrate the textConnection() function as a means of entering data into R.

As shown below, the unstacked data about goats will be hand-entered and then a series of actions will be used to confirm that the data are correct and equivalent to the goats data that were seen previously in stacked format.

```
Goats_Unstacked.df <- read.table(textConnection("
 Regular  Mineral
  80        72
  82        89
  91        86
 100        85
  76        99
  65        47
  85        79
  88        88
  97       100
  55        76
  69        83
  88        94
  75        84
  97        82
  81        93      "), header=TRUE)

getwd()                          # Identify the working directory
ls()                             # List objects
attach(Goats_Unstacked.df)       # Attach the data, for later use
str(Goats_Unstacked.df)          # Identify structure
nrow(Goats_Unstacked.df)         # List the number of rows
ncol(Goats_Unstacked.df)         # List the number of columns
dim(Goats_Unstacked.df)          # Dimensions of the dataframe
names(Goats_Unstacked.df)        # Identify names
colnames(Goats_Unstacked.df)     # Show column names
rownames(Goats_Unstacked.df)     # Show row names
head(Goats_Unstacked.df)         # Show the head
tail(Goats_Unstacked.df)         # Show the tail
Goats_Unstacked.df               # Show the entire dataframe

summary(Goats_Unstacked.df)
  # Summary statistics unstacked data
```

```
    Regular          Mineral
 Min.   : 55.00   Min.   : 47.0
 1st Qu.: 75.50   1st Qu.: 80.5
 Median : 82.00   Median : 85.0
 Mean   : 81.93   Mean   : 83.8
 3rd Qu.: 89.50   3rd Qu.: 91.0
 Max.   :100.00   Max.   :100.0
```

```
tapply(Judgment, Treatment.recode,
  summary, na.rm=TRUE,
  data=Goats.df)
  # Summary statistics stacked data
```

```
$'Regular Feed'
   Min. 1st Qu.  Median    Mean 3rd Qu.    Max.
  55.00   75.50   82.00   81.93   89.50  100.00

$'Added Mineral Supplement'
   Min. 1st Qu.  Median    Mean 3rd Qu.    Max.
   47.0    80.5    85.0    83.8    91.0   100.0
```

After reviewing the summary statistics at the breakout levels of Treatment (i.e., regular feed v regular feed and added mineral supplement), there is assurance that the data are correct. Saying that, use the wilcox.test() function again but now with the R-based syntax needed for unstacked data.

```
wilcox.test(Goats_Unstacked.df$Regular,
  Goats_Unstacked.df$Mineral,
  alternative = c("two.sided"),
  paired=FALSE,    exact=TRUE)
  # Note the use of , between the two object variables
```

```
        Wilcoxon rank sum test with continuity correction

data:  Goats_Unstacked.df$Regular and
       Goats_Unstacked.df$Mineral
W = 98, p-value = 0.5611
alternative hypothesis: true location shift is not equal to 0

Warning message:
In wilcox.test.default(Goats_Unstacked.df$Regular,
  Goats_Unstacked.df$Mineral,   :
  cannot compute exact p-value with ties
```

Both variables (Regular and Mineral) are numeric. There is no grouping variable, such as the role of Treatment and Treatment.recode in Goats.df. This approach, and the use of a comma (i.e., `,`) to separate the two numeric variables for unstacked data, is in contrast to the use of a tilde (i.e., ~) character to separate the two numeric variables for stacked data.

Notice in the output with unstacked data that the calculated p-value is 0.5611, which was the same when the data were in stacked format. Whether stacked or unstacked, the data were consistent and the outcome was equivalent.

Again, the calculated p-value of 0.5611 exceeds the criterion p-value associated with the Null Hypothesis (`p <= 0.05`) and, again, it is confirmed that there is no difference in Judgment for goats fed a regular diet and goats fed a regular diet and an added mineral supplement.

4.9 Prepare to Exit, Save, and Later Retrieve this R Session

```
getwd()                # Identify the current working directory.
ls()                   # List all objects in the working
                       # directory.
ls.str()               # List all objects, with finite detail.
list.files()           # List files at the PC directory.

save.image("R_Mann-Whitney-U-Test.rdata")

getwd()                # Identify the current working directory.
ls()                   # List all objects in the working
                       # directory.
ls.str()               # List all objects, with finite detail.
list.files()           # List files at the PC directory.

alarm()                # Alarm, notice of upcoming action.
q()                    # Quit this session.
                       # Prepare for Save workspace image? query.
```

Use the R Graphical User Interface (GUI) to load the saved rdata file: File -> Load Workspace. Otherwise, use the load() function, keying the full pathname, to load the .rdata file and retrieve the session.

Recall, however, that it may be just as useful to simply use the .R script file (typically saved is a .txt ASCII-type file) and recreate the analyses and graphics, provided the data files remain available.

Chapter 5
Wilcoxon Matched-Pairs Signed-Ranks Test

Abstract The Wilcoxon Matched-Pairs Signed Ranks Test is a nonparametric test that is often viewed as being similar to Student's t-Test for Matched Pairs, but it is used for ordinal data or data that seriously violate any semblance of normal distribution. Of course, there are many who would argue that it is simply too convenient to compare the Wilcoxon Matched-Pairs Signed Ranks Test to Student's t-Test for Matched Pairs even though they serve similar purposes. Group differences for when there are two matched pairs are addressed by both tests, but again, the Wilcoxon Matched-Pairs Signed Ranks Test is often used with ordinal data and/or data that are viewed as being nonparametric (with attention to medians) whereas the Student's t-Test for Matched Pairs is generally used with interval data that rise to the level of parametric distributions (with attention to means). This lesson is interesting in that there is a tied set of values for one of the matched pairs, which introduces some degree of complexity on how values are ranked when there are ties (i.e., for an individual matched pair, there is no difference in the two scores that are being compared).

Keywords Anderson-Darling Test • Bar plot (stacked, side-by-side) • Box plot • Code Book • Comma separator • Comma-separated values (.csv) • Continuous scale • Density plot • Descriptive statistics • Distribution-free • Frequency distribution • Hinge (lower and upper) • Histogram • Interval • Matched pairs • Mean • Median • Mode • Nominal • Nonparametric • Normal distribution • Null Hypothesis • Ordinal • Outlier • Parametric • Percentile • Probability (p-value) • Quantile-Quantile (QQ, Q-Q) • Ranking • Stacked data • Statistical significance • Student's t-Test for Matched Pairs • Tilde separator • Unstacked data • Violin plot • Whisker (lower and upper) • Wilcoxon Matched Pairs Signed Ranks Test

---

Electronic supplementary material The online version of this chapter (doi: 10.1007/978-3-319-30634-6_5) contains supplementary material, which is available to authorized users.

T.W. MacFarland, J.M. Yates, *Introduction to Nonparametric Statistics for the Biological Sciences Using R*, DOI 10.1007/978-3-319-30634-6_5

5.1 Background on this Lesson

As the name suggests, the Wilcoxon Matched-Pairs Signed-Ranks Test uses data from matched pairs. The Wilcoxon Test uses ordinal data and is focused on the magnitude, as well as the direction, of differences for matched pairs. That is to say, the algorithm associated with the Wilcoxon Test considers the degree or amount of difference and accordingly uses an ordered metric scale for this difference.

5.1.1 Description of the Data

This lesson on the Wilcoxon Matched-Pairs Signed Ranks Test is based on a study about young female sheep (*Ovis aries*, where the female is called an ewe and the male is called a ram), with data obtained sometime after weaning but prior to classification as yearlings. In this matched-pairs study, the data are from twin ewes and refer to weight (pounds) measured under field conditions.

A matched-pairs study can be structured as a pretest–posttest design, where data are initially gained from a specific subject as a pretest measure, a treatment is applied, and after a period of time data are then gained again from the same subject as a posttest measure. In this type of matched-pairs design, each individual subject is its own pair.

However, this study represents a matched-pairs design where two closely related (or at least similar) subjects represent the pair. In this specific study, data are gained from twin ewes. Twins of the same gender are used so that genetic variability (i.e., closely related siblings should be genetically similar) and gender variability (i.e., equivalent genders should promote similarity to experimental conditions and outcomes) that may possibly impact weight are controlled, at least to some degree, given the field conditions of this study.

The specific structure for this study is fairly simple and by no means is it suggested that the design is ideal, but that is typically the case for many exploratory studies. To be specific on how the data were obtained:

- From a large flock of sheep sometime after weaning, 20 pairs of recently weaned ewes were selected, resulting in 40 individual ewes—two twin ewes representing each pair.
- Adequate marking (i.e., tags) were used so that each ewe could be identified correctly at all times.
- From each of these 20 pairs of ewes, one ewe was marked as the control ewe and the other ewe (i.e., its twin sibling) was marked as the treatment ewe.
- All subjects were kept with the larger flock, and all sheep generally experienced the same feeding program, exercise, environmental conditions, stress, etc.
- However, the 20 treatment ewes were periodically administered a treatment of some type, and the treatment was administered only to the 20 treatment ewes.
- The initial weight of each ewe was either not attempted or not recorded and is unknown to the researcher assigned with responsibility for data analysis.

- The regularity of treatment (e.g., daily, weekly, etc.) is unknown to the researcher responsible for data analysis. It is only known that treatment was administered as protocols required.
- The nature of the treatment (e.g., mineral supplement, vitamins, extra rations, etc.) is unknown to the researcher assigned responsibility for data analysis.
- The vector for treatment (e.g., feeding supplement, injection, liquid, pill, powder, etc.) is unknown to the researcher assigned responsibility for data analysis.
- The length of time for treatment (e.g., one week, one month, etc.) is unknown to the researcher assigned responsibility for data analysis.
- The number of treatments is unknown to the researcher assigned responsibility for data analysis.

At completion of the treatment period, all subjects were weighed on the same day under field conditions. Because of the harsh realities of weighing sheep out in the field and the difficulty of calibrating a scale to desired levels of accuracy under these conditions, it is assumed that the weights represent ordinal data and that they are not at the level of reliability and validity more appropriately associated with interval data. There is no doubt that a weight of 87 pounds is more than a weight of 86 pounds, but there is limited assurance that the difference between these two measures is consistently equivalent to the difference between 92 pounds and 91 pounds and similar comparisons. Weights are measured to the nearest pound and they are viewed as ordinal data, not interval data.

Further, it was noticed when weights were taken that there may be concerns about normal distribution of weights for subjects in the two breakout groups: Control ewes and Treatment ewes. Accordingly, the data are not only ordinal, but there may also be questions about normal distribution of weights. Both concerns prompt the research staff to consider the use of a nonparametric approach to data analysis.

Be sure to notice once again that this study has not been designed as a pretest–treatment–posttest experiment. Instead, it is assumed that the subjects, because they are gender-equivalent twins in close proximity to each other and experiencing the same field conditions and feeding patterns, are similar to each other at the beginning of the experiment. A treatment is applied to one of the two twins from each pair, and at the end of the treatment all subjects are weighed at the same time: the 20 ewes that did not receive the treatment and the 20 ewes that received the treatment.

Given the nature of the data associated with this study and, specifically, concerns about exact calibration of the scale when used under rough field conditions, it is viewed that the data should be considered ordinal and not internal. There is the additional concern about data distribution and if the data approach normal distribution. With all of these considerations, the Student's t-Test for Matched pairs is not the appropriate test for this study.

Instead, the Wilcoxon Matched-Pairs Signed Ranks Test, which is more appropriately used with ordinal data and/or data that do not show normal distribution, will be used to critically examine differences between the two groups. Again, the weights used in this study represent nonparametric data.

The data are organized as unstacked data and are found in the file EweTwin.csv, which is available on the publisher's Web page associated with this text:

- The first line consists of a header, using descriptive variable names: Pair, Control, Treatment.
- The header is then followed by 20 lines of data, one line of data for each pair of ewe twins.
- Pair: There is a coded identifier (P01–P20) for each pair. Adequate markings and tracking protocols were used to correctly identify each ewe throughout the study: pair number and classification as either the control ewe or the treatment ewe.
- Control: Each datum in the Control column represents the weight (pounds) for the paired ewe viewed as the control subject, with weight taken at end-of-treatment.
- Treatment: Each datum in the Treatment column represents the weight (pounds) for the paired ewe viewed as the treatment subject, with weight taken at end-of-treatment.

As a reminder, there are concerns about the normal distribution of weights for both Control subjects and Treatment subjects. There is equally a concern that the data are ordinal, and not interval. Again, desired precision for the scale was not possible when weights were obtained under field conditions.

This lesson does not demonstrate a biological experiment structured under ideal conditions. However, this lesson gives a glimpse of the conditions for many field studies. At the least, consider how:

- Subjects were selected from a large flock of sheep, but the data are still only from one flock of sheep.
- The researcher assigned responsibility for data analysis has no information about the breed, which may have a role in outcomes.
- There is no pretest measure of weight for either the Control ewes or the Treatment ewes. Instead, it is only possible to assess differences between the two groups (i.e., Control v Treatment) at end-of-treatment.

Again, given the nature of the data the nonparametric Wilcoxon Matched-Pairs Signed Ranks Test is judged the most appropriate inferential test for this analysis of differences between twin ewes and their weights at the end of this study.

5.1.2 Null Hypothesis (Ho)

There is no statistically significant difference (`p <= 0.05`) in weight between ewes that experienced regular field conditions during a treatment period (i.e., the control group) and their gender-equivalent twin counterparts that not only experienced regular conditions but also received an otherwise unidentified supplement during the same treatment period (i.e., the treatment group).

As an exploratory study, the Null Hypothesis (Ho) uses `p <= 0.05`. It is not uncommon for more structured and tightly-controlled studies in the biological sciences to use a more restrictive *p*-level, perhaps `p <= 0.01` or even `p <= 0.001`. However, given the nature of this lesson and how it demonstrates an exploratory study under field conditions, it is appropriate to use `p <= 0.05` as the criterion p-value. Then, with replication and greater controls, more restrictive p-values may have merit—but not for this lesson.

5.2 Data Import of a .csv Spreadsheet-Type Data File into R

The data for this lesson, originally found in EweTwin.csv and later organized in the R session as the object EweTwin.df, are presented in unstacked format. A very brief demonstration, below, shows each of these two methods for organizing data, using a small sample of data from a different study:

```
Unstacked Data

Pair  Control_Height_Inches  Treatment_Height_Inches
1     64                     67
2     61                     62
3     66                     63

Stacked Data

Group                   Pair  Height_Inches
Control                 1     64
Control                 2     61
Control                 3     66
Treatment               1     67
Treatment               2     62
Treatment               3     63
```

It is perhaps more common to experience data in stacked format than to experience data in unstacked format. However, experienced researchers should have the skills needed to work with data in multiple formats, unstacked and stacked. R has some capabilities to transform data, but there are many other software tools that can also be used if it were necessary to reconfigure data to suite production needs.

This lesson was structured to use free desktop software. Given that goal, the dataset for this lesson was originally prepared as a Gnumeric spreadsheet. The data were then also saved in .csv (i.e., comma-separated values) file format as EweTwin.csv. The data are separated by commas, not tabs and not spaces. Similar to the open nature of any .csv file, this file can be easily sent to, and opened by, other researchers without the need for specialized and overly-expensive proprietary software.

Start a new R session and then attend to beginning actions such as removing unwanted files from prior work, declaring the working directory, etc.

```
###############################################################
# Housekeeping                          Use for All Analyses    #
###############################################################
date()              # Current system time and date.
R.version.string    # R version and version release date.
ls()                # List all objects in the working
                    # directory.
rm(list = ls())     # CAUTION: Remove all files in the working
```

```
                      # directory. If this action is not desired,
                      # use the rm() function one-by-one to remove
                      # the objects that are not needed.
ls.str()              # List all objects, with finite detail.
getwd()               # Identify the current working directory.
setwd("F:/R_Nonparametric")
                      # Set to a new working directory.
                      # Note the single forward slash and double
                      # quotes.
                      # This new directory should be the directory
                      # where the data file is located, otherwise
                      # the data file will not be found.
getwd()               # Confirm the working directory.
list.files()          # List files at the PC directory.
################################################################
```

Now that the R session has been initially organized, use R to import the data in the file EweTwin.csv and in turn put the data into an object called EweTwin.df. The object EweTwin.df will be a dataframe, as indicated by the enumerated .df extension to the object name. This object will represent the output of applying the read.table() function against the comma-separated values file called EweTwin.csv. Note the arguments used with the read.table() function, showing that there is a header with descriptive variable names (header = TRUE) and that the separator between fields is a comma (sep = ",").

```
EweTwin.df <- read.table (file =
  "EweTwin.csv",
  header = TRUE,
  sep = ",")                   # Import the .csv file

getwd()                        # Identify the working directory
ls()                           # List objects
attach(EweTwin.df)             # Attach the data, for later use
str(EweTwin.df)                # Identify structure
nrow(EweTwin.df)               # List the number of rows
ncol(EweTwin.df)               # List the number of columns
dim(EweTwin.df)                # Dimensions of the dataframe
names(EweTwin.df)              # Identify names
colnames(EweTwin.df)           # Show column names
rownames(EweTwin.df)           # Show row names
head(EweTwin.df, n=10)         # Show the head
tail(EweTwin.df, n=10)         # Show the tail
EweTwin.df                     # Show the entire dataframe
summary(EweTwin.df)            # Summary statistics
```

By completing this action, an object called EweTwin.df has been created. This R-based object is a dataframe, and it consists of the data originally included in the file EweTwin.csv, a comma-separated values .csv file. To avoid possible conflicts, make sure that there are no prior R-based objects called EweTwin.df. The prior use of rm(list = ls()) accommodates this concern, removing all prior objects in the current R session.

Note how it was only necessary to key the filename for the .csv file and not the full pathname since the R working directory is currently set to the directory and/or subdirectory where this .csv file is located. See the Housekeeping section at the beginning of this lesson.

5.3 Organize the Data and Display the Code Book

The data in EweTwin.csv have been successfully imported into R, now showing as a dataframe-type object called EweTwin.df. It is always a good idea to check the data for format and to then make any changes that may be needed, to be sure that the data are organized as desired. This dataset is fairly small (N = 40 subjects, organized into 20 pairs with data for each pair showing on one line), and there are no missing data. These early lessons purposely use small, but complete, datasets to help build skills and confidence with the use of R.

To support tracking purposes, a rowname will be used with this dataset using the rownames() function. It is not necessary to add rownames, but rownames are helpful when working with large datasets. The rownames() function assigns a unique identifier for each row in the dataset, each beginning with the term Ewe Twin Pair in this example.

```
rownames(EweTwin.df) <- paste('Ewe Twin Pair', 1:20)

head(EweTwin.df)     # Show the first few lines of the dataset
tail(EweTwin.df)     # Show the last few lines of the dataset
EweTwin.df           # Show the entire dataset since it is small
```

For this lesson, the class() function, str() function, and duplicated() function will be used to be sure that data are organized. These actions may seem redundant, but every effort should be made so that the data are organized as desired.

```
class(EweTwin.df)
class(EweTwin.df$Pair)        # DataFrame$ObjectName notation
class(EweTwin.df$Control)     # DataFrame$ObjectName notation
class(EweTwin.df$Treatment)   # DataFrame$ObjectName notation

str(EweTwin.df)               # Structure

duplicated(EweTwin.df)        # Duplicates
```

The class for each object seems to be correct, and there are no duplicate rows of data in the dataframe. Saying this, a Code Book will help with future understanding of this dataset.

A Code Book is a must for practicing researchers. The Code Book is typically brief and only serves as a useful reminder for what can be easily forgotten months (or even weeks) later, to make it easy to decipher what may otherwise be seen as arcane numeric codes. Coding schemes that are intuitively obvious today can easily become forgotten tomorrow.

The Code Book below represents how data are desired before analyses begin. Recoding may be needed to put data into new formats.

```
########################################################
# Code Book for EweTwin.df                             #
########################################################
#                                                      #
# Pair ....................... Factor (i.e., nominal) #
#                  A unique ID ranging from P01 to P20 #
#                                                      #
# Control .................. Numeric (i.e., interval) #
#         Weight (lbs) of a female sheep (e.g., ewe) #
#                     at the end of a treatment program  #
#         Data may also be viewed as ordinal due to  #
#                               measurement issues #
#                                                      #
# Treatment ................ Numeric (i.e., interval) #
#         Weight (lbs) of a female sheep (e.g., ewe) #
#                     at the end of a treatment program #
#         Data may also be viewed as ordinal due to  #
#                               measurement issues #
########################################################
```

The str() function is then again applied against the dataframe to see the nature of each object variable as well as confirmation that the data are collectively viewed as a dataframe:

```
str(EweTwin.df)
```

Recall that the Code Book shows data in their desired formats, as opposed to their original format, which often requires some degree of recoding.

Once there is agreement that the data were brought into R in correct format, it is usually necessary to organize the data to some degree:

- The object variable Pair is only used to identify specific pairs. Each datum for Pair begins with the letter P and this object variable is currently recognized as a factor object variable.
- Values for Control are currently whole numbers and as such they are first treated in R as integers. A simple recode action will instead be used to put these values into decimal format. As needed, review the as.integer() function and the as.numeric() function to see why it is desirable to view the weights for the object Control as a numeric value and not as an integer.
- Values for Treatment are currently whole numbers and as such they are first treated in R as integers. A simple recode action will instead be used to put these values into decimal format. As needed, review the as.integer() function and the as.numeric() function to see why it is desirable to view the weights for the object Treatment as a numeric value and not as an integer.

```
EweTwin.df$Pair      <- as.factor(EweTwin.df$Pair)
EweTwin.df$Control   <- as.numeric(EweTwin.df$Control)
EweTwin.df$Treatment <- as.numeric(EweTwin.df$Treatment)
```

Although it is perhaps redundant, it remains a good idea to place a few actions against the data and to confirm that the data are indeed in correct and desired format.

```
getwd()                   # Identify the working directory
ls()                      # List objects
attach(EweTwin.df)        # Attach the data, for later use
str(EweTwin.df)           # Identify structure
nrow(EweTwin.df)          # List the number of rows
ncol(EweTwin.df)          # List the number of columns
dim(EweTwin.df)           # Dimensions of the dataframe
names(EweTwin.df)         # Identify names
colnames(EweTwin.df)      # Show column names
rownames(EweTwin.df)      # Show row names
head(EweTwin.df)          # Show the head
tail(EweTwin.df)          # Show the tail
EweTwin.df                # Show the entire dataframe
summary(EweTwin.df)       # Summary statistics
```

As a brief recap to how the data have been accommodated so far, note how the data for this lesson were first organized in a Gnumeric spreadsheet. From this spreadsheet (.gnumeric file extension), the data were then saved in .csv format as a comma-separated values file. The .csv file was then imported into R and put into a dataframe-type object with a .df extension. The progression for data format is:

1. EweTwin.gnumeric
2. EweTwin.csv
3. EweTwin.df

Once the data were imported into R, a set of actions was placed against the data to add rownames and to be sure that the data were in desired format, with Pair viewed as a factor-type object and Control and Treatment viewed as numeric-type objects.

Throughout this lesson, be sure to follow along with the formal way object variables are identified: DataframeName$ObjectName. This formal nomenclature may call for strong typing and some redundant actions, but it eliminates the chance of introducing error and possibly working with the incorrect object. Time spent in these initial quality assurance actions will assure that later analyses are correct.

5.4 Conduct a Visual Data Check

Now with a fair degree of assurance that the data are in proper format (i.e., specifically, the object variables EweTwin$Control and EweTwin$Treatment are now of numeric data-type), many inexperienced researchers would immediately begin statistical tests, perhaps starting with a few attempts at descriptive statistics and measures of central tendency and then quickly moving on to the test in question, or the Wilcoxon Matched-Pairs Signed Ranks Test in this lesson. Although this approach is only too common, it should be avoided. Instead, it is always best to prepare a few graphical displays of the data and then reinforce understanding of the data with descriptive statistics and measures of central tendency.

Avoiding that rushed approach, in these lessons the data are first examined visually, using the strong graphical features supported by R. The images can be simple throwaway graphics, designed only to offer a general sense of the data. Or, the images can be fully embellished, of high quality, and suitable for presentation or publication. Regardless of details in the final view, graphics provide a more complete understanding of the data that may be difficult to grasp when only statistics are viewed.

For initial purposes the graphical functions of primary interest are plot() and barplot(table()) for factor-type object variables. For numeric-type object variables, a few of the leading graphics use the following R functions: boxplot(), hist(), plot(density()), vioplot(), and qqnorm(). Although there are far more specialized functions available, these functions should be more than sufficient to provide an initial visual representation of the data.

The par(ask=TRUE) function and argument are used to freeze the presentation on the screen, one figure at a time. When viewing a R-generated figure, note how the top line of the figure, under *File – Save as*, provides a variety of graphical formats to save each figure: Metafile, Postscript, PDF, PNG, BMP, TIFF, and JPEG. It is also possible to perform a simple copy and paste against each graphical image. Graphical images can also be saved by using R syntax.

Visual Presentation of Factor-Type Object Variables

The dataset for this lesson on Ewes is fairly simple, with Pairs as the only factor-type object variable. It is unlikely that the graphics for the object variable Pair will ever be published, but it is still attempted as a quality assurance measure to be sure that data have been imported for each of the 20 pairs of ewes.

```
par(ask=TRUE)
plot(EweTwin.df$Pair,
  main="Ewe Pair (N = 20 Pairs) - Subject(s)",
  xlab="Pairs", ylab="N",
  col=c("red"),  cex.lab=1.25, font=2)
```

Although it may seem somewhat redundant, the barplot() function can be used to generate the same figure by wrapping the barplot() function around the table() function. As is nearly always the case with R, there are usually multiple ways to achieve desired aims.

```
par(ask=TRUE)
barplot(table(EweTwin.df$Pair),
  main="Ewe Pair (N = 20 Pairs) - Subject(s)",
  xlab="Pairs", ylab="N",
  col=c("red"),  cex.lab=1.25, font=2)
```

Visual Presentation of Numeric-Type Object Variables

While viewing and then preparing graphical presentations of the numeric-type object variables EweTwin.df$Control and EweTwin.df$Treatment, recall that the data for these object variables are considered ordinal—not interval. Both object variables are certainly numbers given how they represent weight in pounds. However, use some degree of caution and keep in mind that the scale is not as consistent as would be expected if the data followed along a more parametric perspective.

The boxplot is one of the most frequently used tools for graphically representing measures of central tendency, descriptive statistics, and overall dispersion of a numerical variable.[1] A few text-based (i.e., not graphical) functions that go along with the boxplot() function are the boxplot.stats() function and the fivenum() function:

- boxplot.stats() function
  - lower whisker
  - lower hinge
  - median
  - upper hinge
  - upper whisker
  - N
  - outliers
- fivenum() function
  - minimum
  - lower hinge
  - median
  - upper hinge
  - maximum

```
par(ask=TRUE)
boxplot(EweTwin.df$Control,
  main="Boxplot of Control Ewes (Weight - Pounds)",
  ylab="Weight - Pounds",     # Label
  ylim=c(40,100),             # Range of Y axis
  font=2,                     # Bold text
  cex.lab=1.15,               # Large font
  cex.axis=1.25,              # Large axis text
  lwd=2,                      # Thick line
  col="red")                  # Vibrant color
```

[1] As a reminder on the boxplot, the bottom line (i.e., lower hinge) in the box represents the 25th percentile, the middle line represents the 50th percentile (i.e., median), and the top line (i.e., upper hinge) represents the 75th percentile. The whiskers are drawn as horizontal lines that represent data that go beyond values for the 25th percentile (i.e., bottom whisker) and the 75th percentile (i.e., top whisker). Exceptionally divergent data are often represented as small circles that go beyond the whiskers and are typically termed *outliers*.

```
boxplot.stats(EweTwin.df$Control)
fivenum(EweTwin.df$Control)

par(ask=TRUE)
boxplot(EweTwin.df$Treatment,
  main="Boxplot of Treatment Ewes (Weight - Pounds)",
  ylab="Weight - Pounds",     # Label
  ylim=c(40,100),             # Range of Y axis
  font=2,                     # Bold text
  cex.lab=1.15,               # Large font
  cex.axis=1.25,              # Large axis text
  lwd=2,                      # Thick line
  col="red")                  # Vibrant color
mtext("Notice the outlier, at 50 or so pounds.",
  line=2.5, side=1, cex=1.25, col=c("darkblue"),
  font=2)
  # The mtext() function has been used to place a
  # comment, not a label, below the X axis.  The line
  # argument was very useful, to place the text a few
  # lines below the X axis, to improve presentation.

boxplot.stats(EweTwin.df$Treatment)
fivenum(EweTwin.df$Treatment)
```

If it would help, place both boxplot figures side-by-side while using the same scale, to gain another view of central tendency and distribution for the two numeric object variables, Control and Treatment. By using the mfrow() function as presented below, the two graphics will be placed in a 1 row by 2 column format (Fig. 5.1).

```
par(ask=TRUE)
par(mfrow=c(1,2))             # 1 row by 2 column format
boxplot(EweTwin.df$Control,
  ylab="Weight (Pounds):  Control Ewes",
  ylim=c(0,115), font=2, cex.lab=1.15, cex.axis=1.25,
  lwd=2, col="red")
mtext("Ewes:  Control", line=0.5, side=3, cex=1.25,
  col=c("darkblue"), font=2)
boxplot(EweTwin.df$Treatment,
  ylab="Weight (Pounds):  Treatment Ewes",
  ylim=c(0,115), font=2, cex.lab=1.15, cex.axis=1.25,
  lwd=2, col="red")
mtext("Ewes:  Treatment", line=0.5, side=3, cex=1.25,
  col=c("darkblue"), font=2)
```

The histogram is also a standard graphical tool for showing the dispersion of values for a specific numeric object variable. When looking (below) at the R syntax for the histogram observe how the arguments are similar to what has been seen previously with other functions.

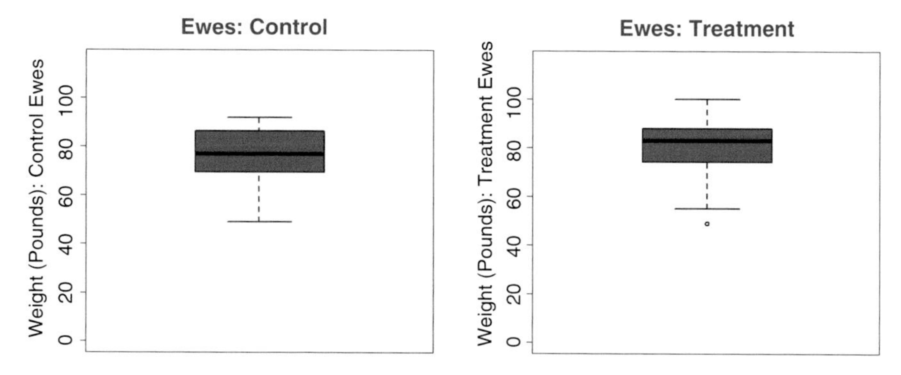

Fig. 5.1 Comparative boxplots of separate object variables in one common graphic

```
par(ask=TRUE)
hist(EweTwin.df$Control,
  main="Histogram of Control Ewes (Weight - Pounds)",
  xlab="Weight - Pounds",     # Label
  font=2,                     # Bold text
  cex.lab=1.15,               # Large font
  cex.axis=1.25,              # Large axis text
  lwd=2,                      # Thick line
  col="red")                  # Vibrant color
mtext("Do Control weights show normal distribution?",
  line=1.75, side=1, cex=0.95, col=c("darkblue"),
  font=2)

par(ask=TRUE)
hist(EweTwin.df$Treatment,
  main="Histogram of Treatment Ewes (Weight - Pounds)",
  xlab="Weight - Pounds",     # Label
  font=2,                     # Bold text
  cex.lab=1.15,               # Large font
  cex.axis=1.25,              # Large axis text
  lwd=2,                      # Thick line
  col="red")                  # Vibrant color
mtext("Do Treatment weights show normal distribution?",
  line=1.75, side=1, cex=0.95, col=c("darkblue"),
  font=2)
```

Following along with the desire to show graphical images for EweTwin.df$Control and EweTwin.df$Treatment, side-by-side, review outcomes for the following syntax:

```
par(ask=TRUE)
par(mfrow=c(1,2))                # 1 row by 2 column format
hist(EweTwin.df$Control,
  main="Ewes:  Control",
  xlab="Weight", ylab="Weight (Pounds):  Control Ewes",
```

```
  ylim=c(0,10), xlim=c(0,115), font=2, cex.lab=1.15,
  cex.axis=1.25, lwd=2, col="red")
hist(EweTwin.df$Treatment,
  main="Ewes:  Treatment",
  xlab="Weight", ylab="Weight (Pounds):  Treatment Ewes",
  ylim=c(0,10), xlim=c(0,115), font=2, cex.lab=1.15,
  cex.axis=1.25, lwd=2, col="red")
```

A density plot is equally used to show the distribution of values for a numerical object variable.[2] Notice below how the density plot is prepared for each object variable in question (EweTwin.df$Control and EweTwin.df$Treatment) and then how these two object variables show side-by-side. Give attention to the plot() function and how it is wrapped around the density() function (Fig. 5.2).

```
par(ask=TRUE)
plot(density(EweTwin.df$Control,
  na.rm=TRUE),     # Required for the density() function
  main="Density Plot of Control Ewes (Weight - Pounds)",
  xlab="Weight (Pounds)",
  font=2,          # Bold text
  cex.lab=1.15,    # Large font
  cex.axis=1.25,   # Large axis text
  lwd=6,           # Thick line
  col="red")       # Vibrant color

par(ask=TRUE)
plot(density(EweTwin.df$Treatment,
  na.rm=TRUE),     # Required for the density() function
  main="Density Plot of Treatment Ewes (Weight - Pounds)",
  xlab="Weight (Pounds)",
  font=2,          # Bold text
  cex.lab=1.15,    # Large font
  cex.axis=1.25,   # Large axis text
  lwd=6,           # Thick line
  col="red")       # Vibrant color

par(ask=TRUE)
par(mfrow=c(1,2))                   # 1 row by 2 column format
plot(density(EweTwin.df$Control,   na.rm=TRUE),
  main="Ewes:  Control", xlab="Weight (Pounds)",
  ylim=c(0, 0.05), xlim=c(0,115), font=2, cex.lab=1.15,
  cex.axis=1.25, lwd=6, col="red")
plot(density(EweTwin.df$Treatment, na.rm=TRUE),
  main="Ewes:  Treatment", xlab="Weight (Pounds)",
  ylim=c(0, 0.05), xlim=c(0,115), font=2, cex.lab=1.15,
  cex.axis=1.25, lwd=6, col="red")
```

[2]The density plot provides a graphical summary of density estimates for a given set of data. Density estimation is a data smoothing tool, with inferences made about a population based on provided data.

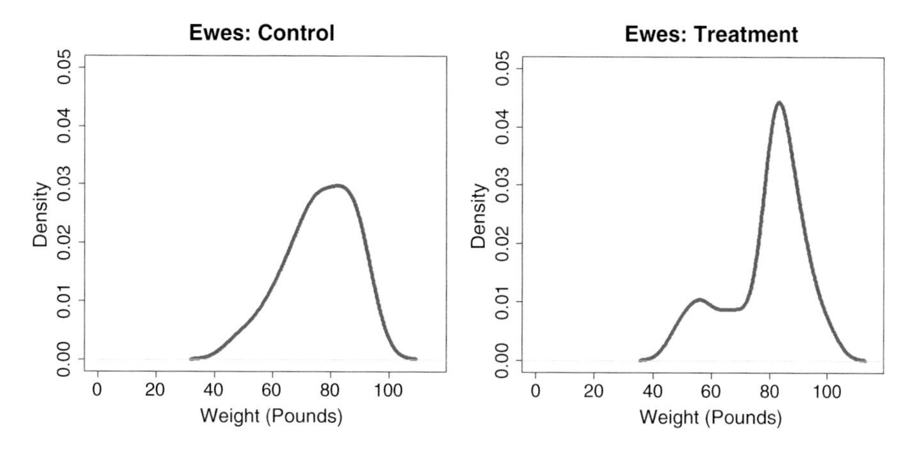

Fig. 5.2 Comparative density plots of separate object variables in one common graphic

Violin plots are not as well-known as boxplots, but their use should be considered. Consider, below, how the violin plot complements what is also shown in the boxplot.

```
install.packages("vioplot")
library(vioplot)              # Load the vioplot package.
help(package=vioplot)         # Show the information page.
sessionInfo()                 # Confirm all attached packages.
# Select the most local mirror site using Set CRAN mirror.

save.cexaxis  <- par(cex.axis=1.25)        # Expand axis size
par(ask=TRUE)
vioplot::vioplot(EweTwin.df$Control,
  names=c("Control Ewes Weight - Pounds"), ylim=c(40,100),
  col="red", horizontal=FALSE, lwd=3, lty=6)
  title("Violin Plot of Control Ewes (Weight - Pounds)")
par(save.cexaxis)                        # Toggle back.

save.cexaxis  <- par(cex.axis=1.25)        # Expand axis size
par(ask=TRUE)
vioplot::vioplot(EweTwin.df$Treatment,
  names=c("Treatment Ewes Weight - Pounds"), ylim=c(40,100),
    col="red", horizontal=FALSE, lwd=3, lty=6)
  title("Violin Plot of Treatment Ewes (Weight - Pounds)")
par(save.cexaxis)                        # Toggle back.
```

Place both violin plots side-by-side, to better understand patterns of central tendency and distribution for the two numeric object variables, Control and Treatment. By using mfrow(), the two graphics will be placed in a 1 row by 2 column format.

```
save.cexaxis  <- par(cex.axis=1.25)        # Expand axis size
par(ask=TRUE)
par(mfrow=c(1,2))                          # 1 row by 2 column format
vioplot::vioplot(EweTwin.df$Control,
  names=c("Weight (Pounds):  Control Ewes"), ylim=c(0,115),
  col="red", horizontal=FALSE, lwd=3, lty=6)
mtext("Ewes:  Control", line=0.5, side=3, cex=1.25,
  col=c("darkblue"), font=2)
vioplot::vioplot(EweTwin.df$Treatment,
  names=c("Weight (Pounds):  Treatment Ewes"), ylim=c(0,115),
  col="red", horizontal=FALSE, lwd=3, lty=6)
par(save.cexaxis)                          # Toggle back.
mtext("Ewes:  Treatment", line=0.5, side=3, cex=1.25,
  col=c("darkblue"), font=2)
```

Along with the graphical tools (i.e., functions) found with the R software obtained at first download, there are many similar tools in the thousands of external packages associated with R. Look below how the descr package and specifically the descr::histkdnc() function combines many different graphical tools in one convenient figure (Fig. 5.3).

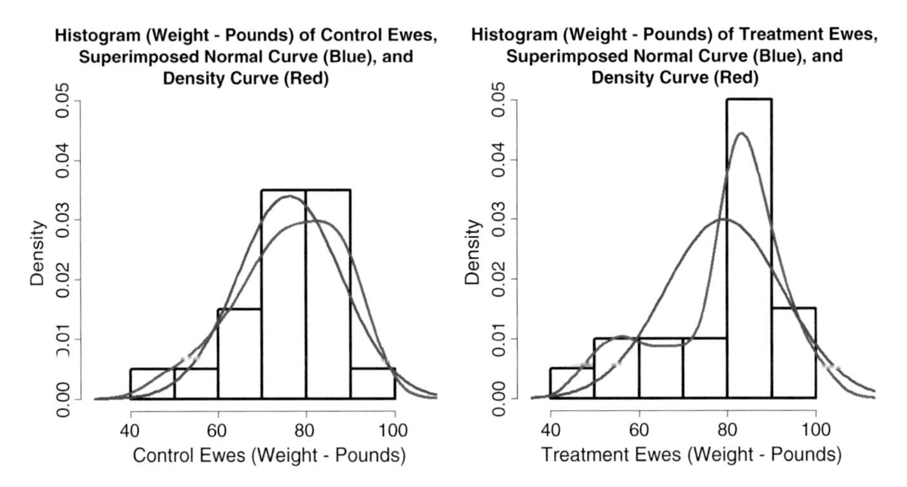

Fig. 5.3 Comparative histograms, normal curves, and density curves of separate object variables using the descr::histkdnc() function placed into one common graphic

```
install.packages("descr")
library(descr)              # Load the descr package.
help(package=descr)         # Show the information page.
sessionInfo()               # Confirm all attached packages.
# Select the most local mirror site using Set CRAN mirror.

save.lwd      <- par(lwd=4)          # Heavy line
save.font     <- par(font=2)         # Bold
save.cexlab   <- par(cex.lab=1.25)   # Label
save.cexaxis  <- par(cex.axis=1.25)  # Axis
par(ask=TRUE)
descr::histkdnc(EweTwin.df$Control,
  main="Histogram (Weight - Pounds) of Control Ewes,
  Superimposed Normal Curve (Blue), and
  Density Curve (Red)",
  xlab="Control Ewes (Weight - Pounds)",
  col=grey(0.95))           # Allow contrast with lines
par(save.lwd); par(save.font); par(save.cexlab);
par(save.cexaxis) # Use ; to move to next line

save.lwd      <- par(lwd=4)          # Heavy line
save.font     <- par(font=2)         # Bold
save.cexlab   <- par(cex.lab=1.25)   # Label
save.cexaxis  <- par(cex.axis=1.25)  # Axis
par(ask=TRUE)
descr::histkdnc(EweTwin.df$Treatment,
  main="Histogram (Weight - Pounds) of Treatment Ewes,
  Superimposed Normal Curve (Blue), and
  Density Curve (Red)",
  xlab="Treatment Ewes (Weight - Pounds)",
  col=grey(0.95))           # Allow contrast with lines
par(save.lwd); par(save.font); par(save.cexlab);
par(save.cexaxis) # Use ; to move to next line

par(ask=TRUE)
par(mfrow=c(1,2))           # 1 row by 2 column format
save.lwd      <- par(lwd=4)          # Heavy line
save.font     <- par(font=2)         # Bold
save.cexlab   <- par(cex.lab=1.25)   # Label
save.cexaxis  <- par(cex.axis=1.25)  # Axis
par(ask=TRUE)
descr::histkdnc(EweTwin.df$Control,
  main="Histogram (Weight - Pounds) of Control Ewes,
  Superimposed Normal Curve (Blue), and
  Density Curve (Red)",
  xlab="Control Ewes (Weight - Pounds)",
 ylim=c(0.0, 0.05),  # Force ylim to have equal scales
  col=grey(0.95))           # Allow contrast with lines
par(save.lwd); par(save.font); par(save.cexlab);
par(save.cexaxis) # Use ; to move to next line
save.lwd      <- par(lwd=4)          # Heavy line
save.font     <- par(font=2)         # Bold
save.cexlab   <- par(cex.lab=1.25)   # Label
```

```
save.cexaxis  <- par(cex.axis=1.25)  # Axis
par(ask=TRUE)
descr::histkdnc(EweTwin.df$Treatment,
  main="Histogram (Weight - Pounds) of Treatment Ewes,
  Superimposed Normal Curve (Blue), and
  Density Curve (Red)",
  xlab="Treatment Ewes (Weight - Pounds)",
 ylim=c(0.0, 0.05),  # Force ylim to have equal scales
  col=grey(0.95))          # Allow contrast with lines
par(save.lwd); par(save.font); par(save.cexlab);
par(save.cexaxis) # Use ; to move to next line
```

As always, remember how R syntax can be used and then reused in multiple ways, in the current session and in future sessions. With a slight change to the syntax, typically the dataframe name, object names, and axis scales, considerable development time can be saved when preparing figures by the simple reuse of existing syntax.

Regarding data distribution for the object variables Control and Treatment, there seems to be some deviation away from normal distribution, especially for the Treatment ewes, but it is cautioned that they key word here is *seems*. From these initial views toward the data it is judged, again, that the use of a nonparametric approach to statistical analysis of the matched pairs seems entirely appropriate.

5.5 Descriptive Analysis of the Data

The dataset for this lesson is fairly small (N = 20 pairs, or 40 subjects) and it is easy to visually scan the data. A casual review confirms that there are no missing data. Even so, it is still best to use R to check for missing data by using the is.na() function and the complete.cases() function against the entire dataset. Both functions return a TRUE or FALSE response, depending on the function and the outcome of whether data are missing or not.

```
is.na(EweTwin.df)             # Check for missing data
complete.cases(EweTwin.df)    # Check for complete cases
```

Before Mode, Median, Mean, Standard Deviation, and any other descriptive statistics are applied against EweTwin.df$Control and EweTwin.df$Treatment, it is important to again recall that a judgment has been made that the data are ordinal, not interval. Equally, there is a concern that the data do not exhibit normal distribution. Given these conditions, the application and interpretation of descriptive statistics should be viewed with some degree of caution. It will be fairly easy to apply the functions against the data, but their meaning may not be quite as easy to understand as would be the case if the data were interval and if the data came from a dataset with normal distribution.

For this simple dataset, the summary() function may be all that is necessary to understand the data and their possible use with statistical tests. Remember that the summary() function, as shown below, is applied against the entire dataset, thus yielding information about all object variables, including the factor-type object variable Pair.

```
summary(EweTwin.df)
```

```
      Pair         Control          Treatment
 P01     : 1   Min.    :49.00   Min.    : 49.0
 P02     : 1   1st Qu.:70.25   1st Qu.: 76.0
 P03     : 1   Median :77.00   Median : 83.0
 P04     : 1   Mean    :76.15   Mean    : 79.2
 P05     : 1   3rd Qu.:85.75   3rd Qu.: 88.0
 P06     : 1   Max.    :92.00   Max.    :100.0
 (Other):14
```

Measures of Central Tendency of the Numeric Object Variables

Although the summary() function is quite sufficient, descriptive statistics for individual object variables may be desired. To achieve this aim, consider the many functions shown below to gain a complete sense of descriptive statistics for the two numeric object variables in this dataset. Although there are no missing data for either EweTwin.df$Control or EweTwin.df$Treatment, if there were it would be necessary to use the na.rm=TRUE argument or some other similar convention to accommodate missing data.

```
length(EweTwin.df$Control)                # N
length(EweTwin.df$Treatment)              # N

install.packages("asbio")
library(asbio)                   # Load the asbio package.
help(package=asbio)              # Show the information page.
sessionInfo()                    # Confirm all attached packages.
# Select the most local mirror site using Set CRAN mirror.

asbio::Mode(EweTwin.df$Control)           # Mode
asbio::Mode(EweTwin.df$Treatment)         # Mode

median(EweTwin.df$Control, na.rm=TRUE)          # Median
median(EweTwin.df$Treatment, na.rm=TRUE)        # Median

mean(EweTwin.df$Control, na.rm=TRUE)            # Mean
sd(EweTwin.df$Control, na.rm=TRUE )             # SD

mean(EweTwin.df$Treatment,na.rm=TRUE )          # Mean
sd(EweTwin.df$Treatment, na.rm=TRUE)            # SD

summary(EweTwin.df)
```

The epicalc::summ() function is also recommended since it can provide descriptive statistics and a representative figure of individual object variables.

```
install.packages("epicalc")
library(epicalc)              # Load the epicalc package.
help(package=epicalc)         # Show the information page.
sessionInfo()                 # Confirm all attached packages.
# Select the most local mirror site using Set CRAN mirror.

par(ask=TRUE) # Use the epicalc package.
epicalc::summ(EweTwin.df$Control,
  by=NULL, graph=TRUE, box=TRUE,  # Generate a boxplot
  pch=18, ylab="auto",
  main="Sorted Dotplot and Boxplot of Control
  (Weight - Pounds)",
  cex.X.axis=1.15, cex.Y.axis=1.15, font.lab=2,
  dot.col="auto")
  # Note the descriptive statistics that go
  # along with the  epicalc::summ() function.

par(ask=TRUE) # Use the epicalc package.
epicalc::summ(EweTwin.df$Treatment,
  by=NULL, graph=TRUE, box=TRUE,  # Generate a boxplot
  pch=18, ylab="auto",
  main="Sorted Dotplot and Boxplot of Treatment
  (Weight - Pounds)",
  cex.X.axis=1.15, cex.Y.axis=1.15, font.lab=2,
  dot.col="auto")
  # Note the descriptive statistics that go
  # along with the epicalc::summ() function.
```

Although the epicalc::summ() function may be sufficient for production of descriptive statistics, there are many other functions that serve the same purpose. A few will be demonstrated, including the prettyR::describe() function, the psych::describe() function, and the lessR::SummaryStats() function. As time permits, explore the many other R functions that serve a similar purpose.

```
install.packages("prettyR")
library(prettyR)              # Load the prettyR package.
help(package=prettyR)         # Show the information page.
sessionInfo()                 # Confirm all attached packages.
# Select the most local mirror site using Set CRAN mirror.

prettyR::describe(EweTwin.df$Control)
prettyR::describe(EweTwin.df$Treatment)

install.packages("psych")
library(psych)                # Load the psych package.
help(package=psych)           # Show the information page.
sessionInfo()                 # Confirm all attached packages.
# Select the most local mirror site using Set CRAN mirror.

psych::describe(EweTwin.df$Control)
psych::describe(EweTwin.df$Treatment)
```

Comment: Notice how the prettyR package and the psych package both have a function called describe: prettyR::describe() and psych::describe(). Because, in part, of this duplicate naming convention, it is always important to use a formal naming scheme when using a function from an external package: package_name::function_name() and not function_name() only.[3]

```
install.packages("lessR")
library(lessR)                # Load the lessR package.
help(package=lessR)           # Show the information page.
sessionInfo()                 # Confirm all attached packages.
# Select the most local mirror site using Set CRAN mirror.

lessR::SummaryStats(Control, brief=TRUE, data=EweTwin.df)
  # The brief argument may or may not be wanted -- experiment
```

```
--- Control ---
      n   miss     mean       sd      min      mdn      max
     20      0    76.15    11.75    49.00    77.00    92.00
```

```
lessR::SummaryStats(Treatment, brief=TRUE, data=EweTwin.df)
  # The brief argument may or may not be wanted -- experiment
```

```
--- Treatment ---
      n   miss     mean       sd      min      mdn      max
     20      0    79.20    13.34    49.00    83.00   100.00

Number of outliers: 1
Small:  49
Large: none
```

The many functions, shown above, all serve the same general purpose in that they provide a broad selection of measures of central tendency and descriptive statistics. However, the output is not necessarily in a formal and attractive format. The tables::tabular() function can be used to provide even more detail, in a fairly attractive table format that can be easily copied or used in some other fashion in a summary report.

```
install.packages("tables")
library(tables)               # Load the tables package.
help(package=tables)          # Show the information page.
sessionInfo()                 # Confirm all attached packages.
# Select the most local mirror site using Set CRAN mirror.

tables::tabular(Control*(length+min+max+median+mean+sd) ~
  1, data=EweTwin.df)
```

[3]The only exception to this recommendation is to avoid the package name for the few packages made available when R is first downloaded: base, datasets, graphics, grDevices, methods, stats, and utils. Thus, it is common to write mean(SBP) and not base::mean(SBP). However, base::mean(SBP) is perfectly acceptable and produces the same result as mean (SBP).

```
                 All
Control length 20.00
        min    49.00
        max    92.00
        median 77.00
        mean   76.15
        sd     11.75
```

```
tables::tabular(Treatment*(length+min+max+median+mean+sd) ~
  1, data=EweTwin.df )
```

```
                    All
Treatment length  20.00
          min     49.00
          max    100.00
          median  83.00
          mean    79.20
          sd      13.34
```

The tables::tabular() function cannot immediately accommodate missing values, which is not an issue for this dataset but should be considered in future analyses. A simple enumeration of a new set of functions for length, min, max, median, mean, and sd will take care of this concern. Again, there are no missing data in this lesson so this demonstration on how to create and use functions that accommodate missing data may not be needed now, but it will be useful for future lessons.

```
LENGTH <- function(x) base::length(x)
MIN    <- function(x) base::min(x, na.rm=TRUE)
MAX    <- function(x) base::max(x, na.rm=TRUE)
MEDIAN <- function(x) stats::median(x, na.rm=TRUE)
MEAN   <- function(x) base::mean(x, na.rm=TRUE)
SD     <- function(x) stats::sd(x, na.rm=TRUE)
```

Comment. Note how the length(), min(), max(), and mean() functions are associated with the base package. In turn, note how median() and sd() functions are associated with the stats package. Both the base package and the stats package are obtained in the initial download of R.[4]

Note also how, because R is case sensitive. The term MEDIAN does not equal median and therefore MEDIAN is a perfectly acceptable name for an enumerated function.

```
tables::tabular(Control*(LENGTH+MIN+MAX+MEDIAN+MEAN+SD) ~
  1, data=EweTwin.df)
```

[4]Going back to the prior comment about package names and functions, in this listing of enumerated functions, the base and stats package names have been purposely used to demonstrate their inclusion among the packages available when R is first downloaded.

```
                 All
Control LENGTH 20.00
        MIN    49.00
        MAX    92.00
        MEDIAN 77.00
        MEAN   76.15
        SD     11.75
```

```
tables::tabular(Treatment*(LENGTH+MIN+MAX+MEDIAN+MEAN+SD) ~
  1, data=EweTwin.df)
```

```
                    All
Treatment LENGTH   20.00
          MIN      49.00
          MAX     100.00
          MEDIAN   83.00
          MEAN     79.20
          SD       13.34
```

Additional functions could be demonstrated, but the above functions should provide a broad representation of how descriptive statistics and measures of central tendency are determined when using R. The immediate concern for the two object variables in question is again easily viewed by using the summary() function:

```
summary(EweTwin.df)
```

With sufficient experience, preferences and individual choice will help determine which functions to use. For now, it is only necessary to determine if there is a statistically significant difference in EweTwin.df$Control, as compared to EweTwin.df$Treatment.

Application of the Anderson-Darling Test

Graphical images and descriptive statistics certainly help with understanding the data. Still, it is also useful to apply selected statistical tests to serve as an additional support for decision-making on acceptance of nonparametric or parametric views toward the data. To that end, consider application of the Anderson-Darling Test, the Lilliefors (KS) Test, and the Shapiro-Wilk Test. It should be mentioned that these tests may be influenced by sample size and that they provide one view, but not the only view, on the nature of distribution patterns. Experience, needs, and practical judgment, supported by careful review of graphical images, descriptive statistics, and statistical tests, should be used when deciding if variables from a dataset are best viewed from a nonparametric or parametric perspective.

```
install.packages("nortest")
library(nortest)              # Load the nortest package.
help(package=nortest)         # Show the information page.
sessionInfo()                 # Confirm all attached packages.
# Select the most local mirror site using Set CRAN mirror.
```

For this lesson, it will be sufficient to apply the Anderson-Darling Test only. The Null Hypothesis for the Anderson-Darling Test is structured to examine if the data follow a specified distribution:

Anderson-Darling Null Hypothesis: The data follow the normal distribution.

There will be two approaches to the Anderson-Darling Test and subsequent examination of p-values for each approach:

- The Anderson-Darling Test will be applied against the values for EweTwin.df$Control.
- The Anderson-Darling Test will be applied against the values for EweTwin.df$Treatment.

```
nortest::ad.test(EweTwin.df$Control)    # Anderson-Darling Test
```

```
        Anderson-Darling normality test

data:  EweTwin.df$Control
A = 0.3008, p-value = 0.5466
```

```
nortest::ad.test(EweTwin.df$Treatment) # Anderson-Darling Test
```

```
        Anderson-Darling normality test

data:  EweTwin.df$Treatment
A = 0.9531, p-value = 0.01273
```

The calculated Anderson-Darling Test for normality p-value exceeds 0.05 for EweTwin.df$Control but is less than 0.05 for EweTwin.df$Treatment:

- The Anderson-Darling Test EweTwin.df$Control p-value is 0.5466.
- The Anderson-Darling Test EweTwin.df$Treatment p-value is 0.01273.

Based on the calculated Anderson-Darling Test p-value for EweTwin.df$Control (0.5466), which certainly exceeds `p <= 0.05`, the data for this object variable follow the normal distribution and the Null Hypothesis is accepted.

However, based on the calculated Anderson-Darling Test p-value for EweTwin.df$Treatment (0.01273), which is less than `p <= 0.05`, the data for this object variable do not follow the normal distribution and the Null Hypothesis is rejected. Thus, the data for object variable EweTwin.df$Treatment do not display normal distribution.

These p-values (especially the p-value for EweTwin.df$Treatment) and the observation that normal distribution is suspect should not be overly surprising given the graphics (especially the density plots) previously displayed. Accordingly, a nonparametric approach (i.e., Wilcoxon Matched-Pairs Signed Ranks Test) will be used for the inferential analysis associated with this lesson.

The QQ plot and associated graphical features will be presented, below, to further reinforce the decision to reject the Null Hypothesis and to instead declare that the full set of data associated with this lesson do not follow the normal distribution, specifically the data associated with EweTwin.df$Treatment.[5]

The qqnorm() function is often used in conjunction with the qqline() function and the qqplot() function. The Quantile-Quantile (Q-Q) functions take some time to understand, but they serve as excellent graphical tools to understand data distribution and it is worth the effort to learn more about these tools. The Q-Q plot is especially useful as a scatter plot.[6] For all applications of the Q-Q functions, the purpose is to determine if the data in a numerical object variable come from a known population. Review the many ways the Q-Q plot is used, below, and give special attention to how the ends (i.e., tails) of the theoretical distributions show (Fig. 5.4).

```
par(ask=TRUE)
qqnorm(EweTwin.df$Control, main="QQ Ewes:  Control",
  ylim=c(40,115), font=2, cex.lab=1.15,  cex.axis=1.25,
  lwd=8, col="red")
qqline(EweTwin.df$Control, lwd=6, col=c("darkblue"))

par(ask=TRUE)
qqnorm(EweTwin.df$Treatment, main="QQ Ewes:  Treatment",
  ylim=c(40,115), font=2, cex.lab=1.15,  cex.axis=1.25,
  lwd=8, col="red")
qqline(EweTwin.df$Control, lwd=6, col=c("darkblue"))

par(ask=TRUE)
par(mfrow=c(1,2))              # 1 row by 2 column format
qqnorm(EweTwin.df$Control, main="QQ Ewes:  Control",
  ylim=c(40,115), font=2, cex.lab=1.15,  cex.axis=1.25,
  lwd=8, col="red")
qqline(EweTwin.df$Control, lwd=6, col=c("darkblue"))
qqnorm(EweTwin.df$Treatment, main="QQ Ewes:  Treatment",
  ylim=c(40,115), font=2, cex.lab=1.15,  cex.axis=1.25,
  lwd=8, col="red")
qqline(EweTwin.df$Control, lwd=6, col=c("darkblue"))
```

Similar to the other graphical presentations, the distributions for EweTwin.df $Control and EweTwin.df$Treatment seem to be different and EweTwin.df $Treatment seems to negate the assumption of normal distribution. The graphical presentations continue to build a case and then reinforce the decision that it may be best to use nonparametric approaches to statistical analysis for the data in this lesson. As an interesting and final view of the data, go beyond the qqnorm() and qqline() functions and consider distribution of the variables (EweTwin.df$Control and EweTwin.df$Treatment) using the qqplot() function.

[5]Recall the prior comment that QQ and Q-Q are both used as a proxy for the term Quantile-Quantile.

[6]Similar to many other compound words, it is common to see the term(s) *scatter plot* and *scatterplot*.

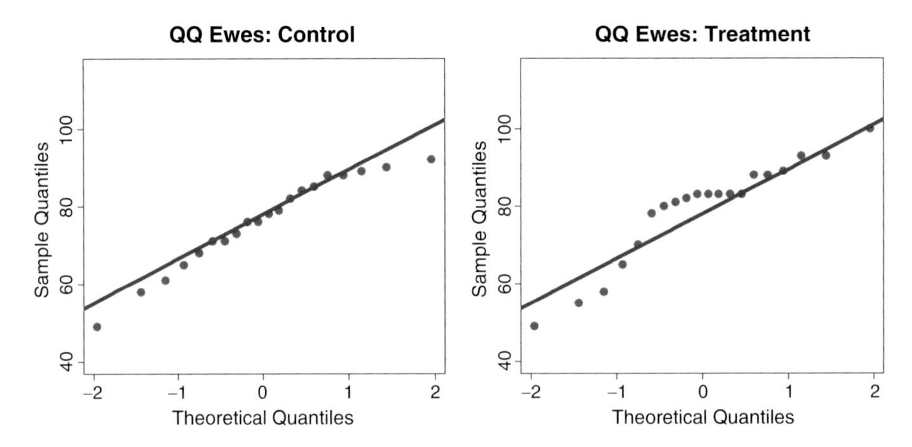

Fig. 5.4 Comparative QQ plots with QQ lines

```
par(ask=TRUE)
qqplot(EweTwin.df$Control, EweTwin.df$Treatment,
  main="QQ Plot of Ewes:  Control v Treatment",
  xlab="Control", ylab="Treatment",
  font=2, cex.lab=1.15,  cex.axis=1.25, lwd=8, col="red")
abline(0,1, lwd=8, col=c("darkblue"))
  # Include a 45-degree reference line
```

Again, there seems to be some degree of concern about data distribution and whether the data follow any reasonable semblance of normal distribution.

5.6 Conduct the Statistical Analysis

The dataset for this part of the lesson was prepared in unstacked format. A brief demonstration of the same data, but presented as a dataset in stacked format, follows later in an addendum to this lesson. Review the help pages for the stack() function and the unstack() function to learn more about this issue.

A fair amount of attention in this lesson has been given to visual presentations of data distribution and descriptive statistics. These two topics help with an understanding of the data and how the data are organized, individually and in league with other variables in the dataset. Yet, the primary emphasis for this lesson involves the Wilcoxon Matched-Pairs Signed Ranks Test and the Null Hypothesis associated with this lesson:

Null Hypothesis (Ho) There is no statistically significant difference (`p <= 0.05`) in weight between ewes that experienced regular field conditions during a treatment period (i.e., the control group) and their gender-equivalent twin counterparts that not only experienced regular conditions but also received an otherwise unidentified supplement during the same treatment period (i.e., the treatment group).

The wilcox.test() function is the primary function used to complete the comparison of the two groups associated with this lesson, ewe weight among members of the control group and ewe weight among twin counterpart members of the treatment group. This lesson does not go into explicit detail on the algorithm for the Wilcoxon Matched-Pairs Signed Ranks Test but is instead focused on the use of R to achieve this analysis. As time permits, read on the Wilcoxon Matched-Pairs Signed Ranks Test and how this test is used to compare medians for two groups (i.e., Control v Treatment). The comparison of medians for two groups (i.e., matched pairs) using the Wilcoxon Matched-Pairs Signed Ranks Test is opposed to the comparison of means for two groups, which is inherent to the Student's t-Test.

As the algorithm for the Wilcoxon Matched-Pairs Signed Ranks Test is reviewed, read also about the way tie scores are accommodated. In the EweTwin.df dataframe, notice how the weight for Pair 17 is tied, Control Weight (pounds) = 88 and Treatment Weight (pounds) = 88. Special accommodations are needed for tied measures. Fortunately, most statistical analysis programs such as R and the leading proprietary programs can accommodate tied scores with matched-pairs.

Clearly, this area is complex and the heuristics of the nonparametric algorithm for matched-pairs is beyond the purpose of this lesson. Instead, this lesson is grounded on the use of R for calculation of the appropriate statistics for the Wilcoxon Matched-Pairs Signed Ranks Test. Saying that, notice immediately below how the wilcox.test() function and related arguments are applied against the EweTwin.df dataframe.

```
wilcox.test(EweTwin.df$Control, EweTwin.df$Treatment,
  alternative=c("two.sided"), paired=TRUE, exact=TRUE,
  correct=TRUE, conf.int=TRUE, conf.level=0.95)
  # Notice how there was no grouping factor.  Instead,
  # Control as a set of numeric weight-type values was
  # compared directly against Treatment which is
  # another set of numeric weight-type values.
```

```
        Wilcoxon signed rank test with continuity correction

data:  EweTwin.df$Control and EweTwin.df$Treatment
V = 79, p-value = 0.5324
alternative hypothesis: true location shift is not equal to 0
95 percent confidence interval:
 -10.999986   4.499993
sample estimates:
(pseudo)median
     -2.500047
```

The important outcome here is that the calculated p-value (`p <= 0.5324`) certainly exceeds the criterion p-value associated with the Null Hypothesis (`p <= 0.05`). There is no statistically significant difference in weight (pounds) between ewes in the Control group and ewes in the Treatment group.

Notice how a comma and not a tilde was used to separate the unstacked object variables EweTwin.df$Control and EweTwin.df$Treatment. There is no grouping variable with unstacked data as there is with stacked data since the two sets of unstacked data represent their own groups. By purposeful design, look at the error message, below, which was generated by R when a ~ (i.e., tilde) instead of a , (i.e., comma) was used with unstacked data.

```
# Purposeful introduction of an error, by using ~ instead of ,
wilcox.test(EweTwin.df$Control ~ EweTwin.df$Treatment,
  alternative=c("two.sided"), paired=TRUE, exact=TRUE,
  correct=TRUE, conf.int=TRUE, conf.level=0.95)
```

```
Error in wilcox.test:  grouping factor must have exactly 2 levels
```

Use the wilcox.test help page to see the many ways this function can be organized. As with all other R functions, first learn the basics and work with default settings and simple confidence-building actions. Then use the R-based help pages and other learning resource materials to develop analyses that are in line with specific needs.

5.7 Summary

The graphics and statistics are helpful and provided a great deal of information (and context) about this lesson on weight differences between the two groups of ewes, those ewes that experienced regular field conditions (i.e., Control) vs those ewes that received some type of supplement (i.e., Treatment) in addition to their exposure to regular field conditions. As useful as this upfront information may be, the purpose of this lesson was to focus on how the Wilcoxon Matched-Pairs Signed Ranks Test can be used to compare differences in the median weight for these two groups of ewes.

As a reminder, the nonparametric Wilcoxon Matched-Pairs Signed Ranks Test was selected for comparison of the two groups instead of Student's t-Test for Matched-Pairs. This selection is justified because:

- Anecdotal information gained during field work raised the concern that the data were ordinal and not interval. Recall how there was an issue about calibration and consistency in measurement.
- There was also compelling graphical evidence that the distribution of data for the two groups did not approximate normal distribution.
- The Anderson-Darling Test equally provided evidence that the data for at least one object variable (EweTwin.df$Treatment) did not follow normal distribution.

Given these three immediate observations, the focus in this lesson has been on comparison of medians, which is shown, in part, below:

```
                   Control    Treatment
Ewes    length     20          20
        min        49.00       49.00
        max        92.00      100.00
        median     77.00       83.00
        mean       76.15       79.20
        sd         11.75       13.34
```

If it is assumed that the data were organized correctly and that the Wilcoxon Matched-Pairs Signed Ranks Test was applied correctly, then there is evidence to support the statement that there is no difference in weights between Control ewes and Treatment ewes since the calculated p-value of 0.5324 exceeded the criterion p-value 0.05 associated with the Null Hypothesis. Again, attention to the p-value is perhaps the easiest way to view differences for this lesson:

- The calculated p-value is 0.5324.
- The criterion (i.e., declared) p-value, from the previously stated Null Hypothesis is 0.05.
- The calculated p-value is greater than the declared p-value.

Therefore, the Null Hypothesis is accepted (or, some may say the Null Hypothesis was not rejected) and it can be claimed that there is no difference (`p <= .05`) between Control ewes and Treatment ewes. That is to say, at the end of the treatment period in this posttest-only study, there was no statistically significant difference (`p <= 0.05`) in the weight of Control ewes and the weight of Treatment ewes. Any observed difference in weights is due to chance and it does not represent a true difference. Regarding weights, the two groups of ewes are from the same population.

R served as a more than useful tool to produce graphical images, to generate descriptive statistics and measures of central tendency, and to apply an appropriate inferential test against the dataset. It is also helpful to use fairly simple ways to view data—especially for a small dataset of only 40 subjects placed into 20 matched pairs. With this challenge, look at the way outcomes are viewed below, after hand-calculation:

```
                     Pair Control Treatment  Control v Treatment
===============================================================
Ewe Twin Pair 1   P01       90          83  Control > Treatment P01
Ewe Twin Pair 2   P02       84          89  Control < Treatment P02
Ewe Twin Pair 3   P03       78          58  Control > Treatment P03
Ewe Twin Pair 4   P04       79          93  Control < Treatment P04
Ewe Twin Pair 5   P05       65          49  Control > Treatment P05
Ewe Twin Pair 6   P06       49          82  Control < Treatment P06
Ewe Twin Pair 7   P07       92          93  Control < Treatment P07
Ewe Twin Pair 8   P08       71         100  Control < Treatment P08
Ewe Twin Pair 9   P09       85          83  Control > Treatment P09
Ewe Twin Pair 10  P10       76          55  Control > Treatment P10
```

```
Ewe Twin Pair 11 P11      68        65  Control > Treatment P11
Ewe Twin Pair 12 P12      71        83  Control < Treatment P12
Ewe Twin Pair 13 P13      88        81  Control > Treatment P13
Ewe Twin Pair 14 P14      89        88  Control > Treatment P14
Ewe Twin Pair 15 P15      76        83  Control < Treatment P15
Ewe Twin Pair 16 P16      61        78  Control < Treatment P16
Ewe Twin Pair 17 P17      88        88  Control = Treatment P17
Ewe Twin Pair 18 P18      58        80  Control < Treatment P18
Ewe Twin Pair 19 P19      73        70  Control > Treatment P19
Ewe Twin Pair 20 P20      82        83  Control < Treatment P20
===============================================================
```

If descriptive statistics, only, were used to compare the two groups it would be easy to assume (falsely) that Treatment ewes were from a different population than Control ewes since the overall median and mean for Treatment ewes is greater than the overall median and mean for Control ewes:

```
                  Control    Treatment
 Ewes    length   20          20
         min      49.00       49.00
         max      92.00      100.00
         median   77.00       83.00
         mean     76.15       79.20
         sd       11.75       13.34
```

Instead, look at the data from a different perspective, recalling that the data are ordinal and the key term here is that ordinal data are ordered:

- Is the Control weight < Treatment weight?
- Is the Control weight > Treatment weight?
- Is the Control weight = Treatment weight (tied)?

With this approach toward the main concern, the summary is fairly easy to determine by hand given how this dataset is small:

- Control < Treatment for 10 pair(s) (Pair 02, 04, 06, 07, 08, 12, 15, 16, 18, 20).
- Control > Treatment for 09 pair(s) (Pair 01, 03, 05, 09, 10, 11, 13, 14, 19).
- Control = Treatment for 01 pair(s) (Pair 17).

From this perspective, it is easier to see justification for acceptance of the Null Hypothesis and the finding that there is no difference in post-treatment weights between Control ewes and Treatment ewes. At the level of individual pairs, Treatment weight was greater than Control weight for only ten of 20 ewe pairs. Conversely, Treatment weight was less than or equal to Control weight for the other ten ewe pairs.

Looking at other issues impacting this lesson, although there is no intention to go into additional details about the strength or weakness of a posttest-only research design, it should also be remembered that there is no knowledge whether breed, environmental conditions, palatability of feedstock, etc., has any possible influence of outcomes. Data were not provided for these factors.

5.8 Addendum 1: Stacked Data and the Wilcoxon Matched-Pairs Signed-Ranks Test

The data in EweTwin.df are in unstacked format, with one column of data reserved for data associated with Control ewes and another column of data reserved for data associated with Treatment ewes. However, go back to the prior statement that researchers should have the skills needed to work with data in multiple formats.

Create a dataframe-type object called EweTwin_Stacked.df directly into the R session. This object will represent the output of wrapping the read.table() function around the textConnection() function and the data that immediately follow. The data are in an easy-to-read fixed-column format. Be sure to note the header=TRUE argument, indicating that the first line is actually a header with descriptive variable names.

```
EweTwin_Stacked.df <- read.table(textConnection("
 SSubject SPair          Group        Weight
 P01C     StackedPair01  Control       90
 P02C     StackedPair02  Control       84
 P03C     StackedPair03  Control       78
 P04C     StackedPair04  Control       79
 P05C     StackedPair05  Control       65
 P06C     StackedPair06  Control       49
 P07C     StackedPair07  Control       92
 P08C     StackedPair08  Control       71
 P09C     StackedPair09  Control       85
 P10C     StackedPair10  Control       76
 P11C     StackedPair11  Control       68
 P12C     StackedPair12  Control       71
 P13C     StackedPair13  Control       88
 P14C     StackedPair14  Control       89
 P15C     StackedPair15  Control       76
 P16C     StackedPair16  Control       61
 P17C     StackedPair17  Control       88
 P18C     StackedPair18  Control       58
 P19C     StackedPair19  Control       73
 P20C     StackedPair20  Control       82
 P01T     StackedPair01  Treatment     83
 P02T     StackedPair02  Treatment     89
 P03T     StackedPair03  Treatment     58
 P04T     StackedPair04  Treatment     93
 P05T     StackedPair05  Treatment     49
 P06T     StackedPair06  Treatment     82
 P07T     StackedPair07  Treatment     93
 P08T     StackedPair08  Treatment    100
 P09T     StackedPair09  Treatment     83
 P10T     StackedPair10  Treatment     55
 P11T     StackedPair11  Treatment     65
 P12T     StackedPair12  Treatment     83
 P13T     StackedPair13  Treatment     81
 P14T     StackedPair14  Treatment     88
 P15T     StackedPair15  Treatment     83
```

```
  P16T     StackedPair16  Treatment     78
  P17T     StackedPair17  Treatment     88
  P18T     StackedPair18  Treatment     80
  P19T     StackedPair19  Treatment     70
  P20T     StackedPair20  Treatment     83    "), header=TRUE)

getwd()                        # Identify the working directory
ls()                           # List objects
attach(EweTwin_Stacked.df)     # Attach the data, for later use
str(EweTwin_Stacked.df)        # Identify structure
nrow(EweTwin_Stacked.df)       # List the number of rows
ncol(EweTwin_Stacked.df)       # List the number of columns
dim(EweTwin_Stacked.df)        # Dimensions of the dataframe
names(EweTwin_Stacked.df)      # Identify names
colnames(EweTwin_Stacked.df) # Show column names
rownames(EweTwin_Stacked.df) # Show row names
head(EweTwin_Stacked.df)       # Show the head
tail(EweTwin_Stacked.df)       # Show the tail
EweTwin_Stacked.df             # Show the entire dataframe
summary(EweTwin_Stacked.df)    # Summary statistics

class(EweTwin_Stacked.df)
class(EweTwin_Stacked.df$SSubject)
class(EweTwin_Stacked.df$SPair)
class(EweTwin_Stacked.df$Group)
class(EweTwin_Stacked.df$Weight)
  # DataFrame$ObjectName notation

str(EweTwin_Stacked.df)                     # Structure

duplicated(EweTwin_Stacked.df$SSubject)     # Duplicates
```

With the dataframe completed, it is only necessary to prepare the Code Book on ewe weights, presented in this addendum in stacked format.

The Code Book below represents how data are desired before analyses begin. Recoding may be needed to put data into new formats.

```
#######################################################
# Code Book for EweTwin_Stacked.df                    #
#######################################################
#                                                     #
# SSubject (Stacked Subject).. Factor (i.e., nominal) #
#              A unique ID ranging from P01C to P20T #
#                     where the C represents Control #
#                         and T represents Treatment #
#                                                     #
# SPair (Stacked Pair) ....... Factor (i.e., nominal) #
#             A unique ID ranging from StackedPair01 #
#                                   to StackedPair20 #
#                                                     #
```

```
# Group ..................... Factor (i.e., nominal) #
#         Breakout identifiers, Control and Treatment #
#                                                      #
# Weight .................. Numeric (i.e., interval) #
#          Weight (lbs) of a female sheep (e.g., ewe) #
#                                      at end-of-program #
#          Data may also be viewed as ordinal due to  #
#                                    measurement issues #
########################################################
```

With a better understanding of desired data formats and assurance that the dataframe is currently in correct format, coerce each object variable into desired format, as a factor object variable, numeric object variable, etc. Each object will be coerced into desired class, even if the action is redundant, just to be sure that all objects are in desired format. In this example, note especially how EweTwin_Stacked.df$Weight was coerced from integer class to numeric class.

```
class(EweTwin_Stacked.df)    # Confirm nature of the dataset
str(EweTwin_Stacked.df)      # Confirm nature of the dataset

EweTwin_Stacked.df$SSubject <- as.factor(
  EweTwin_Stacked.df$SSubject)
EweTwin_Stacked.df$SPair    <- as.factor(
  EweTwin_Stacked.df$SPair)
EweTwin_Stacked.df$Group    <- as.factor(
  EweTwin_Stacked.df$Group)
EweTwin_Stacked.df$Weight   <- as.numeric(
  EweTwin_Stacked.df$Weight)

class(EweTwin_Stacked.df)
class(EweTwin_Stacked.df$SSubject)
class(EweTwin_Stacked.df$SPair)
class(EweTwin_Stacked.df$Group)
class(EweTwin_Stacked.df$Weight)
  # DataFrame$ObjectName notation

str(EweTwin_Stacked.df)                      # Structure

summary(EweTwin_Stacked.df)
```

Confirm that the data in EweTwin_Stacked.df match the data in EweTwin.df by comparing descriptive statistics for each.

Descriptive statistics of ewe weights from EweTwin.df (the dataframe of unstacked data), by Control and by Treatment, follow:

```
summary(EweTwin.df$Control, na.rm=TRUE)
```

```
   Min. 1st Qu.  Median    Mean 3rd Qu.    Max.
  49.00   70.25   77.00   76.15   85.75   92.00
```

```
summary(EweTwin.df$Treatment, na.rm=TRUE)
```

```
   Min. 1st Qu.  Median    Mean 3rd Qu.    Max.
   49.0    76.0    83.0    79.2    88.0   100.0
```

Descriptive statistics of ewe weights from EweTwin_Stacked.df (the dataframe of stacked data), by Weight and by Group, follow:

```
tapply(Weight, Group, summary, na.rm=TRUE,
  data=EweTwin_Stacked.df) # Weight by Group using tapply()
```

```
$Control
   Min. 1st Qu.  Median    Mean 3rd Qu.    Max.
  49.00   70.25   77.00   76.15   85.75   92.00

$Treatment
   Min. 1st Qu.  Median    Mean 3rd Qu.    Max.
   49.0    76.0    83.0    79.2    88.0   100.0
```

The data are now included in this active R session in two separate datasets, with each dataset organized as a dataframe:

```
str(EweTwin.df)                # Unstacked dataframe
EweTwin.df

str(EweTwin_Stacked.df)        # Stacked dataframe
EweTwin_Stacked.df
```

Perform the Wilcoxon Matched-Pairs Signed-Ranks Test on EweTwin.df using the comma as a separator (e.g., Measured_Object_Group1, Measured_Object_Group2). Then perform the Wilcoxon Matched-Pairs Signed Ranks-Test on EweTwin_Stacked.df using the tilde as a separator (e.g., Measured_Object ~ Grouping_Object). Observe similarities and differences, if any, in output and give special attention to the calculated p-value.

wilcox.test() Function with Unstacked Data, Comma Separator

```
wilcox.test(EweTwin.df$Control,
  EweTwin.df$Treatment,
  alternative=c("two.sided"), paired=TRUE, exact=TRUE,
  correct=TRUE, conf.int=TRUE, conf.level=0.95)
```

```
        Wilcoxon signed rank test with continuity correction

data:  EweTwin.df$Control and EweTwin.df$Treatment
V = 79, p-value = 0.5324
alternative hypothesis: true location shift is not equal to 0
95 percent confidence interval:
```

```
 -10.999986   4.499993
sample estimates:
(pseudo)median
     -2.500047
```

Outcome: The calculated p-value is 0.5324, and this value exceeds the criterion p-value associated with the Null Hypothesis (`p <= 0.05`). Therefore there is no statistically significant difference in weight (pounds) between Control ewes and Treatment ewes.

wilcox.test() Function With Stacked Data, Tilde Separator

```
wilcox.test(EweTwin_Stacked.df$Weight ~
  EweTwin_Stacked.df$Group,
  alternative=c("two.sided"), paired=TRUE, exact=TRUE,
  correct=TRUE, conf.int=TRUE, conf.level=0.95)
```

```
        Wilcoxon signed rank test with continuity correction

data:  EweTwin_Stacked.df$Weight by EweTwin_Stacked.df$Group
V = 79, p-value = 0.5324
alternative hypothesis: true location shift is not equal to 0
95 percent confidence interval:
 -10.999986   4.499993
sample estimates:
(pseudo)median
     -2.500047
```

Outcome: The calculated p-value is 0.5324, and this value exceeds the criterion p-value associated with the Null Hypothesis (`p <= 0.05`). Therefore there is no statistically significant difference in weight (pounds) between Control ewes and Treatment ewes.

As demonstrated in this addendum, the results of the inferential test (i.e., Wilcoxon Matched-Pairs Signed-Ranks Test, using the wilcox.test() function) are equivalent for when the data are organized in an unstacked format and later for when the data are organized in a stacked format. As will be seen in a later addendum, there may be slight differences in calculated p-values for when different functions are used, all due to variance in how algorithms are employed, rounding, and presentation.

5.9 Addendum 2: Similar Functions from Different Packages

The wilcox.test() function is associated with the stats package, which is obtained when R is first downloaded. However, there are thousands of external packages available to the R community and in these many packages are what may seem to be countless numbers of functions. It is therefore not overly surprising that a few of these functions would address the Wilcoxon Matched-Pairs Signed-Ranks Test. Below is a repeat of the wilcox.test() function and, similarly, demonstrations of how the Wilcoxon Matched-Pairs Signed Ranks Test is approached when functions in other packages are used:

- stats::wilcox.test() function[7]
- afex::compare.2.vectors() function
- coin::wilcox_test() function
- exactRankTests::wilcox.exact() function

As these different functions (all related to the Wilcoxon Matched-Pairs Signed-Ranks Test) are attempted, notice some degree of variation in calculated p-values:

- Either the calculated p-value for Control v Treatment is approximately 0.5.
- Or, the calculated p-value for control v Treatment is approximately 0.3.

The reasons for this variation in calculated p-values for the different R-based functions is largely due to the way each function accommodates tied values. For teaching purposes, this lesson was purposely based on a dataset where there was one tied value. In this lesson, notice how there are tied values for Ewe Twin Pair 17: Control Weight is 88 pounds and Treatment Weight is 88. Tied values can be a bit problematic when the mechanical part of matched-pairs analyses are attempted. For those with a special interest in the way tied values and their impact on algorithm design are accommodated with the Wilcoxon Matched-Pairs Signed-Ranks Test, conduct an Internet search on the term *nonparametric tests and fuzzy p-values* and similar descriptive phrases dealing with tied pairs and nonparametric tests.

The important outcome here is that the calculated p-value (approximately 0.3–0.5) certainly exceeds the p-value associated with the Null Hypothesis (`p <= 0.05`). As demonstrated immediately below, there is no statistically significant difference in weight (pounds) between ewes in the Control group and ewes in the Treatment group. This finding is consistent for all functions used to address the Wilcoxon Matched-Pairs Signed-Ranks Test. The impact of ties on matched-pairs ranked data should not be underestimated.

stats::wilcox.test() Function with Unstacked Data

```
stats::wilcox.test(EweTwin.df$Control,
  EweTwin.df$Treatment,
  alternative=c("two.sided"), paired=TRUE, exact=TRUE,
  correct=TRUE, conf.int=TRUE, conf.level=0.95)
```

```
p-value = 0.5324
```

[7]By convention, it is not necessary to write stats::functionname() or base::functionname() since the stats package and base package are part of the full set of packages associated with R when it is first downloaded. The formal term stats::wilcox.test is used merely to reinforce the origin (i.e., package) for this function.

stats::wilcox.test() Function with Stacked Data

```
stats::wilcox.test(EweTwin_Stacked.df$Weight ~
  EweTwin_Stacked.df$Group,
  alternative=c("two.sided"), paired=TRUE, exact=TRUE,
  correct=TRUE, conf.int=TRUE, conf.level=0.95)
```

```
p-value = 0.5324
```

afex::compare.2.vectors() Function with Unstacked Data—Two Vectors

```
install.packages("afex")
library(afex)                  # Load the afex package.
help(package=afex)             # Show the information page.
sessionInfo()                  # Confirm all attached packages.
# Select the most local mirror site using Set CRAN mirror.

afex::compare.2.vectors(EweTwin.df$Control,
  EweTwin.df$Treatment,
  paired=TRUE,                 # Data are paired
  na.rm=TRUE,                  # Accommodate missing values
  tests=c("parametric", "nonparametric"),
  coin=TRUE,                   # Multiple test results
  alternative="two.sided",     # Two-sided test
  wilcox.exact=TRUE,           # Exact p-value reported
  wilcox.correct=TRUE)         # Continuity correction
  # Both parametric and nonparametric
```

```
$parametric
  test test.statistic test.value test.df         p
1    t              t -0.9228219      19 0.3676712

$nonparametric
            test test.statistic test.value test.df         p
1 stats::Wilcoxon              V 79.0000000      NA 0.5324156
2     permutation              Z -0.9262647      NA 0.3776800
3  coin::Wilcoxon              Z -1.2247449      NA 0.2353100
4          median              Z  1.6329932      NA 0.2196200

Warning messages:
1: In wilcox.test.default(x, y, paired = paired, exact =
wilcox.exact,  : cannot compute exact p-value with ties
2: In wilcox.test.default(x, y, paired = paired, exact =
wilcox.exact,  :cannot compute exact p-value with zeroes
```

Be sure to see how the afex::compare.2.vectors() function, when using the tests=c("parametric", "nonparametric") argument, supports both a parametric (Student's t-Test) and nonparametric (Wilcoxon) view for analyses.

Tie scores are often problematic with nonparametric statistics. Notice the warning message and go back to how tied scores (i.e., Pair 17 in this lesson on ewes) are accommodated by the various algorithms used to calculate the Wilcoxon Matched-Pairs Signed-Ranks Test.

coin::wilcox_test() Function

When using the coin::wilcox_test() function, note the many options for the distribution argument and the ties.method argument. Each argument selection will alter to some degree the calculated p-value so experimentation and good judgment, along with experience, will help with the best selection for specific needs.

```
install.packages("coin")
library(coin)                  # Load the coin package.
help(package=coin)             # Show the information page.
sessionInfo()                  # Confirm all attached packages.
# Select the most local mirror site using Set CRAN mirror.

coin::wilcox_test(Weight ~ Group,
  data=EweTwin_Stacked.df,
  distribution="approximate",      # Note distribution argument.
  ties.method="mid-ranks",         # Note ties.method argument.
  conf.int=TRUE,
  conf.level=0.95,)
```

```
        Approximative Wilcoxon Mann-Whitney Rank Sum Test

data:  Weight by Group (Control, Treatment)
Z = -0.8943, p-value = 0.353
alternative hypothesis: true mu is not equal to 0
95 percent confidence interval:
 -12   5
sample estimates:
difference in location
                 -4
```

Outcome: p-value = 0.353

```
coin::wilcox_test(Weight ~ Group,
  data=EweTwin_Stacked.df,
  distribution="asymptotic",       # Note distribution argument.
  ties.method="mid-ranks",         # Note ties.method argument.
  conf.int=TRUE,
  conf.level=0.95,)
```

Outcome: p-value = 0.3712

```
coin::wilcox_test(Weight ~ Group,
  data=EweTwin_Stacked.df,
  distribution="exact",            # Note distribution argument.
  ties.method="mid-ranks",         # Note ties.method argument.
  conf.int=TRUE,
  conf.level=0.95,)
```

Outcome: p-value = 0.3789

```
coin::wilcox_test(Weight ~ Group,
  data=EweTwin_Stacked.df,
  distribution="approximate",      # Note distribution argument.
  ties.method="average-scores",    # Note ties.method argument.
  conf.int=TRUE,
  conf.level=0.95, )
```

Outcome: p-value = 0.376

```
coin::wilcox_test(Weight ~ Group,
  data=EweTwin_Stacked.df,
  distribution="asymptotic",       # Note distribution argument.
  ties.method="average-scores",    # Note ties.method argument.
  conf.int=TRUE,
  conf.level=0.95,)
```

Outcome: p-value = 0.3712

```
coin::wilcox_test(Weight ~ Group,
  data=EweTwin_Stacked.df,
  distribution="exact",            # Note distribution argument.
  ties.method="average-scores",    # Note ties.method argument.
  conf.int=TRUE,
  conf.level=0.95,)
```

Outcome: p-value = 0.3789

Although the p-value is slightly different each time, all depending on selected arguments, in each case the outcome is consistent in terms of how the calculated p-value validates acceptance or rejection of the Null Hypothesis.

exactRankTests::wilcox.exact() Function with Stacked Data

```
install.packages("exactRankTests")
library(exactRankTests)       # Load the exactRankTests package.
help(package=exactRankTests)  # Show the information page.
sessionInfo()                 # Confirm all attached packages.
# Select the most local mirror site using Set CRAN mirror.

exactRankTests::wilcox.exact(Weight ~ Group,
  data=EweTwin_Stacked.df,
  alternative=c("two.sided"),
  paired=TRUE,
  exact=TRUE,
  conf.int=TRUE,
  conf.level=0.95)
```

```
        Exact Wilcoxon signed rank test

data:  Weight by Group
V = 79, p-value = 0.5343
alternative hypothesis: true mu is not equal to 0
95 percent confidence interval:
 -11.0   4.5
sample estimates:
(pseudo)median
         -2.75
```

Compare the calculated p-value when using the exactRankTests::wilcox.exact() function (0.5343) to the calculated p-value when using the stats::wilcox.test() function (0.5324). Then, compare these p-values to the calculated p-value when using another function, such as the coin::wilcox_test() function (0.3712, depending on selected arguments). Or, consider the multiple p-values generated by use of the afex::compare.2.vectors() function. Each function provides a slightly different p-value, depending on how ties are accommodated and the use of selected arguments, but the net outcome is the same in this lesson in terms of acceptance or rejection of the Null Hypothesis. The calculated p-value for all selected functions supports acceptance of the Null Hypothesis and the conclusion that there is no difference in weights (pounds) between Control ewes and Treatment ewes.

5.10 Addendum 3: Nonparametric vs Parametric Confirmation of Outcomes

Based on anecdotal comments by those who weighed the sheep associated with this lesson, and the challenges of obtaining precise measurements during field conditions, it has been declared that the data are ordinal and that they are not interval. There is also a degree of suspicion, based on visual presentations of weights for Control ewes and Treatment ewes, that the data seriously violate normal distribution—at least for Treatment ewes. Concern about distribution patterns were also evident when applying the Anderson-Darling Test. Given these three issues, it was judged that a nonparametric inferential test was the most appropriate approach to determine if there were a statistically significant difference between weights of the two groups, Control v Treatment.

However, what if the weighing process had been better organized in terms of obtaining more precise measures? What if there were greater assurance that data were interval? What if there were no concerns about violation of normal distribution? If these conditions were somehow of no direct concern, then would it be appropriate to use Student's t-Test for Matched Pairs for the selected inferential test? Look at the two analyses presented immediately below and give special notice to the calculated p-value for each.

Student's t-Test for Matched Pairs, Against Unstacked Data

```
# Default selections.
t.test(EweTwin.df$Control,                # Measured variable
  EweTwin.df$Treatment,                   # Measured variable
  paired=TRUE,                            # Matched pairs
  na.rm=TRUE)                             # Missing data
```

```
        Paired t-test

data:  EweTwin.df$Control and EweTwin.df$Treatment
t = -0.9228, df = 19, p-value = 0.3677
alternative hypothesis: true difference in means is not equal
to 0
95 percent confidence interval:
 -9.967612  3.867612
sample estimates:
mean of the differences
                 -3.05
```

Student's t-Test for Matched Pairs, Against Stacked Data

```
# Default selections.
t.test(EweTwin_Stacked.df$Weight ~        # Measured variable
  EweTwin_Stacked.df$Group,               # Grouping variable
  paired=TRUE,                            # Matched pairs
  na.rm=TRUE)                             # Missing data
```

```
        Paired t-test

data:  EweTwin_Stacked.df$Weight by EweTwin_Stacked.df$Group
t = -0.9228, df = 19, p-value = 0.3677
alternative hypothesis: true difference in means is not equal
to 0
95 percent confidence interval:
 -9.967612  3.867612
sample estimates:
mean of the differences
                 -3.05
```

For both analyses, against unstacked data and stacked data, the calculated p-value was 0.3677, which is in parity with the prior p-value when the data were subjected to the Wilcoxon Matched-Pairs Signed-Ranks Test in terms of acceptance or rejection the Null Hypothesis.

As a caution, confirm this comparison of two sets of matched weights by using the previously demonstrated afex::compare.2.vectors() function, but now change the tests argument to parametric only.

```
afex::compare.2.vectors(EweTwin.df$Control,
  EweTwin.df$Treatment,
  paired=TRUE,                # Data are paired
  na.rm=TRUE,                 # Accommodate missing values
  tests=c("parametric"),      # Student's t-Test, only
  alternative="two.sided")    # Two-sided test
```

```
$parametric
  test test.statistic test.value test.df         p
1    t              t -0.9228219      19 0.3676712
```

For the way the afex::compare.2.vectors() function accommodates tied values (i.e., Pair 17), and when using a parametric perspective to the data, the calculated p-value is 0.3676712, which exceeds the criterion p-value associated with the Null Hypothesis, `p <= 0.05`. Viewing the data from a parametric perspective and using Student's t-Test for Matched Pairs, there is further confirmation that there is no statistically significant difference between Control weights and Treatment Weights (`p <= 0.05`).

There may be those who insist that it is wrong, or at least neither necessary nor desirable, to perform a confirming parametric test against data that can be defended as being more appropriately subjected to a nonparametric inferential analysis. Although this view can be rationalized, experienced researchers always challenge the data and conduct all manner of confirming quality assurance tests. Although these confirming tests may never be published, it only seems reasonable that some may want to use as many tools as are available for quality assurance purposes, including the use of both parametric as well as nonparametric inferential tests. This view is not necessarily recommended, but its use should not be unexpected.

5.11 Prepare to Exit, Save, and Later Retrieve this R Session

```
getwd()               # Identify the current working directory.
ls()                  # List all objects in the working
                      # directory.
ls.str()              # List all objects, with finite detail.
list.files()          # List files at the PC directory.

save.image("R_Wilcoxon_Matched-Pairs_Test.rdata")

getwd()               # Identify the current working directory.
ls()                  # List all objects in the working
                      # directory.
ls.str()              # List all objects, with finite detail.
list.files()          # List files at the PC directory.

alarm()               # Alarm, notice of upcoming action.
q()                   # Quit this session.
                      # Prepare for Save workspace image? query.
```

Use the R Graphical User Interface (GUI) to load the saved rdata file: File -> Load Workspace. Otherwise, use the load() function, keying the full pathname, to load the .rdata file and retrieve the session.

Recall, however, that it may be just as useful to simply use the .R script file (typically saved is a .txt ASCII-type file) and recreate the analyses and graphics, provided the data files remain available.

Chapter 6
Kruskal–Wallis H-Test for Oneway Analysis of Variance (ANOVA) by Ranks

Abstract The Kruskal–Wallis H-Test for Oneway Analysis of Variance (ANOVA) by Ranks is often viewed as the nonparametric equivalent of the parametric Oneway Analysis of Variance (ANOVA). Both the Kruskal–Wallis Test (often using ordinal data) and Oneway ANOVA (typically using interval data) are used to determine if there are statistically significant differences for comparisons of three or more groups. However, avoid seeing these tests as being mere complements of each other. The Kruskal–Wallis Test, as a nonparametric test, is used with ranked data, particularly for when: (1) the data are ordinal and do not meet the precision of interval data, (2) there are serious concerns about extreme deviation from normal distribution, and (3) there is considerable difference in the number of subjects for each comparative group. This lesson addresses the many quality assurance measures that should be attempted before actual implementation of this type of multiple-group comparative inferential analysis.

Keywords Anderson-Darling Test • Bar plot (stacked, side-by-side) • Box plot • CamelCase • Code Book • Comma-separated values (.csv) • Continuous scale • Density plot • Descriptive statistics • Distribution-free • Dot plot • Factor • Frequency distribution • Hinge (lower and upper) • Histogram • Interval • Kruskal–Wallis H-Test for Oneway Analysis of Variance (ANOVA) by Ranks • Mean • Median • Mode • Multiple comparisons (Bonferroni • Hochberg • Holm • Least Significant Difference (LSD) • Scheffé • and Tukey) • Nominal • Nonparametric • Normal distribution • Null Hypothesis • Oneway Analysis of Variance (ANOVA) • Ordinal • Outlier • Parametric • Percentile • Probability (p-value) • Quantile-Quantile (QQ, Q-Q) • Ranking • Sample (quota, convenience) • Stacked data • Statistical significance • Unstacked data • Violin plot • Whisker (lower and upper)

Electronic supplementary material The online version of this chapter (doi: 10.1007/978-3-319-30634-6_6) contains supplementary material, which is available to authorized users.

T.W. MacFarland, J.M. Yates, *Introduction to Nonparametric Statistics for the Biological Sciences Using R*, DOI 10.1007/978-3-319-30634-6_6

6.1 Background on this Lesson

The Kruskal–Wallis H-Test for Oneway Analysis of Variance (ANOVA) by Ranks is a frequently-used nonparametric test for when it is necessary to determine if three or more independent samples are from the same population or from different populations. The Kruskal–Wallis test is typically used with data that have a continuous distribution, but the data are ordinal and not interval. As a conservative choice, the Kruskal–Wallis Test may also be used if there are grave concerns about distribution patterns of the data or if differences in the number of subjects in the multiple breakout groups are extreme.

6.1.1 Description of the Data

This lesson on the Kruskal–Wallis Test is based on adult human subjects who agreed to participate in a study about Systolic Blood Pressure (SBP). The focus of this study is on differences in SBP by Race-Ethnicity, as Race-Ethnicity is often organized in the United States. Along with SBP and Race-Ethnicity, the Gender of each subject has also been identified but Gender is not a primary focus of this study. To be specific, the dataset consists of 5000 subjects organized along the following:

```
Representation of Adult Subjects Participating
in a Study of Systolic Blood Pressure (SBP)
by Race-Ethnicity and Gender

Race-Ethnicity                      N          %
==============================================
Black Female                      500       10.0
Black Male                        500       10.0
Hispanic Female                   750       15.0
Hispanic Male                     750       15.0
Other Female                      250       05.0
Other Male                        250       05.0
White Female                    1,000       20.0
White Male                      1,000       20.0
Total                           5,000      100.0
----------------------------------------------
Race-Ethnicity Breakouts
Total Black                     1,000       20.0
Total Hispanic                  1,500       30.0
Total Other                       500       10.0
Total White                     2,000       40.0
Total                           5,000      100.0
----------------------------------------------
```

```
Gender Breakouts
Total Female                     2,500          50.0
Total Male                       2,500          50.0
Total                            5,000         100.0
==============================================
```

Other than what is presented in this table, only a limited amount of information about the research design, conditions for data acquisition, etc., has been revealed to the researcher assigned responsibility for this set of analyses:

- It is unknown if the 5000 subjects are representative of the population, or if the data were from the 5000 subjects by means of a quota sample, a convenience sample, or some other non-representative sampling process.
- It is also important to note the extreme difference in sample size for the four breakout groups in this lesson, ranging from 500 subjects classified as Other to 2000 subjects classified as White. This extreme difference in sample size between breakout groups may (or may not) be representative of the population, but it does represent a challenge for inferential test selection and justification of data organization, suggesting that a nonparametric approach may be needed for later statistical analyses.
- The qualifications and skill set of the individual(s) who obtained the data were equally unknown: Student Intern, Technician III, Registered Nurse, Nurse Practitioner, Physician's Assistant, Doctor, etc.
- There is equally no information about the instrument(s) used to obtain SBP data, either the type of instrument or the process used to calibrate the instrument. Was the same instrument or type of instrument used to obtain data for all 5000 subjects? How was calibration of the instrument(s) accommodated, and how often were baseline data against a known value obtained? To be brief, were the data valid and consistent (i.e., reliable)?
- There is no other information about the dataset associated with this lesson. Further, there is no context for SBP readings. That is to say, there is no information about:
  - The time-of-day for when SBP data were obtained is unknown and it is also unknown if the time-of-day for data acquisition was consistent for all subjects.
  - The circumstance for when SBP data were obtained (e.g., measurement after vigorous exercise, measurement after rest, measurement after smoking or consumption of alcohol, measurement after eating, etc.) is also unknown.
  - It is equally unknown if some subjects were on a regime (e.g., exercise, diet, medications, etc.) to control blood pressure whereas other subjects make no attempt to control blood pressure and perhaps have no idea of possible concerns about the effect of blood pressure on general health.

Even before any graphing techniques or statistical analyses are attempted, because this information on background and context is unavailable to the researcher assigned responsibility for analyses, and, in an abundance of caution, it is best to question if the SBP data are truly interval. Or, are the SBP data for this lesson ordinal? Questioning the scale and the issue of interval v ordinal, the nonparametric

Kruskal–Wallis Test will be used instead of the parametric Oneway Analysis of Variance (ANOVA) to determine if there are differences in SBP by the four Race-Ethnicity groups associated with this lesson.

The dataset is fairly simple and the entire dataset is found as stacked data in the comma-separated values file SBPbyRaceEthnicGender.csv:

- The first line consists of a header, using descriptive variable names: ID, RaceEthnic, Gender, and SBP. Notice how there are no spaces or hyphens for variable names and that a CamelCase uppercase and lowercase technique was used to identify the object variable RaceEthnic.[1]
- The header is then followed by 5000 lines (i.e., rows) of data, one line of data for each subject.
  - ID: There is a coded identifier (S0001–S5000) for each subject. IDs are sequential and there is no coded scheme or organizational hierarchy to assigned IDs. IDs are merely continuous and are used to track, if needed, individual subjects.
  - RaceEthnic: Numerical codes have been avoided and instead the four different Race-Ethnicity groups are identified in full-text English, in alphabetical order, as Race-Ethnicity is commonly viewed in the United States:
    * Black (i.e., African-American)
    * Hispanic (i.e., Latino)
    * Other (i.e., American Indian or Alaskan Native, Asian or Pacific Islander, Declined Response, etc.)
    * White
  - Gender: Numeric codes have been avoided, and, instead the two Gender groups are identified in full-text English, in alphabetical order:
    * Female
    * Male
  - SBP: Systolic Blood Pressure has been recorded for each subject. Due to unknown quality assurance concerns about the staff member(s) responsible for obtaining SBP data, concern about consistency, calibration of the instruments, and other research design issues, SBP data will be viewed as ordinal data, and not interval data. That is to say, a SBP reading of 126 is definitely greater than a SBP reading of 124, but there is a concern that the difference in values between these two readings may not be consistent throughout the entire data collection process.

Given these conditions and the view that SBP represents ordinal data, the nonparametric Kruskal–Wallis Test is viewed as the most appropriate inferential test to determine if there is a statistically significant difference (`p <= 0.05`) in Systolic Blood Pressure (SBP) by the four Race-Ethnicity breakout groups:

[1]CamelCase is a common technique used to easily identify object variables that represent compound names. Many consider it better to write ObjectName or objectName, as an example of CamelCase, instead of using hyphens or underscores to separate compound names.

Black, Hispanic, Other, and White. This approach and the use of a nonparametric inferential test is based on concerns about data measurement (i.e., ordinal vs interval), but the issue of normal distribution and possible violation of assumptions associated with normal distribution should also be considered. Throughout these lessons, data are constantly examined for distribution patterns. There is also a concern about the extreme difference in sample size for the four Race-Ethnicity breakout groups, ranging from N = 500 for Other subjects to N = 2000 for White subjects. These extreme differences in breakout sample sizes may be entirely appropriate considering the overall population, but these differences still demand consideration.

6.1.2 *Null Hypothesis (Ho)*

There is no statistically significant difference (`p <= 0.05`) in the Systolic Blood Pressure (SBP) of adult subjects between the four Race-Ethnicity breakout groups: Black, Hispanic, Other, and White.

Notice how the Null Hypothesis (Ho) uses `p <= 0.05`. The expression `p <= 0.05` is used to identify the criterion (i.e., declared) probability level specific to the Null Hypothesis, or the acceptance of a five percent, or less, probability of an incorrect inference related to differences associated with this test.

Many exploratory inferential analyses in the biological sciences and social sciences are conducted at `p <= 0.05`. However, you will see some problems set at the more restrictive `p <= 0.01` and even `p <= 0.001`. Along with the use of p, you will also see the term *alpha* in some discussions about the level of probability, but p will be used in this lesson.

Review SBPbyRaceEthnicGender.csv to see how numerical codes for Race-Ethnicity and Gender have been avoided in this lesson. The two factor-type object variables in this lesson (i.e., RaceEthnic and Gender) collectively use English text to identify breakout group membership, (i.e., Black Female, Black Male, Hispanic Female, Hispanic Male, Other Female, Other Male, White Female, White Male).

6.2 Data Import of a .csv Spreadsheet-Type Data File into R

The dataset for this lesson was originally prepared as spreadsheet, using Gnumeric—which is free desktop software. The data were then also saved in .csv (i.e., comma-separated values) file format as SBPbyRaceEthnicGender.csv. The data are separated by commas, not tabs and not spaces. As a .csv file, the data can be easily sent to and opened by other researchers without the need for specialized software or proprietary software that may be cost prohibitive for many.

Start a new R session and then attend to beginning actions such as removing unwanted files from prior work, declaring the working directory, etc.

```
###############################################################
# Housekeeping                              Use for All Analyses  #
###############################################################
date()               # Current system time and date.
R.version.string     # R version and version release date.
ls()                 # List all objects in the working
                     # directory.
rm(list = ls())      # CAUTION: Remove all files in the working
                     # directory. If this action is not desired,
                     # use the rm() function one-by-one to remove
                     # the objects that are not needed.
ls.str()             # List all objects, with finite detail.
getwd()              # Identify the current working directory.
setwd("F:/R_Nonparametric")
                     # Set to a new working directory.
                     # Note the single forward slash and double
                     # quotes.
                     # This new directory should be the directory
                     # where the data file is located, otherwise
                     # the data file will not be found.
getwd()              # Confirm the working directory.
list.files()         # List files at the PC directory.
###############################################################
```

Create an object called SBPRaceEth.df. The object SBPRaceEth.df will be a dataframe, as indicated by the enumerated .df extension to the object name. This object will represent the output of applying the read.table() function against the comma-separated values file called SBPbyRaceEthnicGender.csv. Note the arguments used with the read.table() function, showing that there is a header with descriptive variable names (header = TRUE) and that the separator between fields is a comma (sep = ",").

```
SBPRaceEth.df <- read.table (file =
  "SBPbyRaceEthnicGender.csv",
  header = TRUE,
  sep = ",")                 # Import the .csv file.

getwd()                      # Identify the working directory
ls()                         # List objects
attach(SBPRaceEth.df)        # Attach the data, for later use
str(SBPRaceEth.df)           # Identify structure
nrow(SBPRaceEth.df)          # List the number of rows
ncol(SBPRaceEth.df)          # List the number of columns
dim(SBPRaceEth.df)           # Dimensions of the dataframe
names(SBPRaceEth.df)         # Identify names
colnames(SBPRaceEth.df)      # Show column names
rownames(SBPRaceEth.df)      # Show row names
head(SBPRaceEth.df, n=10)    # Show the head (first 10 rows)
tail(SBPRaceEth.df, n=10)    # Show the tail (last 10 rows)
SBPRaceEth.df                # Show the entire dataframe
summary(SBPRaceEth.df)       # Summary statistics
```

By completing this action, an object called SBPRaceEth.df has been created. This R-based object is a dataframe, and it consists of the data originally included in the file SBPbyRaceEthnicGender.csv, a comma-separated .csv file. To avoid possible conflicts, make sure that there are no prior R-based objects called SBPRaceEth.df. The prior use of rm(list = ls()) accommodates this concern, removing all prior objects in the current R session.

Recall how it was only necessary to key the filename for the .csv file and not the full pathname since the R working directory is currently set to the directory and/or subdirectory where this .csv file is located. See the Housekeeping section at the beginning of this lesson.

6.3 Organize the Data and Display the Code Book

With the data now imported into R, quality assurance practices should be used. It is necessary to check the data for format and to then make any changes that may be needed to organize the data. The few minutes that it takes to initially check and review data are more than worth the effort in the desire to produce only the highest quality graphics and analyses.

In many datasets, it is common for factor-type object variables to use numeric codes (i.e., the use of 1 for Female and 2 for Male to identify the object variable Gender). However, that is not the case in this lesson. Values for the object variables RaceEthnic and Gender are both presented in full-text English, avoiding the need for any type of coding scheme.

For this lesson, the class() function, str() function, and duplicated() function will be used to be sure that data are organized as desired.

```
class(SBPRaceEth.df)
class(SBPRaceEth.df$ID)         # DataFrame$ObjectName notation
class(SBPRaceEth.df$RaceEthnic) # DataFrame$ObjectName notation
class(SBPRaceEth.df$Gender)     # DataFrame$ObjectName notation
class(SBPRaceEth.df$SBP)        # DataFrame$ObjectName notation

str(SBPRaceEth.df)            # Structure

duplicated(SBPRaceEth.df)     # Duplicates
```

The class for each object seems to be correct, and there are no duplicate rows of data in the dataframe. Saying this, a Code Book will help with future understanding this dataset.

With all of these initial tasks completed, it is now necessary to create a Code Book, for current and future use. A Code Book serves the day-to-day activities of the research and statistics process. The Code Book is typically brief and provides a useful reminder for what can be easily forgotten months (or even weeks) later. Coding schemes that are intuitively obvious today can easily become forgotten tomorrow.

Now that the class(), str(), and duplicated() functions have been used for basic diagnostics, consult the Code Book and coerce each object, as needed, into its correct class.

```
#########################################################
# Code Book for SBPRaceEth.df                           #
#########################################################
#                                                       #
# Variable Labels                                       #
# ===============                                       #
# ID          Subject Identification Number             #
# RaceEthnic  Race-Ethnicity Breakout Group             #
# Gender      Gender Breakout Group                     #
# SBP         Systolic Blood Pressure                   #
#########################################################
#                                                       #
# ID........................ Factor (i.e., nominal)     #
#           A unique ID ranging from S0001 to S5000     #
#                                                       #
# RaceEthnic................ Factor (i.e., nominal)     #
#                                              Black    #
#                                           Hispanic    #
#                                              Other    #
#                                              White    #
#                                                       #
# Gender.................... Factor (i.e., nominal)     #
#                                             Female    #
#                                               Male    #
#                                                       #
# SBP....................... Integer (i.e., ordinal)    #
#      Systolic Blood Pressure, ranging from expected   #
#                           values of >= 80 to <= 200   #
#########################################################
```

Good programming practices (gpp) call for self-documentation and readability. A way to achieve that aim is to label all object variables. First, use the epicalc::des() function and the str() function to see the nature of the dataframe. Then, use the epicalc label.var() function to provide descriptive labels for each variable. Of course, be sure to load the epicalc package, if it is not operational from prior analyses.

```
install.packages("epicalc")
library(epicalc)            # Load the epicalc package.
help(package=epicalc)       # Show the information page.
sessionInfo()               # Confirm all attached packages.
# Select the most local mirror site using Set CRAN mirror.

epicalc::des(SBPRaceEth.df)
```

```
str(SBPRaceEth.df)

epicalc::label.var(ID,          "Subject ID",
    dataFrame=SBPRaceEth.df)
epicalc::label.var(RaceEthnic,"Race-Ethnicity",
    dataFrame=SBPRaceEth.df)
epicalc::label.var(Gender,      "Gender",
    dataFrame=SBPRaceEth.df)
epicalc::label.var(SBP,         "SBP",
    dataFrame=SBPRaceEth.df)
```

Confirm the description of each object variable, to be sure that all actions were deployed correctly.

```
epicalc::des(SBPRaceEth.df)
```

```
 No. of observations =  5000
  Variable      Class           Description
1 ID            factor          Subject ID
2 RaceEthnic    factor          Race-Ethnicity
3 Gender        factor          Gender
4 SBP           integer         SBP
```

```
str(SBPRaceEth.df)
```

```
'data.frame':   5000 obs. of  4 variables:
 $ ID          : Factor w/ 5000 levels "S0001","S0002",..
               : 1 2 3 4 5 6 7
 $ RaceEthnic: Factor w/ 4 levels "Black","Hispanic",..
               : 1 1 1 1 1 1 1
 $ Gender      : Factor w/ 2 levels "Female","Male"
               : 1 1 1 1 1 1 1 1 1
 $ SBP         : int  126 132 148 126 132 132 116 118 134 136 ...
 - attr(*, "var.labels")= chr
 "Subject ID" "Race-Ethnicity" "Gender" "SBP"
```

With assurance that the dataframe is in correct format and that labels are correct, coerce all object variables into desired format. Notice how variables are named: DataframeName$ObjectName. At first, this action may seem somewhat cumbersome and perhaps even redundant for a few object variables, but it is actually very useful to ensure that actions are performed against the correct object. Descriptive object variable names promote efficiency and accuracy. Most text editors allow the use of copy-and-paste and find and replace, so it should be a simple operation to organize the syntax.

Note also how the object variable SBPRaceEth.df$SBP is an integer-type object but that it will be coerced into a numeric-type object. Because of this action it will be possible to apply a full range of numeric-type actions against SBP measurements, as needed.

```
SBPRaceEth.df$ID          <- as.factor(SBPRaceEth.df$ID)
SBPRaceEth.df$RaceEthnic <- as.factor(SBPRaceEth.df$RaceEthnic)
SBPRaceEth.df$Gender      <- as.factor(SBPRaceEth.df$Gender)
SBPRaceEth.df$SBP         <- as.numeric(SBPRaceEth.df$SBP)
```

If needed, use the many help resources to learn about the as.integer() function and the as.numeric() function, specifically to see the differences between these two R functions and when it is appropriate to use each.[2]

Again, confirm the structure of the dataset, using both the epicalc::des() function and the str() function.

```
epicalc::des(SBPRaceEth.df)    # After object coerced
```

```
 No. of observations =  5000
  Variable        Class          Description
1 ID              factor         Subject ID
2 RaceEthnic      factor         Race-Ethnicity
3 Gender          factor         Gender
4 SBP             numeric        SBP
```

```
str(SBPRaceEth.df)             # After object coerced
```

```
'data.frame':   5000 obs. of  4 variables:
 $ ID          : Factor w/ 5000 levels "S0001","S0002",..
               : 1 2 3 4 5 6 7
 $ RaceEthnic: Factor w/ 4 levels "Black","Hispanic",..
               : 1 1 1 1 1 1 1
 $ Gender      : Factor w/ 2 levels "Female","Male"
               : 1 1 1 1 1 1 1 1 1 1
 $ SBP         : num  126 132 148 126 132 132 116 118 134 136 ...
 - attr(*, "var.labels")= chr
 "Subject ID" "Race-Ethnicity" "Gender" "SBP"
```

Then, in a somewhat redundant fashion and to merely further confirm the nature of the dataset, use the levels() function (part of the base package obtained when R is first downloaded) against all factor object variables, to reinforce understanding of the data.

```
levels(SBPRaceEth.df$ID)            # N = 5,000 levels

levels(SBPRaceEth.df$RaceEthnic)   # N = 4 levels
```

```
[1] "Black"    "Hispanic" "Other"     "White"
```

[2]When in doubt about a function or any other R feature, at the R prompt key **??** and then the appropriate term to see a set of selections for more information on the topic in question. By keying **??mean** at the R prompt, a Web page appears with a long list of vignettes, code demonstrations, and help pages that relate to the function mean().

```
levels(SBPRaceEth.df$Gender)        # N = 2 levels
```

```
[1] "Female" "Male"
```

Use the summary() function against the object SBPRaceEth.df, which is a dataframe, to again gain an initial sense of descriptive statistics and frequency distributions.

```
summary(SBPRaceEth.df)
```

```
       ID              RaceEthnic        Gender            SBP
 S0001   :   1    Black    :1000    Female:2500    Min.    : 92.0
 S0002   :   1    Hispanic:1500     Male  :2500    1st Qu.:116.0
 S0003   :   1    Other    : 500                   Median :124.0
 S0004   :   1    White    :2000                   Mean   :125.8
 S0005   :   1                                     3rd Qu.:132.0
 S0006   :   1                                     Max.   :184.0
```

The dataset seems to be in correct format. Further, for this dataset the use of numeric codes for factor-type object variables was avoided, and it is not necessary to perform any type of recode action. Saying this, a few graphical images may help with gaining a more complete sense of the data and how the data are organized (Fig. 6.1).

```
par(ask=TRUE)
epicalc::tab1(SBPRaceEth.df$RaceEthnic,
  decimal=2,                         # The epicalc::tab1() function is
  sort.group=FALSE,                  # used to see details about the
  cum.percent=TRUE,                  # selected object variable.  The
  graph=TRUE,                        # 1 of tab1 is the one numeric
  missing=TRUE,                      # character and it is not the
  bar.values=c("frequency"),  # letter l.
  horiz=FALSE,
  cex=1.15, cex.names=1.15, cex.lab=1.15, cex.axis=1.15,
  main="Factor Levels for Object Variable RaceEthnic:
  Race-Ethnicity",
  ylab="Frequency of Race-Ethnicity Levels",
  col=c("red", "blue", "black", "green"), gen=TRUE)
```

```
SBPRaceEth.df$RaceEthnic :
         Frequency Percent Cum. percent
Black         1000      20           20
Hispanic      1500      30           50
Other          500      10           60
White         2000      40          100
  Total       5000     100          100
```

```
par(ask=TRUE)
epicalc::tab1(SBPRaceEth.df$Gender,
```

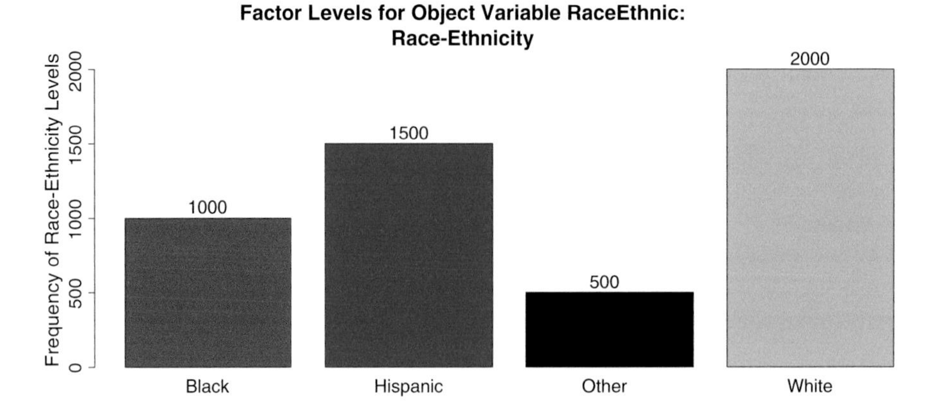

Fig. 6.1 Frequency distribution of four breakout groups using the epicalc::tab1() function

```
  decimal=2,                     # The epicalc::tab1() function is
  sort.group=FALSE,              # used to see details about the
  cum.percent=TRUE,              # selected object variable.  The
  graph=TRUE,                    # 1 of tab1 is the one numeric
  missing=TRUE,                  # character and it is not the
  bar.values=c("frequency"),     # letter l.
  horiz=FALSE,
  cex=1.15, cex.names=1.15, cex.lab=1.15, cex.axis=1.15,
  main="Factor Levels for Object Variable Gender",
  ylab="Frequency of Gender Breakout Groups",
  col=c("red", "blue"), gen=TRUE)
```

```
SBPRaceEth.df$Gender :
        Frequency Percent Cum. percent
Female       2500      50           50
Male         2500      50          100
  Total      5000     100          100
```

Note how the epicalc::tab1() function is quite useful in that it generates both a text-based frequency distribution table as well as a frequency distribution graphic.

Once again as a redundant, but still useful action, use the attach() function to provide assurance that all data are attached to the dataframe.

```
attach(SBPRaceEth.df)
head(SBPRaceEth.df)
tail(SBPRaceEth.df)
summary(SBPRaceEth.df)     # Quality assurance data check.

str(SBPRaceEth.df)         # List all objects, with finite detail
ls.str(SBPRaceEth.df)      # List all objects, with finite detail
```

As an additional data check, use the table() function to see how data have been summarized—just to be assured that data are all in correct format, especially as a check for any possibility of missing data, which in R are marked as NA.

```
table(SBPRaceEth.df$RaceEthnic, useNA = c("always"))
table(SBPRaceEth.df$Gender,     useNA = c("always"))

table(SBPRaceEth.df$RaceEthnic, SBPRaceEth.df$Gender,
  useNA = c("always"))
  # Crosstabs of Race-Ethnicity (rows) by Gender
  # (columns)
```

```
           Female Male <NA>
  Black       500  500    0
  Hispanic    750  750    0
  Other       250  250    0
  White      1000 1000    0
  <NA>          0    0    0
```

Note how the argument useNA = c("always") is used with the table() function, to force identification of missing values.

For far more detail than supported by the table() function, use the gmodels::CrossTable() function for explicit detail on row and column counts, row and column percentages, and contributions of each to total. Again, the need for this type of information may not seem important at first, but it is another quality assurance measure that should be attempted before the dataset is finally accepted and resources are put into graphical presentation and statistical analyses. Anything that can be done to catch a simple oversight at the initial stages of data analysis is more than worth the time-on-task. Attention to quality assurance should be a continuous and pervasive process.

```
install.packages("gmodels")
library(gmodels)              # Load the gmodels package.
help(package=gmodels)         # Show the information page.
sessionInfo()                 # Confirm all attached packages.
# Select the most local mirror site using Set CRAN mirror.

gmodels::CrossTable(SBPRaceEth.df$RaceEthnic,
  SBPRaceEth.df$Gender,
  digits=2, expected=TRUE, prop.r=TRUE, prop.c=TRUE,
  prop.t=TRUE, prop.chisq=TRUE, missing.include=TRUE,
  chisq=TRUE, format="SPSS")
```

Be sure to note how there are four breakout groups for the rows (SBPRaceEth.df$RaceEthnic) and two breakout groups for the columns (SBPRaceEth.df$Gender). As a general approach to organization of a X (rows) by Y (columns) table, it is usually best to place as rows the object variable with the greatest number of breakout groups and to place as columns the object variable with the fewest number of breakout groups. By following this action the table will have a greater length than width which may be useful if the table is copied from R and placed into a word processed document. Of course, experiment with this type of configuration to put output to the best advantage.

6.4 Conduct a Visual Data Check

With the data currently in proper format, it would be common to immediately attempt the appropriate inferential analysis, the Kruskal–Wallis Test for this lesson. However, it is best to first prepare a few graphical displays of the data and to then reinforce comprehension of the data with descriptive statistics and measures of central tendency.

The summary() function, min() function, and max() function are all certainly useful for data checking, but there are also many advantages to a visual data check process. In this case, simple plots can be very helpful in looking for data that may be either illogical or out-of-range. These initial graphics will be, by design, simple and should be considered throwaways as they are intended only for initial diagnostic purposes. More complex figures, often of publishable quality, can then be prepared from these initial throwaway graphics by careful selection of functions and arguments.

Although the emphasis in this lesson is on the Kruskal–Wallis Test for the factor-type object variable RaceEthnic (four breakout groups) and the numeric-type object variable SBP (values can range from >= 80 to <= 200), a simple graphic will be prepared for each variable, largely as a quality assurance check against the entire dataset (Figs. 6.2 and 6.3).

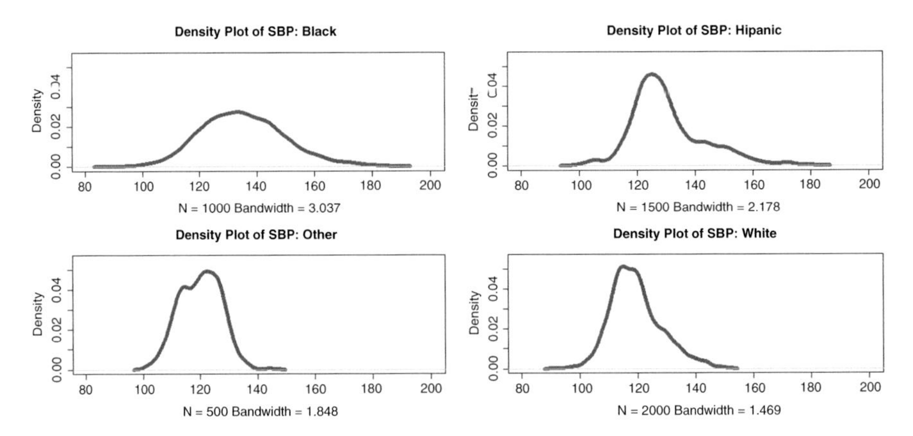

Fig. 6.2 Multiple (two rows by two columns) density plots using the which() function for Boolean selection

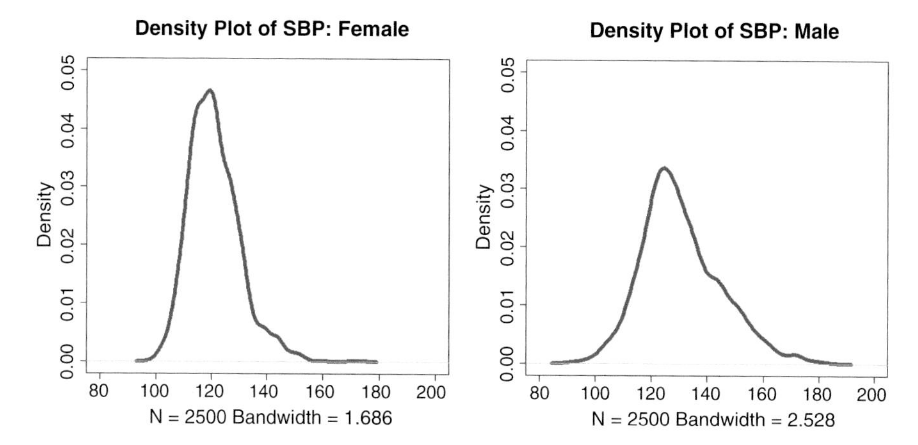

Fig. 6.3 Multiple (one row by two columns) density plots using the which() function for Boolean selection

```
names(SBPRaceEth.df)      # Confirm all object variables.

par(ask=TRUE)
plot(SBPRaceEth.df$ID,
  main="SBPRaceEth.df$ID Visual Data Check")

par(ask=TRUE)
plot(SBPRaceEth.df$RaceEthnic,
  main="SBPRaceEth.df$RaceEthnic Visual Data Check")

par(ask=TRUE)
plot(SBPRaceEth.df$Gender,
  main="SBPRaceEth.df$Gender Visual Data Check")

par(ask=TRUE)
plot(density(SBPRaceEth.df$SBP,
  na.rm=TRUE),    # Required for the density() function
  main="Density Plot of SBP",
  lwd=6, col="red", font.axis=2, font.lab=2)

par(ask=TRUE)          # Side-by-Side Density Plots
par(mfrow=c(2,2))      # of SBP by RaceEthnic
plot(density(SBPRaceEth.df$SBP[
  which(SBPRaceEth.df$RaceEthnic=="Black")],
  na.rm=TRUE), xlim=c(080,200), ylim=c(0,0.055),
  main="Density Plot of SBP:  Black",
  lwd=6, col="red", font.axis=2, font.lab=2)
plot(density(SBPRaceEth.df$SBP[
  which(SBPRaceEth.df$RaceEthnic=="Hispanic")],
  na.rm=TRUE), xlim=c(080,200), ylim=c(0,0.055),
  main="Density Plot of SBP:  Hispanic",
  lwd=6, col="red", font.axis=2, font.lab=2)
```

```
plot(density(SBPRaceEth.df$SBP[
  which(SBPRaceEth.df$RaceEthnic=="Other")],
  na.rm=TRUE), xlim=c(080,200), ylim=c(0,0.055),
  main="Density Plot of SBP:  Other",
  lwd=6, col="red", font.axis=2, font.lab=2)
plot(density(SBPRaceEth.df$SBP[
  which(SBPRaceEth.df$RaceEthnic=="White")],
  na.rm=TRUE), xlim=c(080,200), ylim=c(0,0.055),
  main="Density Plot of SBP:  White",
  lwd=6, col="red", font.axis=2, font.lab=2)
# The which() function is used to make selection.
```

```
par(ask=TRUE)          # Side-by-Side Density Plots
par(mfrow=c(1,2))      # of SBP by Gender
plot(density(SBPRaceEth.df$SBP[
  which(SBPRaceEth.df$Gender=="Female")],
  na.rm=TRUE), xlim=c(080,200), ylim=c(0,0.05),
  main="Density Plot of SBP:  Female",
  lwd=6, col="red", font.axis=2, font.lab=2)
plot(density(SBPRaceEth.df$SBP[
  which(SBPRaceEth.df$Gender=="Male")],
  na.rm=TRUE), xlim=c(080,200), ylim=c(0,0.05),
  main="Density Plot of SBP:  Male",
  lwd=6, col="red", font.axis=2, font.lab=2)
# The which() function is used to make selection.
```

The purpose of these initial plots is to gain a general sense of the data and to equally look for outliers. In an attempt to look for outliers, the xlim argument and ylim argument have either been avoided or expanded, so that all data are plotted. Extreme values may or may not be outliers, but they are certainly interesting and demand attention. Experienced researchers do not look only at expected data but instead consider all data.

This sample lesson has been designed to look into the nature of the numeric-type object variable SBP and the factor-type object variable RaceEthnic. Given the nature of SBP values, it may also be a good idea to supplement the plot(density()) functions with the hist() function and the boxplot() function to gain a another view of the distribution pattern for this object variable. There is a concern that the numeric values for object variable SBP do not show normal distribution along a bell-shaped curve, and there is a question, given the nature of how data were obtained, if the distribution of SBP approximates those conditions needed for correct use of Oneway ANOVA, which is commonly applied using data that meet parametric assumptions.

```
par(ask=TRUE)
hist(SBPRaceEth.df$SBP,
  main="Histogram of Systolic Blood Pressure",
  nclass=50,         # Number of bins
  font=2,            # Bold text
  cex.lab=1.15,      # Large font
  col="red")         # Vibrant color
```

```
par(ask=TRUE)
boxplot(SBPRaceEth.df$SBP,
  horizontal=TRUE,
  main="Horizontal Boxplot of Systolic Blood Pressure",
  xlab="Systolic Blood Pressure:  Expanded Range",
  ylim=c(0,245),    # Note the selection for ylim.
  cex.lab=1.15, cex.axis=1.15, border="blue", col="red")
box()

par(ask=TRUE)
boxplot(SBPRaceEth.df$SBP ~ SBPRaceEth.df$RaceEthnic,
  horizontal=FALSE,
  main="Vertical Boxplot of Systolic Blood Pressure (SBP) by
  Race-Ethnicity",
  ylim=c(0,245), # Note the selection for ylim.
  ylab="Systolic Blood Pressure:  Expanded Range",
  xlab="Race-Ethnicity Breakout Groups",
  cex.lab=1.15, cex.axis=1.15, border="blue", col="red")
box()
```

If all group names do not appear in the graphic, adjust the cex.axis setting to a lower value. As is nearly always the case with R, settings are generally a matter of balance between personal preferences and presentation requirements. Many graphic-type settings can be reviewed by keying help(par) at the R prompt, to learn more about the many arguments and options supported by R graphics.

Note: It is largely a personal preference to display a boxplot in either horizontal mode or vertical mode. To meet the needs of various readers, it is common to use both orientations.

The use of par(mfrow=c(2,2)) and par(mfrow=c(1,2)) was previously demonstrated, in an attempt to place multiple images of breakout values into one composite graphic. Consider the lattice package, also, as a useful resource to prepare a composite graphic that provides a sense of all breakout groups in one easy-to-visualize presentation. Preparing comparisons by breakout groups, all in one graphical presentation, makes comprehension far easier than if the many graphical presentations were in separate images, often over several pages in a final report (Figs. 6.4 and 6.5).[3]

```
install.packages("lattice")
library(lattice)             # Load the lattice package.
help(package=lattice)        # Show the information page.
sessionInfo()                # Confirm all attached packages.
# Select the most local mirror site using Set CRAN mirror.

par(ask=TRUE) # 1 Column by 4 Rows Histogram
lattice::histogram(~ SBPRaceEth.df$SBP |
  SBPRaceEth.df$RaceEthnic, # Pipe, not ~ or ,
```

[3]The ggplot package, which is gaining attention in the R community and which serves as a complement to the lattice package, will be presented in a later lesson.

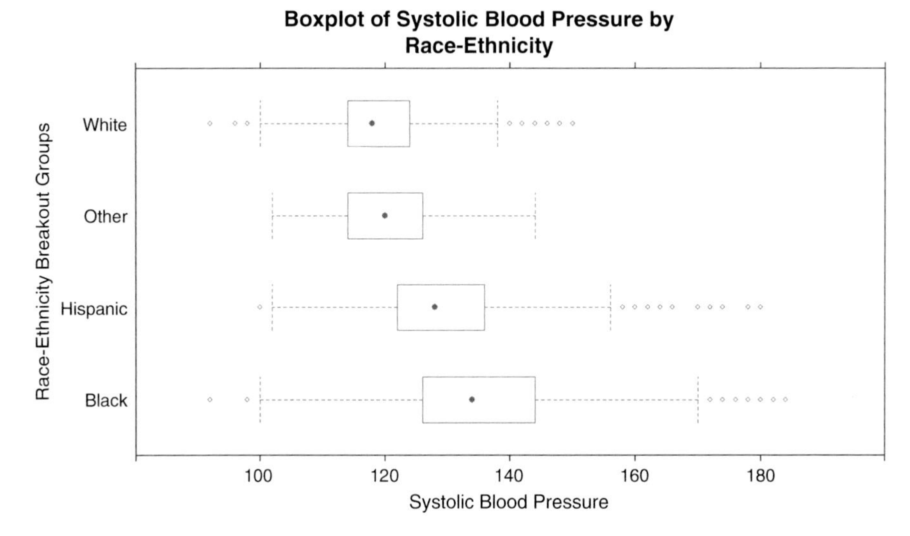

Fig. 6.4 Boxplots of four breakout groups using the lattice::bwplot() function with emphasis on outliers

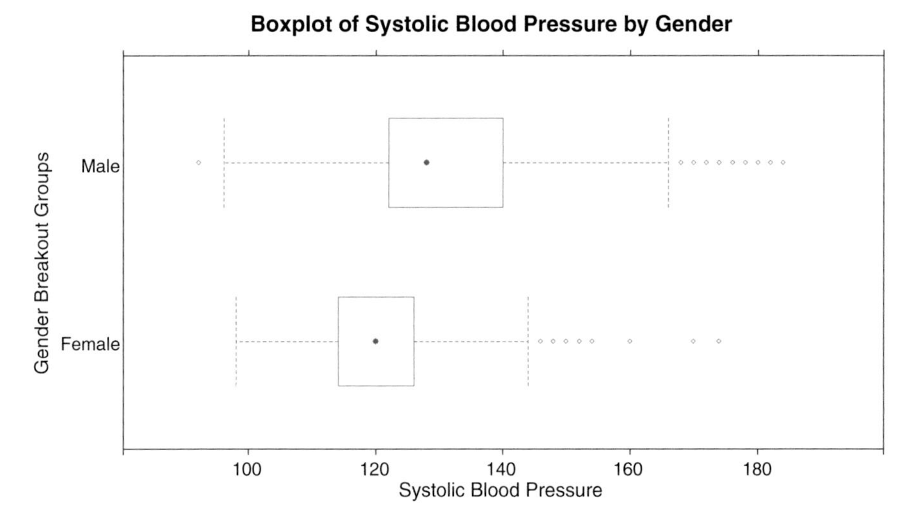

Fig. 6.5 Boxplots of two breakout groups using the lattice::bwplot() function with emphasis on outlines

```
type="count", # Note: count
par.settings=simpleTheme(lwd=2),
par.strip.text=list(cex=1.15, font=2),
scales=list(cex=1.15),
main="Histograms (Count) of Systolic Blood Pressure by
Race-Ethnicity",
xlab=list("Systolic Blood Pressure", cex=1.15, font=2),
```

```
  xlim=c(080,200),            # Note the range.
  ylab=list("Count", cex=1.15, font=2),
  aspect=0.25, breaks=20,
  layout = c(1,4), # Note: 1 Column by 4 Rows.
  col="red")

par(ask=TRUE) # 1 Column by 4 Rows Histogram
lattice::histogram(~ SBPRaceEth.df$SBP |
  SBPRaceEth.df$RaceEthnic, # Pipe, not ~ or ,
  type="percent", # Note: percent
  par.settings=simpleTheme(lwd=2),
  par.strip.text=list(cex=1.15, font=2),
  scales=list(cex=1.15),
  main="Histograms (Percent) of Systolic Blood Pressure by
  Race-Ethnicity",
  xlab=list("Systolic Blood Pressure", cex=1.15, font=2),
  xlim=c(080,200),            # Note the range.
  ylab=list("Percent", cex=1.15, font=2),
  aspect=0.25, breaks=20,
  layout = c(1,4), # Note: 1 Column by 4 Rows.
  col="red")

par(ask=TRUE) # Breakout group by measured object.
lattice::bwplot(SBPRaceEth.df$RaceEthnic ~
  SBPRaceEth.df$SBP,          # Tilde, not | or ,
  par.settings = simpleTheme(lwd=2),
  par.strip.text=list(cex=1.15, font=2),
  scales=list(cex=1.15),
  main="Boxplot of Systolic Blood Pressure by
  Race-Ethnicity",
  xlab=list("Systolic Blood Pressure", cex=1.15, font=2),
  xlim=c(080,200),
  ylab=list("Race-Ethnicity Breakout Groups", cex=1.15,
  font=2), aspect=0.5, layout=c(1,1), col="red")
```

```
par(ask=TRUE) # 1 Column by 4 Rows Histogram
lattice::densityplot(~ SBPRaceEth.df$SBP |
  SBPRaceEth.df$RaceEthnic, # Pipe, not ~ or ,
  type="density", # Note: density
  par.settings=simpleTheme(lwd=4),
  par.strip.text=list(cex=1.15, font=2),
  scales=list(cex=1.15),
  main="Density Plot of Systolic Blood Pressure by
  Race-Ethnicity",
  xlab=list("Systolic Blood Pressure", cex=1.15, font=2),
  xlim=c(080,200),            # Note the range.
  ylab=list("Density", cex=1.15, font=2),
  aspect=0.25, breaks=20,
  layout = c(1,4), # Note: 1 Column by 4 Rows.
  col="red")

par(ask=TRUE) # 1 Column by 2 Rows Histogram
lattice::histogram(~ SBPRaceEth.df$SBP |
```

```
  SBPRaceEth.df$Gender, # Pipe, not ~ or ,
  type="count", # Note: count
  par.settings=simpleTheme(lwd=2),
  par.strip.text=list(cex=1.15, font=2),
  scales=list(cex=1.15),
  main="Histograms (Count) of Systolic Blood Pressure by
  Gender",
  xlab=list("Systolic Blood Pressure", cex=1.15, font=2),
  xlim=c(080,200),           # Note the range.
  ylab=list("Count", cex=1.15, font=2),
  aspect=0.25, breaks=20,
  layout = c(1,2), # Note: 1 Column by 2 Rows.
  col="red")

par(ask=TRUE) # 1 Column by 2 Rows Histogram
lattice::histogram(~ SBPRaceEth.df$SBP |
  SBPRaceEth.df$Gender, # Pipe, not ~ or ,
  type="percent", # Note: percent
  par.settings=simpleTheme(lwd=2),
  par.strip.text=list(cex=1.15, font=2),
  scales=list(cex=1.15),
  main="Histograms (Percent) of Systolic Blood Pressure by
  Gender",
  xlab=list("Systolic Blood Pressure", cex=1.15, font=2),
  xlim=c(080,200),           # Note the range.
  ylab=list("Percent", cex=1.15, font=2),
  aspect=0.25, breaks=20,
  layout = c(1,2), # Note: 1 Column by 2 Rows.
  col="red")

par(ask=TRUE) # Breakout group by measured object.
lattice::bwplot(SBPRaceEth.df$Gender ~
  SBPRaceEth.df$SBP,         # Tilde, not | or ,
  par.settings = simpleTheme(lwd=2),
  par.strip.text=list(cex=1.15, font=2),
  scales=list(cex=1.15),
  main="Boxplot of Systolic Blood Pressure by Gender",
  xlab=list("Systolic Blood Pressure", cex=1.15, font=2),
  xlim=c(080,200),
  ylab=list("Gender Breakout Groups", cex=1.15,
  font=2), aspect=0.5, layout=c(1,1), col="red")
```

```
par(ask=TRUE) # 1 Column by 2 Rows Histogram
lattice::densityplot(~ SBPRaceEth.df$SBP |
  SBPRaceEth.df$Gender, # Pipe, not ~ or ,
  type="density", # Note: density
  par.settings=simpleTheme(lwd=4),
  par.strip.text=list(cex=1.15, font=2),
  scales=list(cex=1.15),
  main="Density Plot of Systolic Blood Pressure by Gender",
  xlab=list("Systolic Blood Pressure", cex=1.15, font=2),
  xlim=c(080,200),           # Note the range.
  ylab=list("Density", cex=1.15, font=2),
```

```
aspect=0.25, breaks=20,
layout = c(1,2), # Note: 1 Column by 2 Rows.
col="red")
```

These lattice-based graphical images would make a good presentation for a large group, or they would be generally acceptable for inclusion in a report or other publication. Again, similar graphical images generated by using the ggplot package are presented in a later lesson.

6.5 Descriptive Analysis of the Data

There are no known missing data in this dataset. Given the different ways missing data can impact analyses, it is still helpful to first check for missing data by using the is.na() function and the complete.cases() function against the entire dataset. Both functions return a TRUE or FALSE response, depending on the function and the outcome of whether data are missing or not. Again, these actions may not be needed, but they are still desired as part of a constant and pervasive attempt to consider quality assurance and how data quality impacts later statistical analyses and eventually decision-making.

```
is.na(SBPRaceEth.df)          # Check for missing data
complete.cases(SBPRaceEth.df) # Check for complete cases
```

After this review of the data, the summary() function is likely all that is needed to gain a first sense of the data. Note how the summary() function is applied against the entire dataset, thus yielding information about all object variables.

```
summary(SBPRaceEth.df)
```

Although the summary() function is generally sufficient, descriptive statistics for individual object variables may be desired, and in this dataset attention will be directed toward the object variable SBPRaceEth.df$SBP, overall and by Race-Ethnicity breakout groups. Although it is not needed for this lesson given how there are no missing data, as a good programming practice (gpp), the na.rm=TRUE argument or some other similar convention will be used to accommodate missing data. Because the nonparametric Kruskal–Wallis Test will be used to determine if there is a statistically significant difference (`p <= 0.05`) for Systolic Blood Pressure by the four Race-Ethnicity breakout groups, give special attention to outcomes from the median() function as well as the mean() function.

Descriptive Statistics of SBPRaceEth.df$SBP—Overall

```
length(SBPRaceEth.df$SBP)                        # N

install.packages("asbio")
library(asbio)                    # Load the asbio package.
help(package=asbio)               # Show the information page.
sessionInfo()                     # Confirm all attached packages.
# Select the most local mirror site using Set CRAN mirror.
```

```
asbio::Mode(SBPRaceEth.df$SBP)                   # Mode
```

```
[1] 120
```

```
median(SBPRaceEth.df$SBP, na.rm=TRUE)      # Median
```

```
[1] 124
```

```
mean(SBPRaceEth.df$SBP, na.rm=TRUE)        # Mean
```

```
[1] 125.8316
```

```
sd(SBPRaceEth.df$SBP,na.rm=TRUE )          # SD
```

```
[1] 12.87823
```

```
summary(SBPRaceEth.df$SBP, na.rm=TRUE)     # Summary
```

```
   Min. 1st Qu.  Median    Mean 3rd Qu.    Max.
   92.0   116.0   124.0   125.8   132.0   184.0
```

Descriptive Statistics of SBPRaceEth.df$SBP – by Race-Ethnicity Breakout Groups

Descriptive statistics at the summary level are certainly needed, but breakout statistics are also needed to gain a more complete understanding of the data. There are many ways to obtain breakout statistics, but the tapply() function, epicalc::summ() function, prettyR::brkdn() function, psych::describeBy() function, Hmisc::bystats() function, and the lessR::SummaryStats() function are among the most detailed and easiest to use to discern differences between breakout groups for SBPRaceEth.df$RaceEthnic: (1) Black, (2) Hispanic, (3) Other, and (4) White. Experiment with all of these different functions to see similarities and differences of how information is placed on the screen, level of detail, etc. Then, make a choice on which function meets requirements and preferences (Figs. 6.6 and 6.7).

```
tapply(SBP, RaceEthnic, summary, na.rm=TRUE,
  data=SBPRaceEth.df)
  # SBP by RaceEthnic, using tapply()
```

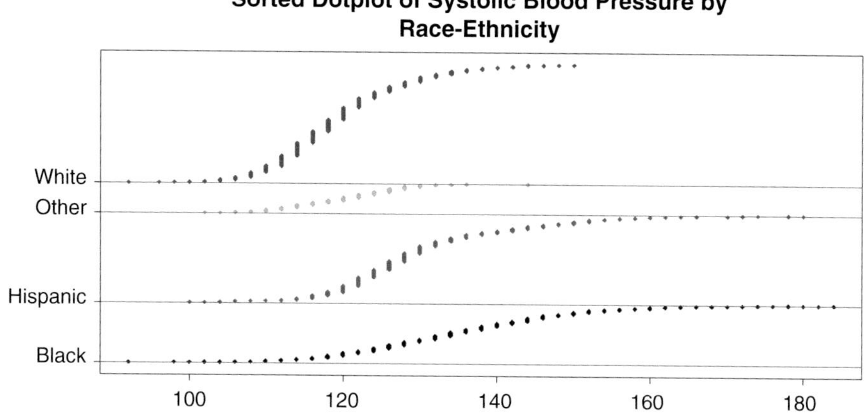

Fig. 6.6 Color-coded sorted dot plots of four breakout groups using the epicalc::summ() function

```
$Black
   Min. 1st Qu.  Median    Mean 3rd Qu.    Max.
   92.0   126.0   134.0   135.2   144.0   184.0

$Hispanic
   Min. 1st Qu.  Median    Mean 3rd Qu.    Max.
  100.0   122.0   128.0   130.2   136.0   180.0

$Other
   Min. 1st Qu.  Median    Mean 3rd Qu.    Max.
  102.0   114.0   120.0   119.9   126.0   144.0

$White
   Min. 1st Qu.  Median    Mean 3rd Qu.    Max.
   92.0   114.0   118.0   119.4   124.0   150.0
```

```
par(ask=TRUE) # Use the epicalc package for breakout analyses
epicalc::summ(SBPRaceEth.df$SBP, by=SBPRaceEth.df$RaceEthnic,
  graph=TRUE, pch=18, ylab="auto",
  main="Sorted Dotplot of Systolic Blood Pressure by
  Race-Ethnicity",
  cex.X.axis=1.15, cex.Y.axis=1.15, font.lab=2, dot.col="auto")
  # Note the descriptive statistics and not only the graphic
  # that go along with the  epicalc::summ() function.
```

```
For SBPRaceEth.df$RaceEthnic = Black
 obs. mean   median  s.d.   min.   max.
 1000 135.2  134     14.336 92     184

For SBPRaceEth.df$RaceEthnic = Hispanic
 obs. mean   median  s.d.   min.   max.
 1500 130.2  128     12.333 100    180
```

```
For SBPRaceEth.df$RaceEthnic = Other
 obs. mean   median  s.d.   min.   max.
 500  119.9  120     7.117  102    144

For SBPRaceEth.df$RaceEthnic = White
 obs. mean   median  s.d.   min.   max.
 2000 119.4  118     8.754  92     150
```

```
install.packages("prettyR")
library(prettyR)                # Load the prettyR package.
help(package=prettyR)           # Show the information page.
sessionInfo()                   # Confirm all attached packages.
# Select the most local mirror site using Set CRAN mirror.

prettyR::brkdn(SBP ~ RaceEthnic, SBPRaceEth.df,
  num.desc=c("median","mean","sd","valid.n"))
```

```
Breakdown of SBP by RaceEthnic
Level      median       mean          sd    valid.n
Black         134      135.2       14.34       1000
Hispanic      128      130.2       12.33       1500
Other         120      119.9        7.12        500
White         118      119.4        8.75       2000
```

```
install.packages("psych")
library(psych)                  # Load the psych package.
help(package=psych)             # Show the information page.
sessionInfo()                   # Confirm all attached packages.
# Select the most local mirror site using Set CRAN mirror.

psych::describeBy(SBPRaceEth.df$SBP,
  SBPRaceEth.df$RaceEthnic,
  digits=2, mat=TRUE) # Matrix output
```

```
group1       n   mean    sd median  min max
Black     1000 135.16 14.34    134   92 101
Hispanic  1500 130.22 12.33    128  100 180
Other      500 119.88  7.12    120  102 144
White     2000 119.36  8.75    118   92 150
```

```
install.packages("Hmisc")
library(Hmisc)                  # Load the Hmisc package.
help(package=Hmisc)             # Show the information page.
sessionInfo()                   # Confirm all attached packages.
# Select the most local mirror site using Set CRAN mirror.

Hmisc::bystats(SBPRaceEth.df$SBP, SBPRaceEth.df$RaceEthnic,
  nmiss=TRUE, fun=median)
```

```
 median of SBPRaceEth.df$SBP by SBPRaceEth.df$RaceEthnic

            N Missing median
Black     1000       0    134
Hispanic 1500       0    128
Other      500       0    120
White     2000       0    118
ALL       5000       0    124
```

```
install.packages("lessR")
library(lessR)                 # Load the lessR package.
help(package=lessR)            # Show the information page.
sessionInfo()                  # Confirm all attached packages.
# Select the most local mirror site using Set CRAN mirror.

lessR::SummaryStats(SBP, by=RaceEthnic, data=SBPRaceEth.df,
  digits.d=2, brief=TRUE)  # Reduced output, to improve final
  # presentation
```

```
SBP - by levels of - RaceEthnic
             n  miss     mean       sd      min      mdn      max
Black     1000     0  135.16   14.34    92.00   134.00   184.00
Hispanic  1500     0  130.22   12.33   100.00   128.00   180.00
Other      500     0  119.88    7.12   102.00   120.00   144.00
White     2000     0  119.36    8.75    92.00   118.00   150.00

Number of outliers: 122
```

Because the focus of this lesson is on the nonparametric Kruskal–Wallis Test and not the parametric Oneway Analysis of Variance, it would be useful to graphically reinforce output from the median() function in proximity to output from the mean() function, presented in this case as a graphical image based on the barplot() function. From among the many possible ways that the breakout statistics could be obtained, the prettyR::brkdn() function will be used to obtain median and mean statistics of Systolic Blood Pressure for each Race-Ethnicity breakout group. These statistics will then be used to create new barplots, side-by-side, to allow for easy comparison of median values to mean values.

```
prettyR::brkdn(SBP ~ RaceEthnic, SBPRaceEth.df,
  num.desc=c("median","mean","sd","valid.n"))
```

```
Breakdown of SBP by RaceEthnic
Level      median       mean        sd    valid.n
Black         134      135.2     14.34       1000
Hispanic      128      130.2     12.33       1500
Other         120      119.9      7.12        500
White         118      119.4      8.75       2000
```

After gaining these descriptive statistics, prepare a set of self-generated bar plots for the Median and Mean of Systolic Blood Pressure by Race-Ethnicity breakout

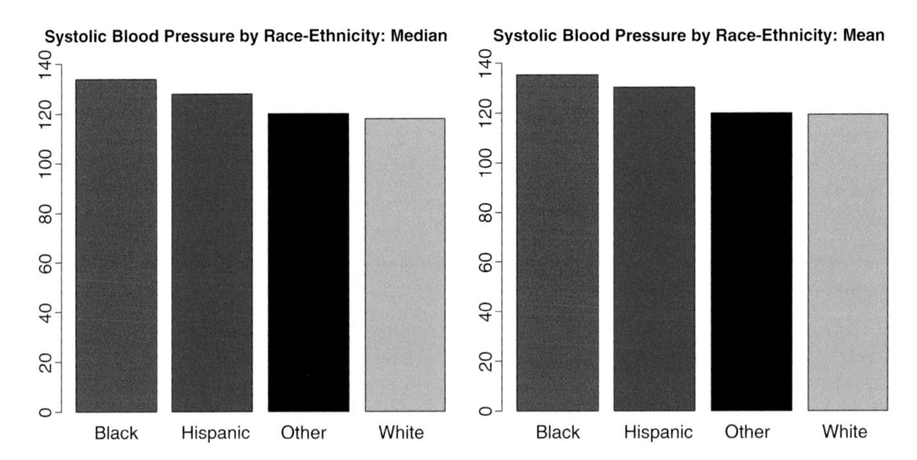

Fig. 6.7 Multiple bar plots in one graphic based on enumerated values

groups. Use the barplot() function and know that this approach is a *kludge* (i.e., review this term since it is commonly used in computing) that is presented merely to show another way to visualize outcomes in R. This method works, and it provides a good sense of comparative outcomes—especially for ranking purposes.

```
par(ask=TRUE)
par(mfrow=c(1,2))          # Side-by-Side of Median and Mean
barplot(c(134, 128, 120, 118),
  names.arg=c("Black", "Hispanic", "Other", "White"),
  col=c("red", "blue", "black", "green"),
  main="Systolic Blood Pressure by Race-Ethnicity:  Median",
  font=2, cex.lab=1.25, ylim=c(0,140))
barplot(c(135.2, 130.2, 119.9, 119.4),
  names.arg=c("Black", "Hispanic", "Other", "White"),
  col=c("red", "blue", "black", "green"),
  main="Systolic Blood Pressure by Race-Ethnicity:  Mean",
  font=2, cex.lab=1.25, ylim=c(0,140))
```

Application of the Anderson-Darling Test

Graphical images and descriptive statistics are helpful in understanding the data. It is also useful to apply selected statistical tests to serve as additional supports for decision-making on acceptance of nonparametric or parametric views toward the data. The Anderson-Darling Test, the Lilliefors (KS) Test, and the Shapiro-Wilk Test are often used to support this type of decision-making. These tests may be influenced by sample size. Overall, these tests provide one view, but not the only view, on the nature of distribution patterns. Experience, needs, and practical judgment, supported by careful review of graphical images, descriptive statistics, and statistical tests, should be used when deciding if variables from a dataset are best viewed from a nonparametric or parametric perspective.

```
install.packages("nortest")
library(nortest)              # Load the nortest package.
help(package=nortest)         # Show the information page.
sessionInfo()                 # Confirm all attached packages.
# Select the most local mirror site using Set CRAN mirror.
```

The Anderson-Darling Test will be used for this lesson. The Null Hypothesis for the Anderson-Darling Test is structured to examine whether the data follow a specified distribution:

Anderson-Darling Null Hypothesis: The data follow the normal distribution.

For this lesson there will be five approaches to the Anderson-Darling Test with subsequent examination of p-values for each approach:

- The Anderson-Darling Test will be applied against the values for SBPRaceEth.df$SBP, overall.
- The Anderson-Darling Test will be applied against the values for SBPRaceEth.df$SBP, where RaceEthnic = Black.
- The Anderson-Darling Test will be applied against the values for SBPRaceEth.df$SBP, where RaceEthnic = Hispanic.
- The Anderson-Darling Test will be applied against the values for SBPRaceEth.df$SBP, where RaceEthnic = Other.
- The Anderson-Darling Test will be applied against the values for SBPRaceEth.df$SBP, where RaceEthnic = White.

```
with(SBPRaceEth.df, nortest::ad.test(SBP))
  # Values of SBPRaceEth.df$SBP for all subjects
  # Wrap the with() function around the nortest::ad.test()
  # function
```

```
        Anderson-Darling normality test

data:  SBP
A = 70.3466, p-value < 0.00000000000000022
```

```
with(SBPRaceEth.df, nortest::ad.test(SBP[RaceEthnic ==
  "Black"]))
  # Values of SBPRaceEth.df$SBP for Black subjects
  # Note use of == and not = in this selection process
```

```
        Anderson-Darling normality test

data:  SBP[RaceEthnic == "Black"]
A = 2.2718, p-value = 0.000009264
```

```
with(SBPRaceEth.df, nortest::ad.test(SBP[RaceEthnic ==
  "Hispanic"]))
  # Values of SBPRaceEth.df$SBP for Hispanic subjects
```

```
        Anderson-Darling normality test

data:  SBP[RaceEthnic == "Hispanic"]
A = 34.5172, p-value < 0.00000000000000022
```

```
with(SBPRaceEth.df, nortest::ad.test(SBP[RaceEthnic ==
  "Other"]))
  # Values of SBPRaceEth.df$SBP for Other subjects
```

```
        Anderson-Darling normality test

data:  SBP[RaceEthnic == "Other"]
A = 3.0279, p-value = 0.000000131
```

```
with(SBPRaceEth.df, nortest::ad.test(SBP[RaceEthnic ==
  "White"]))
  # Values of SBPRaceEth.df$SBP for White subjects
```

```
        Anderson-Darling normality test

data:  SBP[RaceEthnic == "White"]
A = 19.437, p-value < 0.00000000000000022
```

The calculated Anderson-Darling Test p-value was far less than 0.05, overall, and for each Race-Ethnicity breakout group:

- Anderson-Darling Test SBPRaceEth.df$SBP p-value was less than 0.00000000000000022 for all subjects.
- Anderson-Darling Test SBPRaceEth.df$SBP p-value was equal to 0.000009264 for Black subjects.
- Anderson-Darling Test SBPRaceEth.df$SBP p-value was less than 0.00000000000000022 for Hispanic subjects.
- Anderson-Darling Test SBPRaceEth.df$SBP p-value was equal to 0.000000131 for Other subjects.
- Anderson-Darling Test SBPRaceEth.df$SBP p-value was less than 0.00000000000000022 for White subjects.

The p-values associated with these five separate attempts at the Anderson-Darling Test are all less that the p-value of 0.05, and it could be stated that the Null Hypothesis is rejected. For all five iterations of the Anderson-Darling Test for SBP values, overall and by Race-Ethnicity breakout groups, the Null Hypothesis is rejected and there is a question if the data follow the normal distribution.

The QQ plot (i.e., normal probability plot) provides additional confirmation that the data are best viewed from a nonparametric perspective (Fig. 6.8).

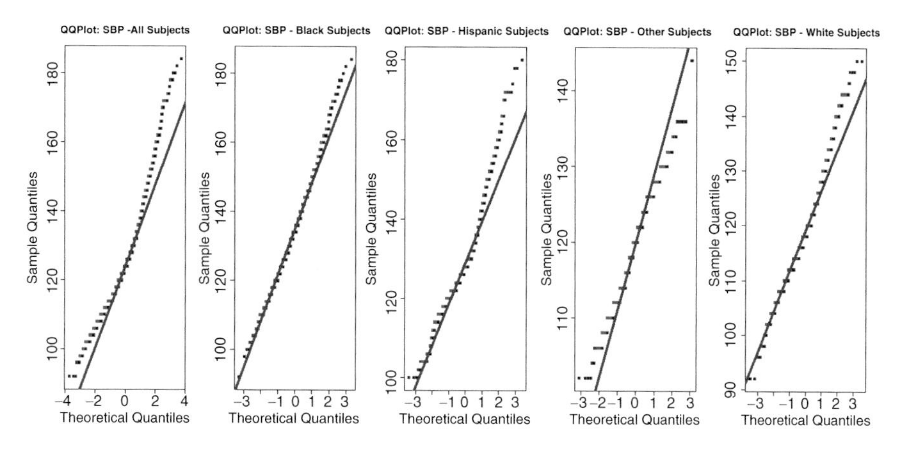

Fig. 6.8 Multiple side-by-side QQ plots based on use of the with() function for Boolean selection

```
par(ask=TRUE)
par(mfrow=c(1,5))              # Multiple Side-by-Side QQ Plots
with(SBPRaceEth.df, qqnorm(SBP,
  pch=22, col="red", bg="black", font=2, font.lab=2,
  cex.axis=1.5,                 # Adjust points in the QQ Plot
  main="QQPlot:  SBP - All Subjects"))
with(SBPRaceEth.df, qqline(SBP,
  lwd=4, col="darkblue"))                   # Adjust the QQ Line
with(SBPRaceEth.df, qqnorm(SBP[RaceEthnic == "Black"],
  pch=22, col="red", bg="black", font=2, font.lab=2,
  cex.axis=1.5, main="QQPlot:  SBP - Black Subjects"))
with(SBPRaceEth.df, qqline(SBP[RaceEthnic == "Black"],
  lwd=4, col="darkblue"))                   # Adjust the QQ Line
with(SBPRaceEth.df, qqnorm(SBP[RaceEthnic == "Hispanic"],
  pch=22, col="red", bg="black", font=2, font.lab=2,
  cex.axis=1.5, main="QQPlot:  SBP - Hispanic Subjects"))
with(SBPRaceEth.df, qqline(SBP[RaceEthnic == "Hispanic"],
  lwd=4, col="darkblue"))                   # Adjust the QQ Line
with(SBPRaceEth.df, qqnorm(SBP[RaceEthnic == "Other"],
  pch=22, col="red", bg="black", font=2, font.lab=2,
  cex.axis=1.5, main="QQPlot:  SBP - Other Subjects"))
with(SBPRaceEth.df, qqline(SBP[RaceEthnic == "Other"],
  lwd=4, col="darkblue"))                   # Adjust the QQ Line
with(SBPRaceEth.df, qqnorm(SBP[RaceEthnic == "White"],
  pch=22, col="red", bg="black", font=2, font.lab=2,
  cex.axis=1.5, main="QQPlot:  SBP - White Subjects"))
with(SBPRaceEth.df, qqline(SBP[RaceEthnic == "White"],
  lwd=4, col="darkblue"))                   # Adjust the QQ Line
```

When viewing the QQ plot, note placement of the data along the qqline, especially at the tails.

6.6 Conduct the Statistical Analysis

The preceding graphical images and descriptive statistics, both summary descriptive statistics and breakout descriptive statistics, provide a fairly good idea of Systolic Blood Pressure, overall and by the four Race-Ethnicity breakout groups as follows:

```
Breakout Descriptive Statistics of Systolic Blood
Pressure by Race-Ethnicity
==================================================
                 N    Missing      Median      Mean
Black         1000          0      134         135.1600
Hispanic      1500          0      128         130.2200
Other          500          0      120         119.8840
White         2000          0      118         119.3630
ALL           5000          0      124         125.8316
==================================================
```

With these breakout statistics (especially Median) as a guide, it is a fairly easy transition to use the kruskal.test() function to gain a more complete sense of the Kruskal–Wallis Test as it is applied against Systolic Blood Pressure and the four Race-Ethnicity breakout groups:

```
kruskal.test(SBP ~ RaceEthnic, data=SBPRaceEth.df)
```

```
        Kruskal-Wallis rank sum test

data:  SBP by RaceEthnic
Kruskal-Wallis chi-squared = 1379.141, df = 3,
                  p-value < 0.00000000000000022
```

As seen by application of the kruskal.test() function, the calculated p-value is less than 0.00000000000000022 which is certainly less than the criterion `p-value <= 0.05`. From this one test, at the overall level of comparison, it is evident that there are statistically significant differences in SBP values between the four Race-Ethnicity breakout groups.

For additional quality assurance, use a different R-based function specific to the Kruskal–Wallis Test against the data (SBPRaceEth.df$SBP and SBPRaceEth.df$RaceEthnic), merely to see if results are consistent. This type of action may not be necessary, but attention to these seemingly redundant quality assurance measures provides confirmation that outcomes are consistent and ostensibly correct. For this additional action, use the muStat::mu.kruskal.test() function.

```
install.packages("muStat")
library(muStat)              # Load the muStat package.
help(package=muStat)         # Show the information page.
sessionInfo()                # Confirm all attached packages.
```

```
# Select the most local mirror site using Set CRAN mirror.

muStat::mu.kruskal.test(SBPRaceEth.df$SBP,
  SBPRaceEth.df$RaceEthnic)
```

```
  Prentice (Wilcoxon/Kruskal-Wallis/Friedman) rank sum test

data:   'SBPRaceEth.df$SBP' (y)  by
        'SBPRaceEth.df$RaceEthnic' (groups)
statistic: chi-square = 1379.141, df = 3,
           p-value < 0.00000000000000022
alternative hypothesis: two.sided
```

Using both the kruskal.test() function and the muStat::mu.kruskal.test() function, the calculated p-value is less than 0.00000000000000022, indicating a significant difference in SBP values by Race-Ethnicity.

Accordingly, there is a statistically significant difference in Systolic Blood Pressure by Race-Ethnicity breakout groups, but where is the difference? It would be reasonable to suggest that there is a statistically significant difference (p <= 0.05) between Black subjects (Median = 134, the Median with the highest value) and White subjects (Median = 118, the Median with the lowest value), but it would only be conjecture to speculate about comparisons for other Race-Ethnicity breakout groups. Quite simply, the kruskal.test() function and the muStat::mu.kruskal.test() function do not support that type of detailed comparison, but this challenge will be addressed in the addendum for this lesson.

6.7 Summary

In this lesson, the graphics and statistics provided a great deal of information. Of immediate importance, however, it is necessary to focus on the Null Hypothesis statement and the calculated p-value in comparison to the criterion p-value:

Null Hypothesis (Ho) There is no statistically significant difference (p <= 0.05) in the Systolic Blood Pressure (SBP) of adult subjects between the four Race-Ethnicity breakout groups: Black, Hispanic, Other, and White.

```
Calculated p-value  < 0.00000000000000022
Criterion p-value  <= 0.05
```

The calculated p-value (0.00000000000000022) is less than the criterion p-value (0.05), and there is a statistically significant difference in Systolic Blood Pressure by the four Race-Ethnicity breakout groups:

```
Median SBP Black ..... 134
Median SBP Hispanic .. 128
Median SBP Other ..... 120
```

```
Median SBP White ..... 118
===========================
Median SBP ALL ....... 124
```

It is assumed that there is a difference in Black SBP (highest median value) and White SBP (lowest median value), but an assumption of significant difference for all other comparisons would be unfounded as these comparisons are not supported by either the kruskal.test() function or the muStat::mu.kruskal.test() function.

6.8 Addendum: Comparison of Kruskal–Wallis Test Differences by Multiple Breakout Groups

An advantage of R is that the user community has contributed literally thousands of additional packages that supplement the many functions available when R is first downloaded. Not surprisingly, the Kruskal–Wallis Test is addressed in some of these additional packages. A few functions from external packages are demonstrated in this addendum, focusing on the functions included in the pgirmess package and the agricolae package.

Use the pgirmess::kruskalmc() Function for Kruskal–Wallis Test Multiple Comparisons

Use the pgirmess::kruskalmc function to prepare a summary of the many breakout comparisons of Systolic Blood Pressure (SBP) by Race-Ethnicity (RaceEthnic).

```
install.packages("pgirmess")
library(pgirmess)             # Load the pgirmess package.
help(package=pgirmess)        # Show the information page.
sessionInfo()                 # Confirm all attached packages.
# Select the most local mirror site using Set CRAN mirror.

pgirmess::kruskalmc(SBPRaceEth.df$SBP,
  SBPRaceEth.df$RaceEthnic, probs=0.05)
```

```
Multiple comparison test after Kruskal-Wallis
p.value: 0.05
Comparisons
                  obs.dif critical.dif difference
Black-Hispanic  422.8452     155.4763       TRUE
Black-Other    1644.0315     208.5934       TRUE
Black-White    1760.9395     147.4978       TRUE
Hispanic-Other 1221.1863     196.6638       TRUE
Hispanic-White 1338.0943     130.0808       TRUE
Other-White     116.9080     190.4189      FALSE
```

As indicated in the column labeled as *difference*, there is no statistically significant difference (`p <= 0.05`) between Other subjects and White subjects regarding Systolic Blood Pressure.

- Note the listing of difference=FALSE for Other-White indicated that it is false to say that there is a difference between Other subjects and White subjects for Systolic Blood Pressure.
- For all other breakout group comparisons, there is a true statistically significant difference (`p <= 0.05`) as indicated by difference=TRUE.

Based on use of the pgirmess::kruskalmc() function against this singular dataset, it is possible to say that:

- There is a statistically significant difference (`p <= 0.05`) in comparison of SBP values between subjects organized in groups marked as Black and Hispanic, Black and Other, Black and White, Hispanic and Other, and Hispanic and White.
- There is no statistically significant difference (`p <= 0.05`) in comparison of SBP values between subjects organized in groups marked as Other and White.

As a general comment, the pgirmess::kruskalmc() function is well received in that the output is organized, easy to read, and easy to interpret.

Use the agricolae::kruskal() Function for Kruskal–Wallis Test Multiple Comparisons

Use the agricolae::kruskal() function to prepare a comparative test of the many breakout comparisons of Systolic Blood Pressure (SBP) by Race-Ethnicity (RaceEthnic).[4]

```
install.packages("agricolae")
library(agricolae)           # Load the agricolae package.
help(package=agricolae)      # Show the information page.
sessionInfo()                # Confirm all attached packages.
# Select the most local mirror site using Set CRAN mirror.

agricolae::kruskal(SBPRaceEth.df$SBP, SBPRaceEth.df$RaceEthnic,
  alpha=0.05, group=FALSE, p.adj="holm",
  main="Kruskal-Wallis Using agricolae::kruskal() Function",
  console=TRUE)
  # Use holm for pairwise comparisons.  Another choice could
  # have been to use bonferroni for pairwise comparisons.
```

```
Study: Kruskal-Wallis Using agricolae::kruskal() Function
Kruskal-Wallis test's
Ties or no Ties

Value: 1379.141
degrees of freedom: 3
Pvalue chisq  : 0
```

[4]Review appropriate literature on multiple comparison techniques for Analysis of Variance. At a minimum, become acquainted with terms such as Bonferroni, Hochberg, Holm, Least Significant Difference (LSD), Scheffé, and Tukey. It is far beyond the purpose of this lesson to go into explicit detail on these, and other, comparative techniques.

```
SBPRaceEth.df$RaceEthnic,  means of the ranks

           SBPRaceEth.df.SBP    r
Black               3496.133 1000
Hispanic            3073.287 1500
Other               1852.101  500
White               1735.193 2000

P value adjustment method: holm
Comparison between treatments mean of the ranks

                  Difference   pvalue sig.        LCL       UCL
Black - Hispanic    422.8452 0.000000  ***  290.65226  555.0381
Black - Other      1644.0315 0.000000  *** 1466.67610 1821.3869
Black - White      1760.9395 0.000000  *** 1635.53030 1886.3487
Hispanic - Other   1221.1863 0.000000  *** 1053.97406 1388.3986
Hispanic - White   1338.0943 0.000000  *** 1227.49381 1448.6949
Other - White       116.9080 0.056732    .  -44.99458  278.8106
```

As indicated in the column labeled *pvalue* and the column labeled *sig*, there is no statistically significant difference (`p <= 0.05`) between Other subjects and White subjects regarding Systolic Blood Pressure. Note how the p-value for this comparison exceeds 0.05, and equally note how there are no asterisks for this comparison, confirming that for a criterion p-value of `p <= 0.05`, there is no statistically significant difference between Other subjects and White subjects regarding Systolic Blood Pressure. For all other breakout group comparisons, there is a statistically significant difference (`p <= 0.05`, actually `p <= 0.001`), as indicated by the values shown in the column labeled *pvalue* and by the three asterisks (i.e., `***`) in the column labeled *sig*.[5]

Whichever test is selected for Kruskal–Wallis Test group comparisons, be sure to consider the concept of data in the large and the meaning of statistically significant differences for when p-values are observed and interpreted. In this example the Other-White p-value was 0.056732, which is greater than 0.05 and therefore indicates that there is no statistically significant difference (`p <= 0.05`) in Systolic Blood Pressure for members of these two breakout groups, but equally observe how a p-value of 0.056732 is in proximity to a p-value of 0.05.

In the ideal world, there would be stringent controls over subject selection, instrumentation, and data collection. It could be argued that it would be best if the data for this lesson were viewed as interval, yet (because of real-world

---

[5]The use of asterisks to indicate statistically significant difference goes back to when papers were typed, not wordprocessed, and a full range of typesetting options was not available. This convention is not used as frequently as it once was, but it is still used to the degree that it deserves review:

- * p <= 0.05
- ** p <= 0.01
- *** p <= 0.001

conditions and in an abundance of caution) the data for this lesson were viewed as ordinal. Would the conclusion that there is no statistically significant difference (p <= 0.05) in Systolic Blood Pressure between Other subjects and White subjects (while there is a statistically significant difference for all other group comparisons) hold if the data had been interval, if there had been more control over subjects, if there had been more control over instrumentation, and if there had been more control over data collection processes, etc.?

It is beyond the purpose of this lesson to respond to those questions, but attention to research design and the command-and-control organization of a study demands attention too. For now, it can only be stated with confidence that based on results from the Kruskal–Wallis Test, there is no statistically significant difference (p <= 0.05) in Systolic Blood Pressure between Other subjects and White subjects, whereas there is a statistically significant difference (p <= 0.05) for all other group comparisons.

6.9 Prepare to Exit, Save, and Later Retrieve this R Session

```
getwd()              # Identify the current working directory.
ls()                 # List all objects in the working
                     # directory.
ls.str()             # List all objects, with finite detail.
list.files()         # List files at the PC directory.

save.image("R_Lesson_Kruskal-Wallis.rdata")

getwd()              # Identify the current working directory.
ls()                 # List all objects in the working
                     # directory.
ls.str()             # List all objects, with finite detail.
list.files()         # List files at the PC directory.

alarm()              # Alarm, notice of upcoming action.
q()                  # Quit this session.
                     # Prepare for Save workspace image? query.
```

Use the R Graphical User Interface (GUI) to load the saved rdata file: File -> Load Workspace. Otherwise, use the load() function, keying the full pathname, to load the .rdata file and retrieve the session.

Recall, however, that it may be just as useful to simply use the .R script file (typically saved is a .txt ASCII-type file) and recreate the analyses and graphics, provided the data files remain available.

Chapter 7
Friedman Twoway Analysis of Variance (ANOVA) by Ranks

Abstract The Friedman Twoway Analysis of Variance (ANOVA) by Ranks Test is often viewed as the nonparametric equivalent of the parametric Twoway Analysis of Variance (ANOVA). Both the nonparametric Friedman Test and parametric Twoway ANOVA are used to determine if there are statistically significant differences for comparisons of multiple groups, with different factors for each group. However, it may be too convenient to view these tests as being mere complements of each other. The Friedman Test, as a nonparametric test, is used with ranked data, particularly for when: (1) the data do not meet the rigor of interval data, (2) there are serious concerns about extreme deviation from normal distribution, and (3) there is considerable difference in the number of subjects for each breakout group. The use of a block-type research design, a factorial design typically associated with ANOVA, is introduced in this lesson. This lesson also reinforces the many quality assurance measures that should be attempted before actual implementation of this type of inferential analysis.

Keywords Anderson-Darling test • Bar plot (stacked, side-by-side) • Block • Block-type research design • Box plot • Breakout groups • Code book • Comma-separated values (.csv) • Continuous scale • Density plot • Descriptive statistics • Distribution-free • Dot plot • Factor • Factorial research design • Frequency distribution • Friedman twoway analysis of variance (ANOVA) by ranks • Hinge (lower and upper) • Histogram • Interaction plot • Interval • Mean • Median • Mode • Multiple comparisons (Bonferroni, Hochberg, Holm, Least significant difference (LSD), Scheffé, and Tukey) • Nominal • Nonparametric • Normal distribution • Null hypothesis • Ordinal • Outlier • Parametric • Percentile • Probability (p-value) • Quantile-Quantile (QQ, Q-Q) • Ranking • Sample (quota, convenience) • Statistical significance • Treatment • Twoway analysis of variance (ANOVA) • Violin plot • Whisker (lower and upper)

Electronic supplementary material The online version of this chapter (doi: 10.1007/978-3-319-30634-6_7) contains supplementary material, which is available to authorized users.

T.W. MacFarland, J.M. Yates, *Introduction to Nonparametric Statistics for the Biological Sciences Using R*, DOI 10.1007/978-3-319-30634-6_7

7.1 Background on This Lesson

The Friedman Twoway Analysis of Variance (ANOVA) by Ranks Test is used with ordinal data that are placed in a factorial two-way table, with N rows and k columns. This type of organization represents, typically, a block design and is easily represented in a group (row) by condition (column) table:

```
                         Condition
                 ----------------------
                     1       2       3
                 ======================
        Group A | Data  | Data  | Data  |
        Group B | Data  | Data  | Data  |
Group   Group C | Data  | Data  | Data  |
        Group D | Data  | Data  | Data  |
        Group E | Data  | Data  | Data  |
                 ======================
```

There are many variations on the way data can be organized in a factorial group (row) by condition (column) format, but the basic theme is that breakouts (i.e., subgroups) and possible differences by breakouts need to be considered for multiple variables. In the above table, that would be consideration of breakouts for Group (Group A to Group E) and breakouts by Condition (Condition 1 to Condition 3).

7.1.1 Description of the Data

This lesson on the Friedman Test is based on a factorial study of alfalfa weevil (*Hypera postica Gyllenhal*) larvae where the incidence of alfalfa weevil larvae is viewed for five different alfalfa varieties (i.e., presented as the block in this factorial design) and four different management practices (i.e., presented as the treatment in this factorial design), using data from a total of 20 separate plots (i.e., presented as the cells or observations in this factorial design):

Alfalfa Varieties (i.e., Block):

- ALPV44NP18
- ALPV54QX13
- ALPV55QX17
- ALPV64TJ19
- ALPV78DG42

A code is used for each alfalfa variety so that it is unknown if the different varieties are experimental, recently introduced, or established alfalfa varieties.

Management Practices (i.e., Treatment):

- None—Alfalfa is cut at regular intervals, but no proactive measures are used to manage the crop.
- Organic—Practices that avoid the use of any agricultural petro-chemicals (e.g., chemical fertilizers, chemical pesticides, etc.) are used to manage the crop.
- IPM—Integrated Pest Management calls for the sound use of various management practices, all in a prudent and appropriate attempt to use a minimal amount of petro-chemicals in support of crop management.
- Conventional—Agricultural petro-chemicals are used in a prescribed approach to crop management.

Given these conditions, the five alfalfa varieties and four management practices were organized into 20 (5 blocks $\star$ 4 treatments = 20 plots) separate plots. For this lesson, there was one case of data collection for each plot.

The number of alfalfa weevil larvae in each plot was determined by using a well planned data collection process:

- By using multiple technicians assigned to field work, all data from the 20 plots were obtained on the same day, within less than 2 hours of other. This action minimizes any possible influence of variance due to humidity, sunlight, temperature, etc., on the incidence of alfalfa weevil larvae in each plot.
- It is assumed that the plots used to grow the alfalfa are equivalent in terms of support for plant growth, minimizing possible variance in growth patterns that are due to soil type, rainfall, sunlight, etc. Ideally, the only difference in final results (i.e., number of alfalfa weevil larvae in each plot) should be due to difference in alfalfa varieties and difference in management practices.
- On the day of data collection, a team of technicians (i.e., field scouts) went into separate plots beginning at approximately 8:00 AM. There was a sufficient number of team members so that data were collected from each of the 20 plots before 10:00 AM, within the 2-hour time frame for data collection.
- Each team member collected data by using a fine-mesh insect collection net on a three foot pole. A previously determined set of protocols was used for data collection (i.e., alfalfa weevil larvae) at random locations throughout each plot.
- Data were collected by making 10 vigorous sweeps in each plot, using the fine mesh net. All sweeps were attempted at prescribed random locations.
- After the 10 sweeps in each plot, technicians went back to their trucks where the entire contents for each net were deposited in a coded collection jar. The collection jar had a fine mesh covering and was kept in a shaded collection bin with a mesh covering. No attempt was made at this time to sort through the contents.
- After all 20 collection jars were obtained, the team met to count the number of alfalfa weevil larvae in each jar, with each jar representing an individual plot.
- The purpose of the post-collection process was to count the number of alfalfa weevil larvae in each jar, with 20 collection jars representing the 20 separate plots. The technicians had adequate training so that they could differentiate between alfalfa weevil larvae and larvae from other insects.

- As an additional point of interest about the established protocols, no attempt was made to distinguish between live larvae and larvae that were dead, for whatever reason. All whole (i.e., not parts) alfalfa weevil larvae were counted, regardless of state. Further, adult alfalfa weevils were not counted. Again, only whole alfalfa weevil larvae were counted.

A schematic of how the plots were organized, the alfalfa variety (i.e., block) grown in each plot, the management practice (i.e., treatment) for each plot, and the number of alfalfa weevil larvae found in each plot might help better describe how this factorial study was organized, but of course the data file associated with this study (which is available at the publisher's Web page for this book) should also be reviewed before any attempt is made to begin analyses:

```
Data Organization of Alfalfa Variety
by Management Treatment

Plot  Variety     Treatment     Larvae
======================================
P01   ALPV44NP18  None          121
P02   ALPV54QX13  None          132
P03   ALPV55QX17  None          148
P04   ALPV64TJ19  None          101
P05   ALPV78DG42  None          153
P06   ALPV44NP18  Organic       104
P07   ALPV54QX13  Organic       115
P08   ALPV55QX17  Organic       136
P09   ALPV64TJ19  Organic       094
P10   ALPV78DG42  Organic       102
P11   ALPV44NP18  IPM           094
P12   ALPV54QX13  IPM           107
P13   ALPV55QX17  IPM           128
P14   ALPV64TJ19  IPM           081
P15   ALPV78DG42  IPM           090
P16   ALPV44NP18  Conventional  088
P17   ALPV54QX13  Conventional  078
P18   ALPV55QX17  Conventional  105
P19   ALPV64TJ19  Conventional  052
P20   ALPV78DG42  Conventional  049
--------------------------------------
```

The purpose of this lesson is to show how R is used for the Friedman Test. Although it is beyond the purpose of this lesson to go into too much detail about research designs, it may be helpful to view the data from the perspective of a factorial table, using the common term *N rows by k columns*.

```
Alfalfa Weevil Larvae Counts by Alfalfa Variety and
by Treatment (i.e., Management Practice)
=====================================================
                          Treatment
            -----------------------------------------
Variety      None   Organic       IPM   Conventional
=====================================================
ALPV44NP18   121       104        094            088
ALPV54QX13   132       115        107            078
ALPV55QX17   148       136        128            105
ALPV64TJ19   101       094        081            052
ALPV78DG42   153       102        090            049
-----------------------------------------------------
Note:  As this complete block design has been
organized, Variety represents blocks and Treatment
represents the manipulated variable, or treatment.
Larvae represent counts of whole alfalfa weevil
larvae, and this datum is viewed as a ranked, or
ordinal, datum.
```

When viewing this table-like schematic of how the data are organized into rows and columns, know that the alfalfa plots are in general proximity but they were not adjacent to each other. This degree of separation was made in an effort to reduce the ease by which insects and pathogens can otherwise easily move from one plot to another. Instead, the 20 plots were distributed throughout a more than five square mile area. For the purpose of this lesson, assume that the soil type, rainfall, sunlight, and all other growing conditions were equivalent at all 20 plots.

By following this data collection method it was possible to gain a sense of the incidence of alfalfa weevil larvae infesting this crop, by variety, and to later investigate possible differences due to alfalfa crop management practices for the five alfalfa varieties included in this lesson. However, by no means is it suggested that the data provide a precise measure of insect infestation:

- Although prescribed protocols were used, it was unknown if the random locations in each plot, where the netting process was used to sweep the alfalfa, were representative of the entire plot.
- There was no differentiation in this process between stages in the life cycle of alfalfa weevil larvae. That is to say, there was no differentiation in the data counting process between live larvae and dead larvae, small larvae and large larvae. All whole larvae were counted and included in total counts for each plot.
- Note also how the emphasis was on larvae and not adults. Only alfalfa weevil larvae were included in final counts for each plot.
- It was equally unknown if the alfalfa weevil larvae data collection process was conducted before the crop was cut for the first time, second time, etc., during the growing season.

- The height and subsequent biomass of the alfalfa at the time of alfalfa weevil larvae data collection was also unknown. Data were not recorded on the height, and it is unknown if the alfalfa was low (had just been cut) or high (waiting to be cut).

Finally, a feature of this fairly simple factorial design is that it represents a one-time assessment of alfalfa variety and crop management treatment and the subsequent number of alfalfa weevil larvae. This lesson is not a repeated measures design, where data are collected at multiple time periods.

Now, with a better understanding of the data associated with this lesson, consider how it is prudent to view the data (specifically, the number of alfalfa weevil larvae counted for each plot) as ordinal data and subsequently why it is necessary to take a nonparametric approach to inferential analysis. That is to say, from an ordered perspective there is a fair degree of assurance that Plot P03 (Variety = ALPV55QX17, Treatment = None, Larvae = 148) had more alfalfa weevil larvae than Plot P20 (Variety = ALPV78DG42, Treatment = Conventional, Larvae = 049). However, given the nature of this design and the emphasis on counted larvae, regardless of state (alive or dead) and size (small or large), it is only prudent to view the counts as ordinal (i.e., ordered) data and not as interval data.

7.1.2 *Null Hypothesis (Ho)*

There is no statistically significant difference (`p <= 0.05`) in the infestation (i.e., number, count) of alfalfa weevil larvae by alfalfa variety (ALPV44NP18, ALPV54QX13, ALPV55QX17, ALPV64TJ19, ALPV78DG42) and by treatment (None, Organic, IPM, Conventional).

As the data are organized, note how numerical codes are not used for the factor-type data in this lesson. The full name for each alfalfa variety (i.e., Variety) is used and equally the proper name for each crop management practice (i.e., Treatment) is also used. Equally, the factorial design is complete and there are no missing data.

7.2 Data Import of a .csv Spreadsheet-Type Data File into R

For this lesson, the dataset has been prepared in .csv (i.e., comma-separated values) file format. The data are separated by commas. The data are not separated by tabs, and the data are not separated by spaces. As a .csv file the data can be easily sent to, and opened by, other researchers without the need for expensive specialized or proprietary software.

Start a new R session and then attend to beginning actions such as removing unwanted files from prior work, declaring the working directory, etc.

```
###############################################################
# Housekeeping                         Use for All Analyses   #
###############################################################
date()               # Current system time and date.
R.version.string     # R version and version release date.
ls()                 # List all objects in the working
                     # directory.
rm(list = ls())      # CAUTION: Remove all files in the working
                     # directory. If this action is not desired,
                     # use the rm() function one-by-one to remove
                     # the objects that are not needed.
ls.str()             # List all objects, with finite detail.
getwd()              # Identify the current working directory.
setwd("F:/R_Nonparametric")
                     # Set to a new working directory.
                     # Note the single forward slash and double
                     # quotes.
                     # This new directory should be the directory
                     # where the data file is located, otherwise
                     # the data file will not be found.
getwd()              # Confirm the working directory.
list.files()         # List files at the PC directory.
###############################################################
```

Create an object called AfWeevil.df. The object AfWeevil.df will be a dataframe, as indicated by the enumerated .df extension to the object name. This object will represent the output of applying the read.table() function against the comma-separated values file called AlfalfaWeevil.csv. Note the arguments used with the read.table() function, showing that there is a header with descriptive variable names (header = TRUE) and that the separator between fields is a comma (sep = ",").

```
AfWeevil.df <- read.table (file =
  "AlfalfaWeevil.csv",
  header = TRUE,
  sep = ",")                  # Import the  csv file

getwd()                       # Identify the working directory
ls()                          # List objects
attach(AfWeevil.df)           # Attach the data, for later use
str(AfWeevil.df)              # Identify structure
nrow(AfWeevil.df)             # List the number of rows
ncol(AfWeevil.df)             # List the number of columns
dim(AfWeevil.df)              # Dimensions of the dataframe
names(AfWeevil.df)            # Identify names
colnames(AfWeevil.df)         # Show column names
rownames(AfWeevil.df)         # Show row names
head(AfWeevil.df)             # Show the head
tail(AfWeevil.df)             # Show the tail
AfWeevil.df                   # Show the entire dataframe
summary(AfWeevil.df)          # Summary statistics
```

With these actions completed, an object called AfWeevil.df has been created and put into acceptable format for current needs. This R-based object is a dataframe and it consists of the data originally included in the file AlfalfaWeevil.csv, a comma-separated values .csv file. To avoid possible conflicts, make sure that there are no prior R-based objects called AfWeevil.df. The prior use of rm(list = ls()) accommodates this concern, removing all prior objects in the current R session.

Note how it was only necessary to key the filename for the .csv file and not the full pathname since the R working directory is currently set to the directory and/or subdirectory where this .csv file is located. See the Housekeeping section at the beginning of this lesson.

7.3 Organize the Data and Display the Code Book

After the data have been imported into R, it is usually necessary to check the data for format and then make any changes that may be needed to organize the data. For this dataset, codes have been avoided, and, instead narrative text has been used to distinguish between factor-type object variable breakouts: Variety (ALPV44NP18, ALPV54QX13, ALPV55QX17, ALPV64TJ19, ALPV78DG42) and Treatment (None, Organic, IPM, Conventional). Recoding is not needed, which is likely the case, however, when numeric codes are used to identify breakout groups.

For this lesson, the class() function, str() function, and duplicated() function will be used to be sure that data are organized as desired.

```
class(AfWeevil.df)
class(AfWeevil.df$Plot)      # DataFrame$ObjectName notation
class(AfWeevil.df$Variety)   # DataFrame$ObjectName notation
class(AfWeevil.df$Treatment) # DataFrame$ObjectName notation
class(AfWeevil.df$Larvae)    # DataFrame$ObjectName notation

str(AfWeevil.df)            # Structure
duplicated(AfWeevil.df)     # Duplicates
```

The class for each object seems to be correct, and there are no duplicate rows of data in the dataframe. A Code Book will help with future understanding of this dataset.

The Code Book is best if it is brief since it serves as a useful reminder for what can be easily forgotten months (or even weeks) later. Coding schemes that are intuitively obvious today can easily become forgotten tomorrow.

Now that the class(), str(), and duplicated() functions have been used for basic diagnostics, consult the Code Book and coerce each object, as needed, into its correct class.

```
#######################################################
# Code Book for AfWeevil.df                           #
#######################################################
#                                                     #
# Plot....................... Factor (i.e., nominal) #
#                A unique plot (e.g., field) ranging #
#                                    from P01 to P20 #
#                                                     #
# Variety ................... Factor (i.e., nominal) #
#                                          ALPV44NP18 #
#                                          ALPV54QX13 #
#                                          ALPV55QX17 #
#                                          ALPV64TJ19 #
#                                          ALPV78DG42 #
#                                                     #
# Treatment ................. Factor (i.e., nominal) #
#                                                None #
#                                             Organic #
#                                                 IPM #
#                                        Conventional #
#                                                     #
# Larvae ........ ........ Integer (i.e., ordinal) #
#      Number (e.g., count) of alfalfa weevil larvae #
#                                collected in each plot #
#######################################################
```

In an effort to promote self-documentation and readability, it is often desirable to label all object variables. First, use the epicalc::des() function and the str() function to see the nature of the dataframe. Then, use the epicalc::label.var() function to provide descriptive labels for each variable. Of course, be sure to load the epicalc package if it is not operational from prior analyses.

```
install.packages("epicalc")
library(epicalc)            # Load the epicalc package.
help(package=epicalc)       # Show the information page.
sessionInfo()               # Confirm all attached packages.
# Select the most local mirror site using Set CRAN mirror.

epicalc::des(AfWeevil.df)
str(AfWeevil.df)

epicalc::label.var(Plot,       "Plot or Field",
  dataFrame=AfWeevil.df)
epicalc::label.var(Variety,    "Alfalfa Variety",
  dataFrame=AfWeevil.df)
epicalc::label.var(Treatment,  "Treatment or Management",
  dataFrame=AfWeevil.df)
epicalc::label.var(Larvae,     "Larvae Count",
  dataFrame=AfWeevil.df)
```

Confirm the description of each object variable to be sure that all actions were deployed correctly.

```
epicalc::des(AfWeevil.df)
```

```
 No. of observations =  20
  Variable      Class         Description
1 Plot          factor        Plot or Field
2 Variety       factor        Alfalfa Variety
3 Treatment     factor        Treatment or Management
4 Larvae        integer       Larvae Count
```

```
ls.str(AfWeevil.df)
```

```
Larvae :  int [1:20] 121 132 148 101 153 104 115 136 94 102 ...
Plot :  Factor w/ 20 levels "P01","P02","P03",..: 1 2 3 4 5 6 7
Treatment :  Factor w/ 4 levels "Conventional",..: 3 3 3 3 3 4
Variety :  Factor w/ 5 levels "ALPV44NP18","ALPV54QX13",..: 1 2
```

The dataframe is now in correct format, and the labels are correct. Coerce objects into correct format. Notice how variables are named: DataFrame-Name$ObjectName. At first this action may seem somewhat cumbersome and perhaps even redundant for a few object variables, but it is actually very useful to ensure that actions are performed against the correct object. Descriptive object variable names promote efficiency and accuracy. Most text editors allow the use of copy-and-paste and find-and-replace, so it should be a simple operation to organize the syntax.

```
AfWeevil.df$Plot       <- as.factor(AfWeevil.df$Plot)
AfWeevil.df$Variety    <- as.factor(AfWeevil.df$Variety)
AfWeevil.df$Treatment  <- as.factor(AfWeevil.df$Treatment)
AfWeevil.df$Larvae     <- as.numeric(AfWeevil.df$Larvae)
```

If needed, review help pages for the as.numeric() function and the as.integer() function to see the differences between these two R functions and when it may be best to use each.

Again, confirm the structure of the dataset, using both the epicalc::des() function and the ls.str() function.

```
epicalc::des(AfWeevil.df)

ls.str(AfWeevil.df)
```

```
Larvae :  num [1:20] 121 132 148 101 153 104 115 136 94 102 ...
Plot :  Factor w/ 20 levels "P01","P02","P03",..: 1 2 3 4 5 6 7
Treatment :  Factor w/ 4 levels "Conventional",..: 3 3 3 3 3 4
Variety :  Factor w/ 5 levels "ALPV44NP18","ALPV54QX13",..: 1 2
```

After the variables were coerced, see how AfWeevil.df$Larvae now shows as numeric and that it is no longer an integer. Although it was unnecessary to coerce the factor-type object variables, this redundant action was put into place to have full assurance that all data were organized as desired.

Use the summary() function against the object AfWeevil.df, which is a dataframe, to gain an initial sense of descriptive statistics and frequency distributions.

```
summary(AfWeevil.df)
```

To have full assurance about the data, use the attach() function again so that all data are attached to the dataframe.

```
attach(AfWeevil.df)
head(AfWeevil.df)
tail(AfWeevil.df)
summary(AfWeevil.df) # Quality assurance data check
```

```
      Plot          Variety           Treatment        Larvae
 P01     : 1   ALPV44NP18:4   Conventional:5   Min.   : 49.0
 P02     : 1   ALPV54QX13:4   IPM         :5   1st Qu.: 89.5
 P03     : 1   ALPV55QX17:4   None        :5   Median :103.0
 P04     : 1   ALPV64TJ19:4   Organic     :5   Mean   :103.9
 P05     : 1   ALPV78DG42:4                    3rd Qu.:122.8
 P06     : 1                                   Max.   :153.0
 (Other):14
```

```
str(AfWeevil.df)      # List all objects, with finite detail
ls.str(AfWeevil.df)   # List all objects, with finite detail
```

7.4 Conduct a Visual Data Check

With the data in proper format, it would be common to immediately attempt the appropriate inferential analyses, the Friedman Test for this lesson. However, it is best to first prepare a few graphical displays of the data and to then reinforce comprehension of the data with descriptive statistics and measures of central tendency.

The summary() function, min() function, and max() function are all certainly useful for data checking, but there are also many advantages to a visual data check process. In this case, simple plots can be very helpful in looking for data that may be either illogical or out-of-range. These initial plots will be, by design, simple and should be considered throwaways as they are intended only for initial diagnostic purposes. More complex figures, often of publishable quality, can then be prepared from these initial throwaway graphics by careful selection of functions and arguments.

The emphasis in this lesson is on the Friedman Test for the factor-type object variables Variety (five breakout groups), Treatment (four breakout groups), and the ordinal variable Larvae. The object variable Larvae was coerced into a numeric-type format, ranging from a count of 0–200 or more. With this background, a simple graphic will be prepared for each variable, largely as a quality assurance check against the entire dataset.

```
names(AfWeevil.df)      # Confirm all object variables.

par(ask=TRUE)
plot(AfWeevil.df$Plot,
  main="AfWeevil.df$Plot Visual Data Check",
  col=rainbow(length(AfWeevil.df$Plot)),
  lwd=6, font.axis=2, font.lab=2)
  # Note how rainbow was used to select a continuum
  # of colors.  Then, note how the length function
  # was applied against the AfWeevil.df$Plot object
  # variable, to determine the number of colors to
  # use.

par(ask=TRUE)
plot(AfWeevil.df$Variety,
  main="AfWeevil.df$Variety Visual Data Check",
  col=c("red", "black", "green", "blue", "cyan"),
  lwd=6, font.axis=2, font.lab=2)
  # Note how an alpha ordering is seen with output.

par(ask=TRUE)
plot(AfWeevil.df$Treatment,
  main="AfWeevil.df$Treatment Visual Data Check",
  col=c("red", "black", "green", "blue"),
  lwd=6, font.axis=2, font.lab=2)
  # Note how an alpha ordering is seen with output.

par(ask=TRUE)
plot(density(AfWeevil.df$Larvae,
  na.rm=TRUE),    # Required for the density() function
  main="Density Plot of AfWeevil.df$Larvae",
  lwd=6, col="red", font.axis=2, font.lab=2)
```

The purpose of these initial plots is to gain a general sense of the data and to equally look for outliers or any data that may be unexpected or possibly out-of-range. In an attempt to look for outliers, the ylim argument has been avoided, so that all data are plotted. Extreme values may or may not be outliers, but they are certainly interesting and demand attention (Fig. 7.1).

Boxplot (i.e., Box-and-Whiskers Plot)

Although the data for AfWeevil.df$Larvae are viewed from an ordinal perspective, it is still useful to complete a few graphical images typically associated with interval data to gain a broad sense of the ordinal data. Graphics, such as the boxplot, histogram, density plot, and violin plot, are valued and should be used, even if never published in a memo, report, or article.

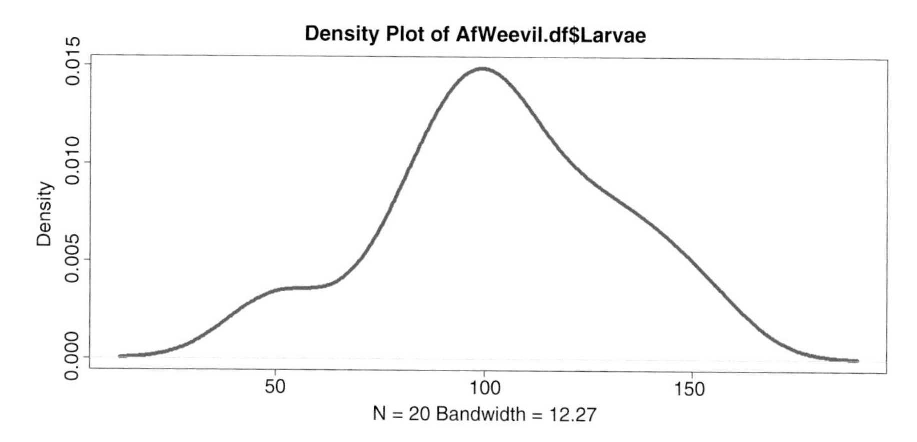

Fig. 7.1 Simple density plot of a single object variable

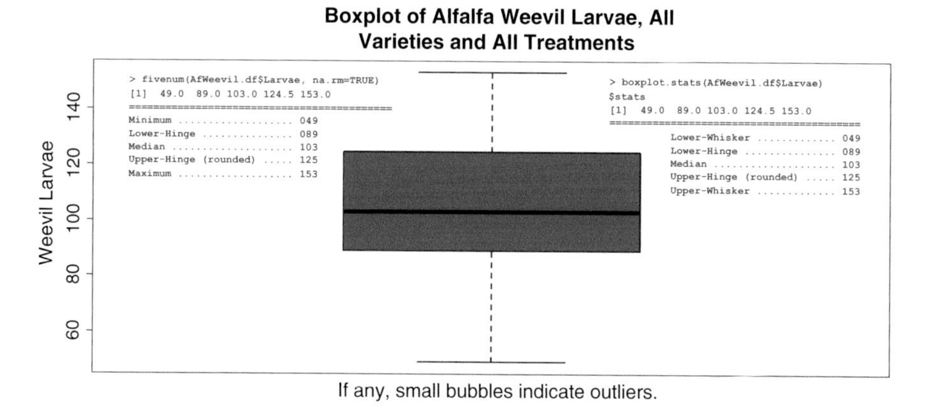

Fig. 7.2 Box plot with descriptive enumerated legends

As an interesting addition to the boxplot() function, add output from the fivenum() function (Tukey's 5: minimum, lower-hinge, median, upper-hinge, maximum) in a legend. Then, add output from the boxplot.stats() function (lower-whisker, lower-hinge, median, upper-hinge, upper-whisker) as an additional legend (Fig. 7.2)

```
fivenum(AfWeevil.df$Larvae, na.rm=TRUE)
```

```
[1]  49.0  89.0 103.0 124.5 153.0
```

```
boxplot.stats(AfWeevil.df$Larvae)
```

```
$stats
[1]  49.0  89.0 103.0 124.5 153.0

$n
[1] 20

$conf
[1]  90.45789 115.54211

$out
numeric(0)
```

```
par(ask=TRUE)
boxplot(AfWeevil.df$Larvae,
  main="Boxplot of Alfalfa Weevil Larvae, All
  Varieties and All Treatments",
  col="red",  lwd=2, cex.axis=1.25,
  ylab="Weevil Larvae", cex.lab=1.25)
savefamily <- par(family="mono") # Courier font
savefont   <- par(font=2)        # Bold
legend("topleft",
  legend = c(
  "> fivenum(AfWeevil.df$Larvae, na.rm=TRUE)",
  "[1]  49.0  89.0 103.0 124.5 153.0        ",
  "=========================================",
  "Minimum .................. 049",
  "Lower-Hinge .............. 089",
  "Median ................... 103",
  "Upper-Hinge (rounded)..... 125",
  "Maximum .................. 153"),
  ncol=1, locator(1), xjust=1,
  text.col="darkblue",
  cex=1.05, inset=0.02, bty="n")
par(savefamily)
par(savefont)
savefamily <- par(family="mono") # Courier font
savefont   <- par(font=2)        # Bold
legend("topright",
  legend = c(
  "> boxplot.stats(AfWeevil.df$Larvae)      ",
  "$stats                                   ",
  "[1]  49.0  89.0 103.0 124.5 153.0        ",
  "========================================",
  "          Lower-Whisker ............ 049",
  "          Lower-Hinge .............. 089",
  "          Median ................... 103",
  "          Upper-Hinge (rounded)..... 125",
  "          Upper-Whisker ............ 153"),
  ncol=1, locator(1), xjust=1,
  text.col="darkblue",
  cex=1.05,  inset=0.02, bty="n")
par(savefamily); par(savefont)
mtext("If any, small bubbles indicate outliers.",
  side=1, cex=0.75, font=2)
```

```
par(ask=TRUE)
boxplot(AfWeevil.df$Larvae ~ AfWeevil.df$Variety,
  main="Boxplot of Alfalfa Weevil Larvae by Variety",
  col=c("red", "orange", "yellow", "green", "blue"),
  lwd=2, cex.axis=1.25, ylab="Weevil Larvae",
  cex.lab=1.25)
mtext("If any, small bubbles indicate outliers.",
  side=1, cex=0.75, font=2)

par(ask=TRUE)
boxplot(AfWeevil.df$Larvae ~ AfWeevil.df$Treatment,
  main="Boxplot of Alfalfa Weevil Larvae by Treatment",
  col=c("red", "orange", "green", "blue"),
  lwd=2, cex.axis=1.25, ylab="Weevil Larvae",
  cex.lab=1.25)
mtext("If any, small bubbles indicate outliers.",
  side=1, cex=0.75, font=2)
```

Histogram

Due to the low N for each breakout group (N Variety = 5 and N Treatment = 4), use the histogram as a general guide, only. Of course, this syntax is entirely appropriate and should be used for object vectors where there is a much larger N.

```
par(ask=TRUE)
hist(AfWeevil.df$Larvae,
  main="Histogram of Alfalfa Weevil Larvae, All
  Varieties and All Treatments",
  xlab="Weevil Larvae",  col="red", cex.axis=1.25,
  cex.lab=1.25, font=2, nclass=10)

install.packages("lattice")
library(lattice)              # Load the lattice package.
help(package=lattice)         # Show the information page.
sessionInfo()                 # Confirm all attached packages.
# Select the most local mirror site using Set CRAN mirror.

par(ask=TRUE)
lattice::histogram(~ Larvae | Variety,
  data=AfWeevil.df, type="percent",
  main="Histogram (lattice::histogram() Function) of
  Alfalfa Weevil Larvae by Variety:  Percent",
  xlab=list("Variety", cex=1.15, font=2),
  xlim=c(0,250), ylab=list("Larvae", cex=1.15, font=2),
  layout=c(5,1), col="red")

 par(ask=TRUE)
 lattice::histogram(~ Larvae | Variety,
  data=AfWeevil.df, type="density",
  main="Histogram (lattice::histogram() Function) of
  Alfalfa Weevil Larvae by Variety:  Density",
  xlab=list("Variety", cex=1.15, font=2),
  xlim=c(0,250), ylim=c(0,0.03), ylab=list("Larvae",
```

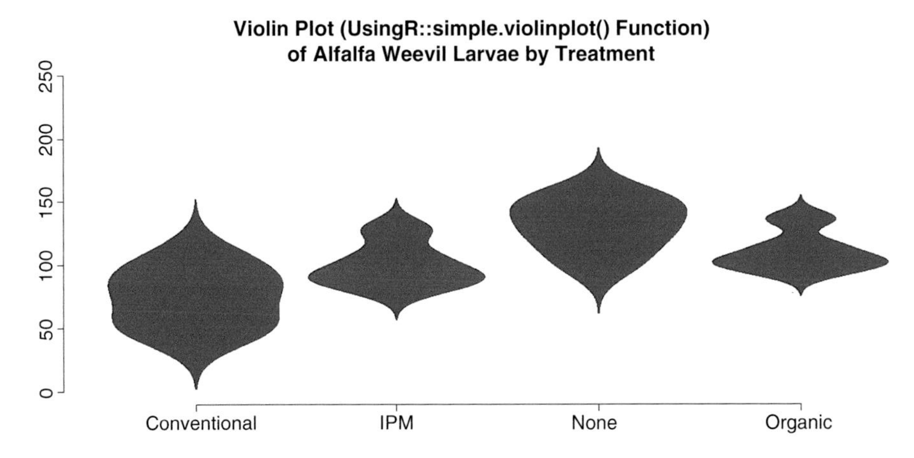

Fig. 7.3 Multiple violin plots using the UsingR::simple.violinplot() function

```
  cex=1.15, font=2), layout=c(5,1), col="red")

par(ask=TRUE)
lattice::histogram(~ Larvae | Treatment,
  data=AfWeevil.df, type="percent",
  main="Histogram (lattice::histogram() Function) of
  Alfalfa Weevil Larvae by Treatment:  Percent",
  xlab=list("Treatment", cex=1.15, font=2),
  xlim=c(0,250), ylab=list("Larvae", cex=1.15, font=2),
  layout=c(4,1), col="red")

par(ask=TRUE)
lattice::histogram(~ Larvae | Treatment,
  data=AfWeevil.df, type="density",
  main="Histogram (lattice::histogram() Function) of
  Alfalfa Weevil Larvae by Treatment:  Density",
  xlab=list("Treatment", cex=1.15, font=2),
  xlim=c(0,250), ylim=c(0,0.03), ylab=list("Larvae",
  cex=1.15, font=2), layout=c(4,1), col="red")
```

Density Curve, Normal Curve, Histogram, and Violin Plot

There is seemingly no limit to the number of R-based functions that support graphics and visualization of the data. Experiment, as time permits, with these and other functions (Fig. 7.3).

```
install.packages("descr")
library(descr)                  # Load the descr package.
help(package=descr)             # Show the information page.
sessionInfo()                   # Confirm all attached packages.
# Select the most local mirror site using Set CRAN mirror.

savelwd      <- par(lwd=4)          # Heavy line
savefont     <- par(font=2)         # Bold
```

```
savecex.lab  <- par(cex.lab=1.25)  # Label
savecex.axis <- par(cex.axis=1.25) # Axis
par(ask=TRUE)
descr::histkdnc(AfWeevil.df$Larvae,
  main="Histogram (descr::histkdnc() Function) of Alfalfa Weevil
  Larvae, All Varieties and All Treatments: Superimposed
  Normal Curve (Blue) and Density Curve (Red)",
  xlab="Weevil Larvae", col=grey(0.95))
  # Allow contrast with lines
par(savelwd); par(savefont); par(savecex.lab);
par(savecex.axis)  # Use ; to move to next line - save space

install.packages("vioplot")
library(vioplot)              # Load the vioplot package.
help(package=vioplot)         # Show the information page.
sessionInfo()                 # Confirm all attached packages.
# Select the most local mirror site using Set CRAN mirror.

savelwd      <- par(lwd=3)        # Heavy line
savefont     <- par(font=2)       # Bold
savecex.lab  <- par(cex.lab=1.25) # Label
savecex.axis <- par(cex.axis=1.25)# Axis
par(ask=TRUE)
vioplot::vioplot(AfWeevil.df$Larvae,
  names=c("Weevil"),  col="red")
title("Violin Plot (vioplot::vioplot() Function) of Alfalfa
Weevil Larvae, All Varieties and All Treatments")
par(savelwd); par(savefont); par(savecex.lab);
par(savecex.axis)

install.packages("UsingR")
library(UsingR)               # Load the UsingR package.
help(package=UsingR)          # Show the information page.
sessionInfo()                 # Confirm all attached packages.
# Select the most local mirror site using Set CRAN mirror.

savelwd      <- par(lwd=3)        # Heavy line
savefont     <- par(font=2)       # Bold
savecex.lab  <- par(cex.lab=1.25) # Label
savecex.axis <- par(cex.axis=1.25)# Axis
par(ask=TRUE)
UsingR::simple.violinplot(AfWeevil.df$Larvae ~
  AfWeevil.df$Variety, lty=1, col="red",  ylim=c(0,250))
  title("Violin Plot (UsingR::simple.violinplot() Function)
  of Alfalfa Weevil Larvae by Variety")
par(savelwd); par(savefont); par(savecex.lab);
par(savecex.axis)

savelwd      <- par(lwd=3)        # Heavy line
savefont     <- par(font=2)       # Bold
savecex.lab  <- par(cex.lab=1.25) # Label
savecex.axis <- par(cex.axis=1.25)# Axis
UsingR::simple.violinplot(AfWeevil.df$Larvae ~
  AfWeevil.df$Treatment, lty=1, col="red", ylim=c(0,250))
```

```
  title("Violin Plot (UsingR::simple.violinplot() Function)
  of Alfalfa Weevil Larvae by Treatment")
par(savelwd); par(savefont); par(savecex.lab);
par(savecex.axis)
```

7.5 Descriptive Analysis of the Data

Given the different ways missing data can impact analyses, it is often helpful to first check for missing data by using the is.na() function and the complete.cases() function against the entire dataset. Both functions return a TRUE or FALSE response, depending on the function and the outcome of whether data are missing or not.

```
is.na(AfWeevil.df)           # Check for missing data
complete.cases(AfWeevil.df)  # Check for complete cases
```

Although there are no missing data in the dataset associated with this lesson, view the output to see how these functions confirm this statement. Notice how the output would be somewhat difficult to scan if the dataset were large. For now, it is only necessary to determine if there are missing data and to use appropriate functions and arguments if there are missing data.

Especially for this small dataset, the summary() function may be all that is necessary to gain a sense of the data. As typically used, the summary() function is applied against the entire dataset, thus yielding information about all object variables, including the object variable Subject.

```
summary(AfWeevil.df)
```

As always, give attention to the listing of NAs, if any, for those object variables with missing data. Again, the summary() function is very useful, and it should always be a first selection when preparing descriptive analyses. If needed (but not always, depending on specific functions), the na.rm=TRUE argument or some other similar convention will be used to accommodate missing data.

The dataset seems to be in correct form, and to conserve space descriptive statistics, frequency distributions, and measures of central tendency will only be provided as needed. Be sure to recall how values for AfWeevil.df$Larvae are provided for what is viewed as an ordinal object variable. Because of the ordinal nature of AfWeevil.df$Larvae, an emphasis will be placed on Median, but it is still good to know Mean and SD for AfWeevil.df$Larvae, as well as a few other useful statistics.

```
install.packages("asbio")
library(asbio)                 # Load the asbio package.
help(package=asbio)            # Show the information page.
sessionInfo()                  # Confirm all attached packages.
# Select the most local mirror site using Set CRAN mirror.
```

```
asbio::Mode(AfWeevil.df$Larvae)                  # Mode
```

```
[1] 94
```

```
median(AfWeevil.df$Larvae, na.rm=TRUE)      # Median
```

```
[1] 103
```

```
mean(AfWeevil.df$Larvae, na.rm=TRUE)        # Mean
```

```
[1] 103.9
```

```
sd(AfWeevil.df$Larvae,na.rm=TRUE )          # SD
```

```
[1] 27.85281
```

```
summary(AfWeevil.df)
```

```
      Plot            Variety            Treatment        Larvae
 P01     : 1   ALPV44NP18:4   Conventional:5   Min.   : 49.0
 P02     : 1   ALPV54QX13:4   IPM         :5   1st Qu.: 89.5
 P03     : 1   ALPV55QX17:4   None        :5   Median :103.0
 P04     : 1   ALPV64TJ19:4   Organic     :5   Mean   :103.9
 P05     : 1   ALPV78DG42:4                    3rd Qu.:122.8
 P06     : 1                                   Max.   :153.0
 (Other):14
```

Descriptive statistics at the summary level are always useful, but breakout statistics are also needed to gain a more complete understanding of the data. A wide variety of functions are presented in this lesson to demonstrate how breakout statistics are obtained when using R. The key here is to discern differences in Larvae counts for the five Variety breakout groups (e.g., ALPV44NP18, ALPV54QX13, ALPV55QX17, ALPV64TJ19, ALPV78DG42) and the four Treatment breakout groups (e.g., None, Organic, IPM, Conventional) (Fig. 7.4).

```
tapply(Larvae, Variety, summary, na.rm=TRUE,
  data=AfWeevil.df) # Weevil by Variety
```

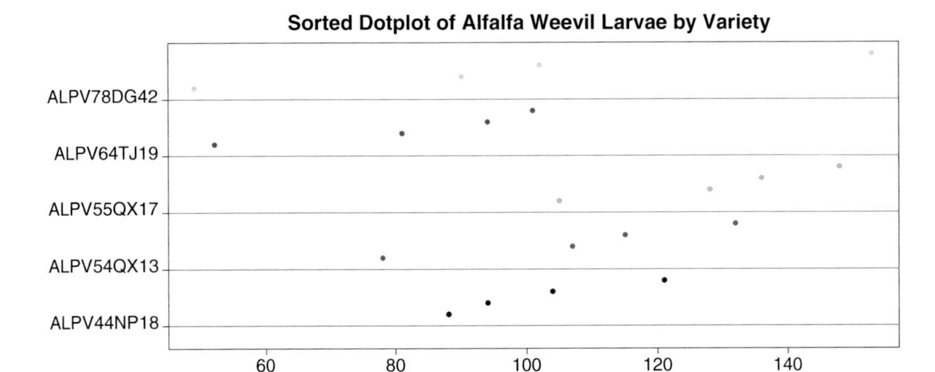

Fig. 7.4 Color-coded sorted dot plots of five breakout groups using the epicalc::summ() function

```
$ALPV44NP18
   Min. 1st Qu.  Median    Mean 3rd Qu.    Max.
   88.0    92.5    99.0   101.8   108.2   121.0

$ALPV54QX13
   Min. 1st Qu.  Median    Mean 3rd Qu.    Max.
  78.00   99.75  111.00  108.00  119.20  132.00

$ALPV55QX17
   Min. 1st Qu.  Median    Mean 3rd Qu.    Max.
  105.0   122.2   132.0   129.2   139.0   148.0

$ALPV64TJ19
   Min. 1st Qu.  Median    Mean 3rd Qu.    Max.
  52.00   73.75   87.50   82.00   95.75  101.00

$ALPV78DG42
   Min. 1st Qu.  Median    Mean 3rd Qu.    Max.
  49.00   79.75   96.00   98.50  114.00  153.00
```

```
par(ask=TRUE) # Use the epicalc package for breakout analyses
epicalc::summ(AfWeevil.df$Larvae, by=AfWeevil.df$Variety,
  graph=TRUE, pch=19, cex=1.25, ylab="auto",
  main="Sorted Dotplot of Alfalfa Weevil Larvae by Variety",
  cex.X.axis=1.15, cex.Y.axis=1.10, font.lab=2, dot.col="auto")
  # Note the descriptive statistics and not only the graphic
  # that go along with the  epicalc::summ() function.
```

```
tapply(Larvae, Treatment, summary, na.rm=TRUE,
  data=AfWeevil.df) # Weevil by Treatment

par(ask=TRUE) # Use the epicalc package for breakout analyses
epicalc::summ(AfWeevil.df$Larvae, by=AfWeevil.df$Treatment,
  graph=TRUE, pch=19, cex=1.25, ylab="auto",
  main="Sorted Dotplot of Alfalfa Weevil Larvae by Treatment",
  cex.X.axis=1.15, cex.Y.axis=1.15, font.lab=2, dot.col="auto")
  # Note the descriptive statistics and not only the graphic
  # that go along with the  epicalc::summ() function.
```

```
For AfWeevil.df$Treatment = Conventional
 obs. mean   median  s.d.   min.   max.
 5    74.4   78      23.881 49     105

For AfWeevil.df$Treatment = IPM
 obs. mean   median  s.d.   min.   max.
 5    100    94      18.235 81     128

For AfWeevil.df$Treatment = None
 obs. mean   median  s.d.   min.   max.
 5    131    132     21.059 101    153

For AfWeevil.df$Treatment = Organic
 obs. mean   median  s.d.   min.   max.
 5    110.2  104     16.254 94     136
```

Frequency Distributions of the Factor-Type Object Variables

Simple frequency distributions and descriptive statistics are needed to gain a general idea of the data. More detail and greater precision can come later. These initial attempts are simple and are only prepared to provide an initial view of the data. For any work in biostatistics consider the many functions found in the epicalc package.

```
par(ask=TRUE)
epicalc::tab1(AfWeevil.df$Variety, # Bar Plot
  decimal=2,                       # Use the tab1() function
  sort.group=FALSE,                # from the epicalc
  cum.percent=TRUE,                # package to see details
  graph=TRUE,                      # about the selected
  missing=TRUE,                    # object variable. (The
  bar.values=c("frequency"),       # 1 of tab1 is the one
  horiz=FALSE,                     # numeric character and
  cex=1.15,                        # it is not the letter
  cex.names=1.15,                  # l).
  cex.lab=1.15, cex.axis=1.15,
  main="Factor Levels for Object Variable Variety",
  ylab="Frequency of Variety, Includings NAs if Any",
  col=c("red", "orange", "yellow", "green", "blue"), gen=TRUE)

par(ask=TRUE)
epicalc::tab1(AfWeevil.df$Treatment, # Bar Plot
```

```
  decimal=2,                        # Use the tab1() function
  sort.group=FALSE,                 # from the epicalc
  cum.percent=TRUE,                 # package to see details
  graph=TRUE,                       # about the selected
  missing=TRUE,                     # object variable. (The
  bar.values=c("frequency"),        # 1 of tab1 is the one
  horiz=FALSE,                      # numeric character and
  cex=1.15,                         # it is not the letter
  cex.names=1.15,                   # l).
  cex.lab=1.15, cex.axis=1.15,
  main="Factor Levels for Object Variable Treatment",
  ylab="Frequency of Treatment, Includings NAs if Any",
  col=c("red", "orange", "yellow", "green"), gen=TRUE)
```

The catspec package and specifically the catspec::ctab() function support a very rich display of frequency distributions. This resource should be used, especially if there is a desire to copy and paste the frequency distribution table from R into a word processed report.

```
install.packages("catspec")
library(catspec)              # Load the catspec package.
help(package=catspec)         # Show the information page.
sessionInfo()                 # Confirm all attached packages.
# Select the most local mirror site using Set CRAN mirror.

catspec::ctab(AfWeevil.df$Variety, AfWeevil.df$Treatment,
  dec.places=2,
  type=c("n", "row", "column", "total"), style="long",
  percentages=TRUE, addmargins=TRUE)

catspec::ctab(AfWeevil.df$Treatment, AfWeevil.df$Variety,
  dec.places=2,
  type=c("n", "row", "column", "total"), style="long",
  percentages=TRUE, addmargins=TRUE)
```

Measures of Central Tendency of the Numeric Object Variables
Along with frequency distributions of selected factor-type variables, it is also necessary to prepare descriptive statistics and measures of central tendency for numeric-type variables. From among the many possibilities, consider the functions from external packages shown immediately below, using the fields::stats() function and the tables::tabular() function.

```
install.packages("fields")
library(fields)               # Load the fields package.
help(package=fields)          # Show the information page.
sessionInfo()                 # Confirm all attached packages.
# Select the most local mirror site using Set CRAN mirror.

fields::stats(AfWeevil.df$Larvae)
```

```
                      [,1]
N                 20.00000
mean             103.90000
Std.Dev.          27.85281
min               49.00000
Q1                89.50000
median           103.00000
Q3               122.75000
max              153.00000
missing values     0.00000
```

```
fields::stats(AfWeevil.df$Larvae, by=AfWeevil.df$Variety)
```

```
         ALPV44NP18 ALPV54QX13 ALPV55QX17 ALPV64TJ19 ALPV78DG42
N           4.00000    4.00000    4.00000    4.00000     4.0000
mean      101.75000  108.00000  129.25000   82.00000    98.5000
Std.Dev.   14.43087   22.55364   18.13606   21.64871    42.8369
min        88.00000   78.00000  105.00000   52.00000    49.0000
Q1         92.50000   99.75000  122.25000   73.75000    79.7500
median     99.00000  111.00000  132.00000   87.50000    96.0000
Q3        108.25000  119.25000  139.00000   95.75000   114.7500
max       121.00000  132.00000  148.00000  101.00000   153.0000
missing     0.00000    0.00000    0.00000    0.00000     0.0000
```

```
fields::stats(AfWeevil.df$Larvae, by=AfWeevil.df$Treatment)
```

```
                     None   Organic       IPM Conventional
N                 5.00000   5.00000   5.00000      5.00000
mean            131.00000 110.20000 100.00000     74.40000
Std.Dev.         21.05944  16.25423  18.23458     23.88095
min             101.00000  94.00000  81.00000     49.00000
Q1              121.00000 102.00000  90.00000     52.00000
median          132.00000 104.00000  94.00000     78.00000
Q3              148.00000 115.00000 107.00000     88.00000
max             153.00000 136.00000 128.00000    105.00000
missing values    0.00000   0.00000   0.00000      0.00000
```

```
install.packages("tables")
library(tables)                # Load the tables package.
help(package=tables)           # Show the information page.
sessionInfo()                  # Confirm all attached packages.
# Select the most local mirror site using Set CRAN mirror.

tables::tabular( (Variety + 1) ~ (n=1) + Format(digits=2)*
  (Larvae)*(min + max + median + mean + sd), data=AfWeevil.df)
```

```
               Larvae
 Variety    n  min    max median mean  sd
 ALPV44NP18  4  88    121  99     102   14
 ALPV54QX13  4  78    132 111     108   23
 ALPV55QX17  4 105    148 132     129   18
```

```
ALPV64TJ19   4  52     101  88      82   22
ALPV78DG42   4  49     153  96      98   43
All         20  49     153 103     104   28
```

```
tables::tabular( (Treatment + 1) ~ (n=1) + Format(digits=2)*
  (Larvae)*(min + max + median + mean + sd), data=AfWeevil.df)
```

```
                      Larvae
Treatment        n    min     max median mean sd
Conventional     5     49     105   78     74   24
IPM              5     81     128   94    100   18
None             5    101     153  132    131   21
Organic          5     94     136  104    110   16
All             20     49     153  103    104   28
```

By judgment, the Anderson-Darling Test is not needed for this set of data, given the way the data were organized into distinct plots and the low N for each grouping variable (N Variety = 5 and N Treatment = 4). It is stated that Larvae represents counted ordinal data, without any degree of assurance of an interval view toward the data.

7.6 Conduct the Statistical Analysis

The preceding graphical images and descriptive statistics, both summary descriptive statistics and breakout descriptive statistics, provide a fairly good idea of Alfalfa Weevil Larvae counts, overall and by Variety and Treatment:

```
Median Alfalfa Weevil Larvae Counts
in Rank Order by Variety
===================================
Variety                    Median
ALPV64TJ19                     88
ALPV78DG42                     96
ALPV44NP18                     99
ALPV54QX13                    111
ALPV55QX17                    132
-----------------------------------
All                           103
===================================

Median Alfalfa Weevil Larvae Counts
in Rank Order by Treatment
===================================
Treatment                  Median
Conventional                   78
```

```
IPM                                94
Organic                           104
None                              132
-------------------------------------
All                               103
=====================================
```

Using the prior graphics (i.e., boxplot, violin plot, etc.), there is certainly a suspicion (but at this point, only a suspicion) that there are differences in Larvae counts between the four Treatment groups from among the five alfalfa varieties.

However, it would be best to use an inferential test to confirm these observations and suspicions on differences. Descriptive statistics and graphical presentations are insufficient to make declarative statements about statistically significant difference.

Because the quantitative data for the object variable Larvae have been declared as ordinal data, the nonparametric Friedman Test is likely the most appropriate inferential test for this lesson, where data have been organized in a factorial block design. The friedman.test() function is used to perform the Friedman Test with blocked data (i.e., a complete block design). It is beyond the purpose of this lesson to go into too much discussion on research design, but recall that in this lesson:

- Block—The object variable Variety (ALPV44NP18, ALPV54QX13, ALPV55QX17, ALPV64TJ19, ALPV78DG42) was viewed as the blocking variable for this design.
- Treatment—The object variable Treatment (None, Organic, IPM, Conventional) was the variable that was manipulated, and, as such, the different management practices are collectively viewed as the treatment for this design.
- Data—Larvae (alfalfa weevil larvae) were counted for each of the 20 block and treatment combinations, and there was one and only one measurement for each block and treatment. This approach represents a blocked design. Note also how there were no missing data, which would present unique challenges to data analysis if there were missing data.

The friedman.test() function is associated with the stats package, which is obtained when R is first downloaded. To use the naming conventions in this set of lessons, it is not necessary to type stats::friedman.test() as the package name is only identified for external packages.

```
friedman.test(AfWeevil.df$Larvae, AfWeevil.df$
Treatment, AfWeevil.df$Variety)
```

```
        Friedman rank sum test

data:  AfWeevil.df$Larvae, AfWeevil.df$Treatment and
       AfWeevil.df$Variety
Friedman chi-squared = 15, df = 3, p-value = 0.001817
```

The immediate interpretation of this Friedman Test of alfalfa weevil Larvae by Variety and Treatment is that:

- There is a statistically significant difference in the number (i.e., count) of alfalfa weevil larvae by the four Treatment breakout groups for the five Variety breakout groups (`p <= 0.05`). The calculated p-value (`p <= 0.001817`) is certainly less than the criterion p-value (`p <= 0.05`) and therefore the Null Hypothesis is rejected.
- With a calculated p-value of 0.001817, which is again certainly less than the criterion p-value of 0.05, there is strong evidence that the number (i.e., count) of alfalfa weevil larvae is not the same for each Variety (i.e., block) and Treatment (i.e., management practice).

For further understanding of outcomes, consider the value of an interaction plot.[1] Recall that interactions can possibly mask main effects. Saying that, an interaction plot is a useful tool to examine the data and visualize outcomes from multiple perspectives. Because the data are ordinal, the focus will be on Median and not Mean.

```
savelwd      <- par(lwd=4)          # Heavy line
savefont     <- par(font=2)         # Bold
savecex.lab  <- par(cex.lab=1.25)   # Label
savecex.axis <- par(cex.axis=1.25) # Axis
par(ask=TRUE)
interaction.plot(AfWeevil.df$Variety, AfWeevil.df$Treatment,
  AfWeevil.df$Larvae,    # Note the ordering of variables.
  main="Interaction Plot (Median) of Alfalfa Weevil Larve
  Counts by Alfalfa Variety and Treatment",
  fun=median,                  # Use median instead of mean.
  legend=TRUE, trace.label="Treatment", fixed=TRUE,
  col=c("red", "black", "green", "blue"),
  lwd=4, lty=c("solid", "dashed", "dotted", "dotdash"),
  xlab="Alfalfa Variety", ylab="Count Alfalfa Weevil Larvae",
  font.lab=2, ylim=c(0,200), xtick=TRUE)
par(savelwd)        # Return to original setting.
par(savefont)       # Return to original setting.
par(savecex.lab)    # Return to original setting.
par(savecex.axis)   # Return to original setting.
```

This interaction plot should be reviewed carefully since it clearly demonstrate the order of Larvae median counts for each Treatment and Variety. Note how there is no visual indication of interaction (Fig. 7.5).

[1] Although it is beyond the purpose of this lesson on applications of R for the Friedman Test, as time permits review interaction and interaction plots as applied to factorial designs. Give special notice to the terms ordinal interactions and disordinal interactions (i.e., crossover interactions). Allow sufficient time to study the complexity of how these two conditions are interpreted when presented in an interaction plot.

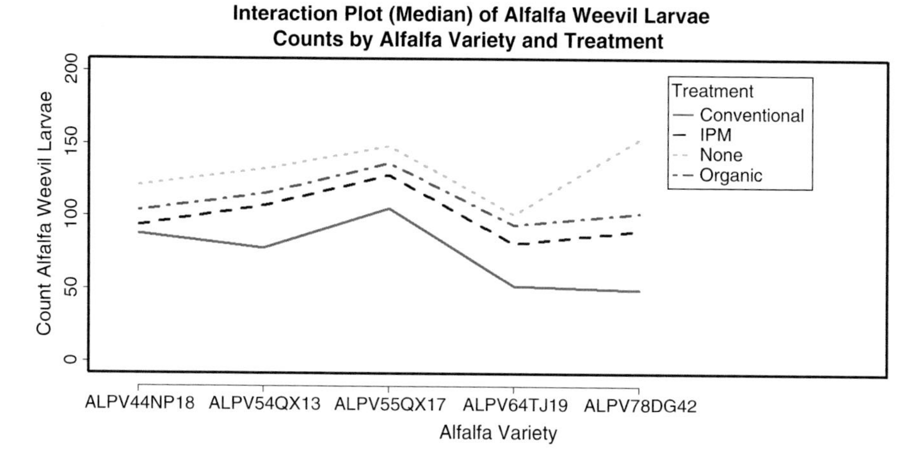

Fig. 7.5 Interaction plot of median values for multiple object variables

7.7 Summary

The graphics and statistics in this lesson provide a great deal of information for this one (but only one) study, about alfalfa weevil larvae and the influence of variety and treatment on larvae counts. For a complete summary, it is perhaps best to first revisit the Null Hypothesis. Recall that this design was organized so that Variety represented block and Treatment represented treatment.

Null Hypothesis (Ho) There is no statistically significant difference (`p <= 0.05`) in the infestation (i.e., number, count) of alfalfa weevil larvae by alfalfa variety (ALPV44NP18, ALPV54QX13, ALPV55QX17, ALPV64TJ19, ALPV78DG42) and by treatment (None, Organic, IPM, Conventional).

Application of the friedman.test() function provided ample evidence to reject the Null Hypothesis. The calculated p-value (`p <= 0.001817`) is certainly less than the criterion p-value (`p <= 0.05`), and therefore the Null Hypothesis is rejected.

Going beyond calculated statistical difference, a graphical interaction plot also provided a general view toward interaction in median larvae counts for Treatment and Variety.

When viewing these conclusions, observe the caution that replication and rigid attention to established protocols are inherent to the research process. This sample is merely one attempt in what is likely a broad assessment of issues answered, in part, by attention to biostatistics.

This lesson makes no attempt to consider the economic impact of the different treatment (i.e., management practices) options to control alfalfa weevil or yields of the selected alfalfa varieties. As readily evident from the descriptive statistics in this lesson, a conventional treatment program resulted in the fewest number of alfalfa weevils. Although it may be desirable to have as few alfalfa weevil larvae as possible, it must be cautioned that conventional management is not inexpensive. Petro-chemicals, such as fertilizers, fungicides, herbicides, and insecticides, are all fairly expensive. The advantage of Integrated Pest Management is that the benefits of petro-chemicals are recognized, but their use is attempted in a more prudent manner.

It may be necessary to also consider the ancillary cost of these petro-chemicals, both immediate and long-term costs. Consumer demand and willingness to pay for organic foods, as well as concern about harm to the environment, are growing concerns in agriculture. Imagine if the aerial application of an insecticide were used to control alfalfa weevil larvae, but in the process the insecticide drifted in the wind to an adjacent field and killed honeybees pollinating cantaloupes. For immediate concern, any gain from reduced alfalfa weevil counts could easily be lost in lower yields from the crop of cantaloupes, which would be the case if they were not adequately pollinated by honeybees. Then, consider the long-term economic cost of lost honeybees and how this has yield implications for years to come. The decision to react to statistical analyses is not always easy, given the many factors that impact the economics of biostatistics.

7.8 Addendum: Similar Functions from External Packages

R has the advantage that the user community has contributed thousands of packages to supplement the many functions available when R is first downloaded. As expected, Twoway ANOVA (using interval and ordinal data) is the focus of some of these additional packages. A few of these other R functions will be demonstrated below. The additional information gained from these external packages provides a rich understanding of the data. Experienced researchers purposely use redundant approaches to test data and to gain perspective from multiple viewpoints.

Although the friedman.test() function and the interaction.plot() function provide a wealth of information, external packages will be used to provide more granularity and a better understanding of outcomes. The agricolae (Statistical Procedures for Agricultural Research) package, the asbio (A Collection of Statistical Tools for Biologists) package, and the pgirmess (Data Analysis in Ecology) package will be emphasized in this addendum. As part of the general search process supported by R, at the R prompt, key `??friedman` to see search results about the term friedman in all R packages.

Friedman Test Using the agricolae Package

```
install.packages("agricolae")
library(agricolae)              # Load the agricolae package.
help(package=agricolae)         # Show the information page.
sessionInfo()                   # Confirm all attached packages.
# Select the most local mirror site using Set CRAN mirror.
```

The agricolae::friedman() function is especially useful in that it can be used to confirm prior use of the friedman.test() function. Perhaps more importantly, it can also be used to examine group comparisons of outcomes by block and by treatment. The general approach for this complete block design is to use agricolae::friedman(block, treatment, datum) and then add appropriate arguments.

The agricolae::friedman() function will also be used to generate a barchart. To better show similarities and differences in alfalfa weevil larvae counts by block and by treatment, an enumerated object variable (Larvae.Difference.Out) will be created to hold output from application of the agricolae::friedman(block, treatment, datum) function.

```
Larvae.Difference.Out <- (
agricolae::friedman(AfWeevil.df$Variety, AfWeevil.df$Treatment,
  AfWeevil.df$Larvae,
  main="Alfalfa Weevil Larvae by Variety and by Treatment",
  alpha=0.05, group=TRUE, console=TRUE)
) # Note placement of ending ) parentheses - rounded bracket
```

Create the object Larvae.Difference.Out, which is shown below in slightly edited format to save space.

```
Larvae.Difference.Out
```

```
Study: Alfalfa Weevil Larvae by Variety and by Treatment

AfWeevil.df$Treatment,  Sum of the ranks

Friedman's Test
===============
Adjusted for ties
Value: 15
Pvalue chisq : 0.001816649
F value : Inf
Pvalue F: 0

Alpha     : 0.05
t-Student : 2.178813
LSD       : 0

Means with the same letter are not significantly different.
GroupTreatment and Sum of the ranks
a         None     20
b         Organic          15
c         IPM      10
d         Conventional    5
```

Using Means and how they are identified by lowercase letters (above), note how each treatment group (None, Organic, IPM, and Conventional) is significantly different from the other.

Information related to the ordinal Sum of Ranks will then be incorporated as part of a legend into a barchart generated from use of the agricolae::bar.group() function. Again, this is all done to have a better understanding of comparative outcomes of alfalfa weevil counts (i.e., Larvae) by the different management practices (i.e., Treatment).

```
savelwd       <- par(lwd=3)         # Heavy line
savefont      <- par(font=2)        # Bold
savecex.lab   <- par(cex.lab=1.25) # Label
savecex.axis  <- par(cex.axis=1.25)# Axis
agricolae::bar.group(Larvae.Difference.Out$groups,
  main="Comparison (Sum of Ranks) of Alfalfa Weevil Larvae
  Counts by Management Practices (e.g, Treatment)",
  col=rainbow(4), # Above output shows four groups
  ylim=c(0,24))
par(savelwd); par(savefont); par(savecex.lab);
par(savecex.axis)
savefamily <- par(family="mono") # Courier font
savefont   <- par(font=2)        # Bold
legend("topright",
  legend = c(
  "==== Alfalfa Weevil Larvae =====",
  "               Mean  r  Min  Max",
  "Conventional   74.4  5   49  105",
  "IPM           100.0  5   81  128",
  "None          131.0  5  101  153",
  "Organic       110.2  5   94  136",
  "                                ",
  "     ==== Group Comparisons ====",
  "                     Sum of     ",
  "          Treatment  ranks     M",
  "     1         None     20     a",
  "     2      Organic     15     b",
  "     3          IPM     10     c",
  "     4 Conventional      5     d",
  "                                ",
  "               p <= 0.001816649 "),
  ncol=1, locator(1), xjust=1,
  text.col="black",
  cex=1.01, inset=0.02, bty="n")
par(savefamily); par(savefont)
```

The agricolae::friedman() function for text output and the agricolae::bar.group() function for graphical output should both be considered when attempting a Friedman Test (Fig. 7.6).

Friedman Test Using the asbio Package

To make this demonstration of how the asbio::pairw.fried() function is used to best advantage for the Friedman Test, purposely restructure the data and create a new dataframe. The dataset is fairly small so this should be a simple task. Note how numeric codes were used to distinguish between the five alfalfa varieties and the four treatment practices. Further, note how a similar naming convention was used for object names, but every object is created in lowercase. Remember that R is case sensitive, so lowercase larvae is not the same as Larvae, where the first letter is in caps.

```
larvae    <-        c(121, 132, 148, 101, 153,
                      104, 115, 136, 094, 102,
                      094, 107, 128, 081, 090,
                      088, 078, 105, 052, 049)
# Create larvae (note the lowercase l of larvae)
variety   <- factor(c( 11,  12,  13,  14,  15,
                       11,  12,  13,  14,  15,
                       11,  12,  13,  14,  15,
                       11,  12,  13,  14,  15))
# Create variety (note the lowercase v of variety)
treatment <- factor(c( 21,  21,  21,  21,  21,
                       22,  22,  22,  22,  22,
                       23,  23,  23,  23,  23,
                       24,  24,  24,  24,  24))
# Create treatment (note the lowercase t of treatment)
```

The object variable variety has been coded as:

- 11 ALPV44NP18
- 12 ALPV54QX13
- 13 ALPV55QX17
- 14 ALPV64TJ19
- 15 ALPV78DG42

The object variable treatment has been coded as:

- 21 None
- 22 Organic

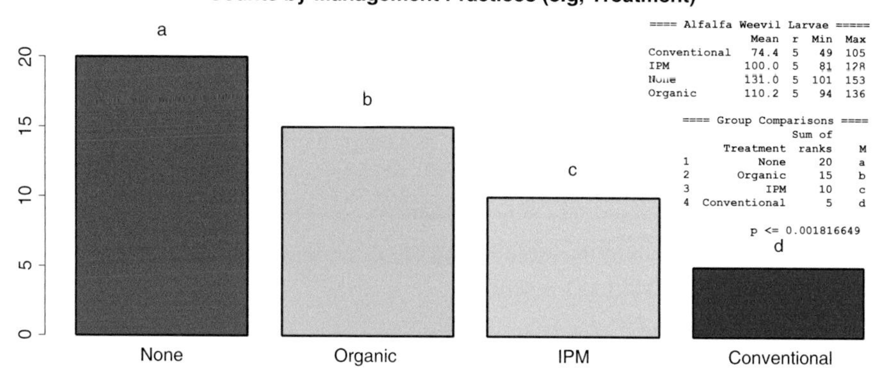

Fig. 7.6 Sum of ranks comparison bar plots of breakout groups using the agricolae::bar.group() function

- 23 IPM
- 24 Conventional

```
afweevil.df <- cbind(larvae, variety, treatment)
class(afweevil.df)
# Combine all three object variables into a matrix.

afweevil.df <- data.frame(afweevil.df)
class(afweevil.df)
# Transform the matrix into dataframe format.

afweevil.df$larvae    <- as.numeric(afweevil.df$larvae)
afweevil.df$variety   <- as.factor(afweevil.df$variety)
afweevil.df$treatment <- as.factor(afweevil.df$treatment)
# Be sure that object variables are in desired format.

attach(afweevil.df)
names(afweevil.df)
str(afweevil.df)
afweevil.df
summary(afweevil.df)
```

Now that the data are in desired format, apply the asbio::pairw.fried() function to obtain a sense of multiple comparisons with the Friedman Test.

```
with(afweevil.df, asbio::pairw.fried(y=larvae,
  x = treatment, blocks = variety, nblocks = 5,
  conf = .95)) # Use with() as a wrapper
```

The text output for the asbio::pairw.fried() function follows. Note here, similar to what was seen previously, the greatest difference in treatment ranks is for comparisons of *Conventional* to *None*. More specifically, the output provides a reminder to Reject Ho and the calculated p-value is listed as 0.001431 which is certainly less that a criterion `p <= 0.05`.

```
95% confidence intervals for Friedman's comparisons

                   Diff    Lower   Upper  Decision Adj. P-value
Avg.rank1-Avg.rank2   1 -1.15413 3.15413    FTR H0            1
Avg.rank1-Avg.rank3   2 -0.15413 4.15413    FTR H0     0.085835
Avg.rank2-Avg.rank3   1 -1.15413 3.15413    FTR H0            1
Avg.rank1-Avg.rank4   3  0.84587 5.15413 Reject H0     0.001431
Avg.rank2-Avg.rank4   2 -0.15413 4.15413    FTR H0     0.085835
Avg.rank3-Avg.rank4   1 -1.15413 3.15413    FTR H0            1
```

The graphical output of the asbio::bplot() function will help reinforce interpretation of the asbio::pairw.fried() function.

```
asbio::bplot(y=afweevil.df$larvae, x=afweevil.df$treatment,
  main="afweevil.df$treatment Visual Data Check (Median)
  With Error Bars",
  bar.col=c("red", "violet", "green", "blue"),
  slwd=6, font.axis=2, font.lab=2, loc.meas= median)
```

Friedman Test Using the pgrimess Package

As a purposefully redundant attempt to confirm prior outcomes, use the pgrimess::friedmanmc() function. Note similarities as well as differences from use of the simple friedman.test() function.

```
friedman.test(AfWeevil.df$Larvae, AfWeevil.df$Treatment,
  AfWeevil.df$Variety)
```

```
        Friedman rank sum test

data:  AfWeevil.df$Larvae, AfWeevil.df$Treatment and
       AfWeevil.df$Variety
Friedman chi-squared = 15, df = 3, p-value = 0.001817
```

Again, the friedman.test() provides overall information that there is a statistically significant difference with a p-value of 0.001817, but a comparison between the different treatment breakout groups is absent.

Use the pgirmess::friedmanmc() function to gain a sense of comparisons, similar to what was obtained by using the asbio::bplot() function.

```
install.packages("pgirmess")
library(pgirmess)            # Load the pgirmess package.
help(package=pgirmess)       # Show the information page.
sessionInfo()                # Confirm all attached packages.
# Select the most local mirror site using Set CRAN mirror.

pgirmess::friedmanmc(AfWeevil.df$Larvae, AfWeevil.df$Treatment,
  AfWeevil.df$Variety)
```

```
Multiple comparisons between groups after Friedman test
p.value: 0.05
Comparisons
                     obs.dif critical.dif difference
Conventional-IPM           5     10.77064      FALSE
Conventional-None         15     10.77064       TRUE
Conventional-Organic      10     10.77064      FALSE
IPM-None                  10     10.77064      FALSE
IPM-Organic                5     10.77064      FALSE
None-Organic               5     10.77064      FALSE
```

Again, there is confirmation that the statistically significant difference in treatment groups is for a comparison of *Conventional* to *None*. There is no statistically significant difference for comparisons of the other treatment groups, listed immediately above in the pgirmess::friedmanmc() output.

And, of course, look at the boxplots below, comparing Larvae by Treatment. Again, visual presentations should be in league with inferential analyses. Clearly as demonstrated by using the Friedman Test and the supporting boxplots, there is a statistically significant difference in Larvae counts between Treatments Conventional—None. But, again, consider the economic cost(s)—both short term and long term. Take into account the cost of management practices, the cost of supplies and application equipment, and the value of management time-on-task—and then factor in the constantly changing price of alfalfa.

```
par(ask=TRUE)
boxplot(AfWeevil.df$Larvae ~ AfWeevil.df$Treatment,
  main="Boxplot of Alfalfa Weevil Larvae by Treatment",
  col=c("red", "orange", "green", "blue"),
  lwd=2, cex.axis=1.25, ylab="Weevil Larvae",
  cex.lab=1.25)
mtext("If any, small bubbles indicate outliers.",
  side=1, cex=0.75, font=2)

savelwd       <- par(lwd=3)         # Heavy line
savefont      <- par(font=2)        # Bold
savecex.lab   <- par(cex.lab=1.25) # Label
savecex.axis  <- par(cex.axis=1.25)# Axis
par(ask=TRUE)
descr::compmeans(AfWeevil.df$Larvae, AfWeevil.df$Treatment,
  sort=TRUE, plot=TRUE, relative.widths=TRUE,
  xlab="Treatment (e.g., Management Practice)",
  ylab="Number of Alfalfa Weevil Larvae",
  main="Boxplot of Number of Alfalfa Weevil Larvae
  by Treatment",
  col=c("red", "orange", "yellow", "green"))
  # Look at the way sort=TRUE was used, to put output into
  # ascending order, from left to right.
par(savelwd); par(savefont); par(savecex.lab);
par(savecex.axis)
```

It is never an easy task to make these management decisions, but these statistical tests provide some degree of guidance and direction (Fig. 7.7).

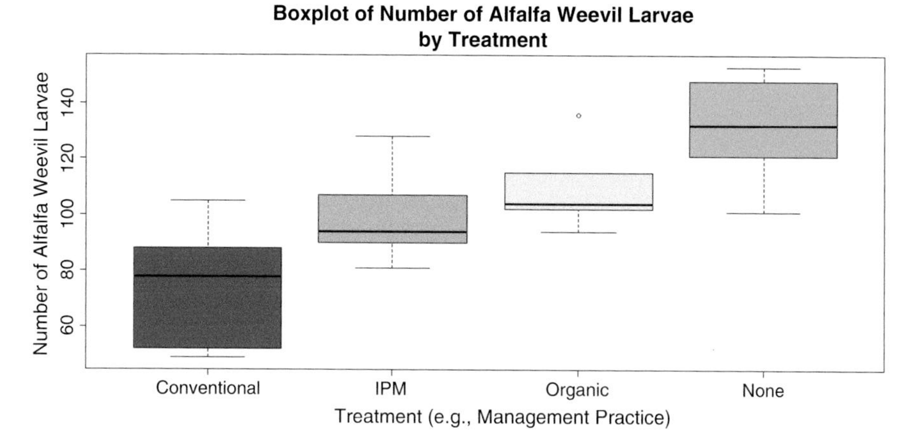

Fig. 7.7 Boxplot of breakout groups using the descr::compmeans() function

7.9 Prepare to Exit, Save, and Later Retrieve This R Session

```
getwd()                # Identify the current working directory.
ls()                   # List all objects in the working
                       # directory.
ls.str()               # List all objects, with finite detail.
list.files()           # List files at the PC directory.

save.image("R_Lesson_Friedman.rdata")

getwd()                # Identify the current working directory.
ls()                   # List all objects in the working
                       # directory.
ls.str()               # List all objects, with finite detail.
list.files()           # List files at the PC directory.

alarm()                # Alarm, notice of upcoming action.
q()                    # Quit this session.
                       # Prepare for Save workspace image? query.
```

Use the R Graphical User Interface (GUI) to load the saved rdata file: File -> Load Workspace. Otherwise, use the load() function, keying the full pathname, to load the .rdata file and retrieve the session.

Recall, however, that it may be just as useful to simply use the .R script file (typically saved is a .txt ASCII-type file) and recreate the analyses and graphics, provided the data files remain available.

Chapter 8
Spearman's Rank-Difference Coefficient of Correlation

Abstract Spearman's Rank-Difference Coefficient of Correlation is often referred to as Spearman's ρ (i.e., the Greek letter rho). It is common to read how Spearman's Correlation is often viewed as the nonparametric counterpart to the parametric Pearson's Correlation. However, that comparison may be somewhat misleading given how Spearman's is used with nonparametric data, whereas Pearson's is used with data that are more reasonably viewed as parametric. The key point to Spearman's Correlation is that this test is used to determine if there is an association between two nonparametric variables. However, as a constant reminder, be sure to recall the often used expression *Correlation does not imply causation*. There may be a correlation (i.e., association) between Variable X and Variable Y, but by no means does that mean that measures for Variable X either cause or influence measures for Variable Y.

Keywords Anderson-Darling test • Association • Bag plot • Bar plot (stacked, side-by-side) • Box plot • Breakout groups • Code book • Comma-separated values (.csv) • Continuous scale • Correlation • Correlation coefficient • Correlation matrix • Density plot • Descriptive statistics • Distribution-free • Factor • Hinge (lower and upper) • Histogram • Institutional Review Board (IRB) • Interval • Kendall's tau • Mean • Median • Mode • Nominal • Nonparametric • Normal distribution • Null hypothesis • Ordinal • Outlier • Parametric • Pearson's product-moment coefficient of correlation • Pearson's r • Percentile • Probability (p-value) • Quantile-Quantile (QQ, Q-Q) • Ranking • Regression line • Sample (quota, convenience) • Scatter plot • Scatter plot matrix (SPLOM) • Spearman's rank-difference coefficient of correlation • Spearman's rho • Statistical significance • Trellis graphics • Whisker (lower and upper)

Electronic supplementary material The online version of this chapter (doi: 10.1007/978-3-319-30634-6_8) contains supplementary material, which is available to authorized users.

T.W. MacFarland, J.M. Yates, *Introduction to Nonparametric Statistics for the Biological Sciences Using R*, DOI 10.1007/978-3-319-30634-6_8

8.1 Background on This Lesson

Spearman's Rank-Difference Coefficient of Correlation, more commonly called Spearman's rho or Spearman's, is one of the earliest nonparametric tests. It was developed in the early 1900s. Spearman's is based on ranks (i.e., data that are ranked in order) and therefore typically uses ordinal data.[1] With Spearman's, two variables are compared, using ordered series (i.e., ranks) to determine if there is an association (i.e., correlation) between them. A constant reminder with Spearman's or any other test of association is the frequently expressed caution that *Correlation does not imply causation*. It is quite possible that two variables may exhibit a strong degree of association—as X increases Y increases and as X decreases Y decreases. However, it should never be assumed, without far more evidence, that X causes Y. This caution applies to all measures of association or correlation.

8.1.1 Description of the Data

This lesson on a nonparametric view toward correlation (i.e., association) is specific to adult human subjects (N = 200) who have recently experienced some type of medical procedure and their self-rating of pain, approximately 24 hours later:

- Self-rating of the degree of pain experienced during bed rest
- Self-rating of the degree of pain experienced when standing up after bed rest
- Self-rating of the degree of pain experienced when walking—immediately after standing up from bed rest

For the purpose of this lesson it is not necessary to know the exact nature of the medical procedure. It is only necessary to know that Institutional Review Board (IRB) policy and procedures were followed and that all subjects (i.e., patients) were subjected to the same medical procedure and that five different protocols were used to provide the procedure.

For each of the 200 subjects, data on weight (expressed as pounds, not kilograms) and a self-rating of pain under three different conditions have been recorded for two factor-type groups, factor F1 (two breakout groups) and factor F2 (five breakout groups):

- Factor F1 (`F1_1 (N = 100)` and `F1_2 (N = 100)`), is represented by two separate breakout groups that constitute the two genders: Female and Male.

[1] Spearman's rho is to ordinal data as Pearson's r is to interval data. Both tests are used to determine association and both tests were developed by contemporaries, Charles Spearman and Karl Pearson. Recognizing the human element to the development of statistical tests, if time permits consult external resources to see the way both men reacted to each other, having developed similar tests for association.

- Factor F2 (F2_1 (N = 40), F2_2 (N = 40), F2_3 (N = 40), F2_4 (N = 40), and F2_5 (N = 40)), is represented by five separate breakout groups that constitute the five protocols used to provide the medical procedure: Protocol A, Protocol B, Protocol C, Protocol D, and Protocol E.

Although it may not be an issue for this specific lesson, it is useful to observe the factorial organization of the data and that there are equal numbers of subjects for each combined breakout group (F1 and F2):

```
Organization of Human Subjects in a Study of Pain
=============================================================
                            Female         Male
                            Group F1_1     Group F1_2     Total

Protocol A   Group F2_1     N =   20       N =   20       N =   40
Protocol B   Group F2_2     N =   20       N =   20       N =   40
Protocol C   Group F2_3     N =   20       N =   20       N =   40
Protocol D   Group F2_4     N =   20       N =   20       N =   40
Protocol E   Group F2_5     N =   20       N =   20       N =   40

Total                       N = 100        N = 100        N = 200
-------------------------------------------------------------
```

Although it is not the primary focus of this lesson, once again observe the factorial design of the data and the equal number of subjects for each cell. This type of organizational structure is certainly convenient for grouping purposes, with equal numbers of subjects in each cell. However, given knowledge of the population and the expected representation of subjects for each breakout group, it is immediately suspected that normal distribution and random selection are not evident for the data in this lesson and that perhaps some type of quota sampling process or other means for subject selection were used so that there would be an equal number of subjects for each cell.

This lesson also looks into the nature of how human subjects view pain. Along with the notion of no pain, imagine a binomial scale of (1) *A little pain* or (2) *A lot of pain* to express the degree of pain a subject experiences after a medical protocol. Other notions of pain could be equally presented to subjects. The important thing to remember for this lesson is that a self-rating is used to describe the degree of pain currently experienced, as opposed to more finite measures gained from some type of device, such as the way a medical scale is used to measure weight or a sphygmomanometer is used to measure blood pressure. There is no such device to accurately and consistently measure pain, thus the need for a self-rating.

Coupled with this concept of self-rating for pain is the observation that human subjects vary widely in how they can tolerate, and therefore self-rate, pain. Some subjects may express intense pain for what other subjects would view as only mild pain.

Given this background on the wide variance in self-ratings of pain, this lesson looks at 200 subjects who received some degree of instruction on a self-rating of pain, using a scale of 0 (no pain) to 100 (excruciating or intense pain). To add greater use to the opportunities presented in this lesson, pain was self-rated approximately 24 hours after a medical protocol under three conditions: (1) the degree of pain experienced during bed rest, (2) the degree of pain experienced when standing up after bed rest, and (3) the degree of pain experienced when walking—immediately after standing up from bed rest.

It has been judged that the three measures for pain in this lesson represent ordinal data, due to concerns about scale (i.e., ordinal v interval) and subject selection (i.e., possible violation of population representation and therefore violation of normal distribution due to sampling and cell population techniques):

- Although all subjects received the same instructions on how to self-rate pain and the meaning of the 0–100 scale, it is recognized that there will be variance in how each subject marks the level of pain. The 0–100 scale represents an attempt at more finite quantification of pain, but by no means is it suggested that the self-rating scale is consistent (reliable) and accurate (valid) for all subjects (N = 200) under all conditions (e.g., bed rest, standing after bed rest, walking after standing).
- Although the process for subject selection is unknown in this lesson, it is suspected that subjects were not selected at random and that some type of quota, convenience, or other process was used to populate this study: subjects who met the conditions needed to be classified as F1_1 by F2_1, F1_1 by F2_2, F1_1 by F2_3, F1_1 by F2_4, F1_1 by F2_5, F1_2 by F2_1, F1_2 by F2_2, F1_2 by F2_3, F1_2 by F2_4, and F1_2 by F2_5.

The measure for weight is definitely a more precise datum, where weight was recorded an hour or so before the medical protocol was provided, using a medical scale. Even though weight is fairly precise and accordingly represented as an interval datum, note how height and subsequently Body Mass Index (BMI) are absent from the dataset associated with this lesson. Is it possible that the pain experienced when standing by someone who is 200 pounds and 5 ft–2 in. tall is different than the degree of pain experienced when standing by someone who is 200 pounds and six feet–two inches tall?

This lesson will focus on Spearman's Rank-Difference Coefficient of Correlation (Spearman's rho). Spearman's rho is perhaps the most common test for determining if there is an association between phenomena when the data do not meet the assumptions associated with Pearson's r, such as when the data are clearly ordinal and not interval or, as some may caution, if there are serious concerns about random selection processes and distribution of the data.

Given all of this background information, the purpose of this lesson on correlation, from a nonparametric perspective, is to provide guidance on how R can be used to determine the association between two variables and then to use this degree of association to gain a sense of future outcomes. *Past behavior is the best predictor of future behavior*. This concept applies in the biological sciences, physical sciences, social sciences, and also in economics. By knowing past relationships between variables (i.e., correlation or association), it is then possible to anticipate future outcomes.

As an additional point of interest, this lesson will also demonstrate how R is used to determine Kendall rank correlation. Kendal also provides an opportunity to make sense of associations, if any, between nonparametric phenomena.

8.1.2 *Null Hypothesis (Ho)*

Because there are more than a few correlations associated with this dataset (e.g., Weight:Bed, Weight:Standing, Weight:Walking, Bed:Standing, Bed:Walking, Standing:Walking), a generic Null Hypothesis (Ho) is presented below, with this Null Hypothesis applying to all possible X:Y associations associated with this lesson.

There is no statistically significant correlation (`p <= 0.05`) between Variable X and Variable Y.

8.2 Data Import of a .csv Spreadsheet-Type Data File into R

The dataset for this lesson was originally prepared as a Gnumeric spreadsheet, based on a desire to use only free desktop software for these lessons. The data were later saved in .csv (i.e., comma-separated values) file format as Pain.csv. The data in the .csv file are separated by commas, not tabs and not spaces. As a .csv file, the data can be easily sent to and opened by other researchers without the need for expensive specialized or proprietary software.

Start a new R session and then attend to beginning actions such as removing unwanted files from prior work, declaring the working directory, etc. After this initial activity, import the data and conduct the first set of quality assurance diagnostics.

```
###############################################################
# Housekeeping                          Use for All Analyses    #
###############################################################
date()                 # Current system time and date.
R.version.string       # R version and version release date.
ls()                   # List all objects in the working
                       # directory.
rm(list = ls())        # CAUTION: Remove all files in the working
                       # directory. If this action is not desired,
                       # use the rm() function one-by-one to remove
                       # the objects that are not needed.
ls.str()               # List all objects, with finite detail.
getwd()                # Identify the current working directory.
setwd("F:/R_Nonparametric")
                       # Set to a new working directory.
                       # Note the single forward slash and double
                       # quotes.
```

```
                    # This new directory should be the directory
                    # where the data file is located, otherwise
                    # the data file will not be found.
getwd()             # Confirm the working directory.
list.files()        # List files at the PC directory.
###############################################################

Pain.df <- read.table (file =
  "Pain.csv",
  header = TRUE,
  sep = ",")                  # Import the  csv file

getwd()                       # Identify the working directory
ls()                          # List objects
attach(Pain.df)               # Attach the data, for later use
str(Pain.df)                  # Identify structure
nrow(Pain.df)                 # List the number of rows
ncol(Pain.df)                 # List the number of columns
dim(Pain.df)                  # Dimensions of the dataframe
names(Pain.df)                # Identify names
colnames(Pain.df)             # Show column names
rownames(Pain.df)             # Show row names
head(Pain.df, n=15)           # Show the head
tail(Pain.df, n=15)           # Show the tail
Pain.df                       # Show the entire dataframe
summary(Pain.df)              # Summary statistics
```

By completing these actions, an object called Pain.df has been created, attached, and initially reviewed for content and structure. The R-based object Pain.df is a dataframe and it consists of the data originally included in the file Pain.csv, a comma-separated values .csv file taken from a directory on an external F drive.[2] To avoid possible conflicts, make sure that there are no prior R-based objects called Pain.df. The use of rm(list = ls()) accommodates this concern, removing all prior objects in the current R session.

Note how it was only necessary to key the filename to read in (i.e., import) the .csv file. It was not necessary to key the full pathname since the R working directory is currently set to the directory and/or subdirectory where this .csv file is located. See the Housekeeping section at the beginning of this lesson.

8.3 Organize the Data and Display the Code Book

Now that the data have been imported into R, it is always best to check the data for format and then make any changes that may be needed to organize the data. Experienced researchers always challenge the data and never assume that the data were imported correctly, without error.

[2] In this lesson and all other lessons in this text, the working directory is consistently on the external F drive. Make accommodations, as needed, for correct directory placement(s).

The object Pain.df was created by importing a dataset that had a header row and 200 rows of data, one row for each subject. The dataset is fairly simple in terms of organization, but note how there is one missing datum for each measured object variable (i.e. WeightLb, Bed, Standing, Walking). It is unknown why these data are missing and although the missing data are few, it may be necessary to make special accommodation for these variables.

Although it may not be necessary, a rowname will be used with this dataset, which will be created by using the rownames() function. For small datasets the use of rownames may not be necessary, but for large datasets rownames are certainly helpful. The rownames() function assigns a unique identifier for each row of data in the dataset, with each row beginning with the term ID.

```
rownames(Pain.df) <- paste('Row ', 1:200)

tail(Pain.df)  # Show the tail, now to confirm rownames
```

For this lesson, the class() function, str() function, and duplicated() function will be used to be sure that data are organized as desired. As stated earlier, experienced researchers always challenge the data and confirm that all data are in good form. The class() function is one quality assurance tool to achieve this aim.

```
class(Pain.df)
class(Pain.df$ID)
class(Pain.df$F1)
class(Pain.df$F2)
class(Pain.df$WeightLb) # Note the CAPITAL L of Lb (pounds)
class(Pain.df$Bed)
class(Pain.df$Standing)
class(Pain.df$Walking)
# Use DataFrame$ObjectName notation for object variables

str(Pain.df, digits.d=6)   # digits.d argument for WeightLb
```

```
'data.frame':   200 obs. of  7 variables:
 $ ID       : Factor w/ 200 levels "Subject_001",..: 1 2 3 4 5 6
 $ F1       : Factor w/ 2 levels "F1_1","F1_2": 1 1 1 1 1 1 1 1
 $ F2       : Factor w/ 5 levels "F2_1","F2_2",..: 1 1 1 1 1 1 1
 $ WeightLb: num  165.14 168.1 167.77 175.04 169.21 176.65
 $ Bed      : int  52 78 61 57 54 61 59 72 NA 70 ...
 $ Standing: int  72 72 69 68 68 72 68 66 61 73 ...
 $ Walking : int  70 81 77 78 77 82 84 84 79 84 ...
```

```
duplicated(Pain.df)      # Duplicates
```

The class for each object seems to be correct, and there are no duplicate rows of data in the dataframe. A Code Book will help with future understanding of this dataset.

The day-to-day activities of the research and statistics process are so demanding that a Code Book is an essential aid. The Code Book is typically brief and it serves as a useful summary of the data and what the data represent.

Now that the class(), str(), and duplicated() functions have been used for basic diagnostics, consult the Code Book and coerce each object, as needed, into its correct class. A recoding-type activity will also be used for the breakout groups in object variables Pain.df$F1 and Pain.df$F2 so that later output is more descriptive and easier to read and understand.

```
#######################################################
# Code Book for Pain.df                               #
#######################################################
#                                                     #
# Variable Values                                     #
# ===============                                     #
# ID ........................ Factor (i.e., nominal) #
#            A unique ID ranging from Subject_001 to #
#                                        Subject_200 #
#                                                     #
# F1 .......................  Factor (i.e., nominal) #
#        100 subjects in breakout group F1_1 - Female #
#        100 subjects in breakout group F1_2 - Male   #
#                                                     #
#       Object variable F1 will be recoded later into #
#                              object variable F1.recode #
#                                                     #
# F2 .......................  Factor (i.e., nominal) #
#    040 subjects in breakout group F2_1 - Protocol A #
#    040 subjects in breakout group F2_2 - Protocol B #
#    040 subjects in breakout group F2_3 - Protocol C #
#    040 subjects in breakout group F2_4 - Protocol D #
#    040 subjects in breakout group F2_5 - Protocol E #
#                                                     #
#       Object variable F2 will be recoded later into #
#                              object variable F2.recode #
#                                                     #
# WeightLb................... Numeric (i.e., interval) #
#       Weight (Lbs or pounds), possibly ranging from #
#             075.00 pounds to 275.00 pounds or more #
#                                                     #
# Bed ......................  Integer (i.e., ordinal) #
#        A self-ranked ordinal measure of pain during #
#          bed rest, on a scale of 0 (no pain) to 100 #
#                          (excruciating or intense pain) #
#                                                     #
# Standing .................  Integer (i.e., ordinal) #
#         A self-ranked ordinal measure of pain, when #
#         standing, immediately after rising from bed #
```

```
#               rest, on a scale of 0 (no pain) to 100 #
#                          (excruciating or intense pain) #
#                                                       #
# Walking ..................  Integer (i.e., ordinal) #
#          A self-ranked ordinal measure of pain, when #
#              walking, soon after rising and standing #
#                   from bed rest, on a scale of 0 (no #
#                        pain) to 100 (excruciating or #
#                                        intense pain) #
########################################################
```

In an effort to promote self-documentation and readability, it is desirable to label all object variables. First, use the epicalc::des() function and the str() function to see the nature of the dataframe. Then, use the epicalc::label.var() function to provide descriptive labels for each variable. Of course, be sure to load the epicalc package, if it is not operational from prior analyses.

```
install.packages("epicalc")
library(epicalc)              # Load the epicalc package.
help(package=epicalc)         # Show the information page.
sessionInfo()                 # Confirm all attached packages.
# Select the most local mirror site using Set CRAN mirror.

epicalc::des(Pain.df)
str(Pain.df, digits.d=6)    # digits.d argument for WeightLb

epicalc::label.var(ID,        "Subject ID",
  dataFrame=Pain.df)
epicalc::label.var(F1,        "Gender",
  dataFrame=Pain.df)
epicalc::label.var(F2,        "Protocol",
  dataFrame=Pain.df)
epicalc::label.var(WeightLb, "Weight - Pounds",
  dataFrame=Pain.df)
epicalc::label.var(Bed,       "Pain - Bed Rest",
  dataFrame=Pain.df)
epicalc::label.var(Standing, "Pain - Standing",
  dataFrame=Pain.df)
epicalc::label.var(Walking,  "Pain - Walking",
  dataFrame=Pain.df)
```

Confirm the description of each object variable to be sure that all labeling actions associated with the epicalc::label.var() function were correct.

```
epicalc::des(Pain.df)
```

```
 No. of observations =  200
  Variable       Class            Description
1 ID             factor           Subject ID
2 F1             factor           Gender
3 F2             factor           Protocol
4 WeightLb       numeric          Weight - Pounds
5 Bed            integer          Pain - Bed Rest
6 Standing       integer          Pain - Standing
7 Walking        integer          Pain - Walking
```

```
str(Pain.df, digits.d=6)   # digits.d argument for WeightLb
```

With assurance that the dataframe is in correct format and that labels are correct, coerce objects into correct format as needed. Notice how variables are named: DataFrameName$ObjectName. The use of DataFrameName$ObjectName may seem overly verbose and too formal, especially for a dataset subjected to the attach() function, but it is actually very useful to ensure that actions are performed against the correct object. Descriptive object variable names promote efficiency and accuracy. Most text editors allow the use of copy-and-paste and find-and-replace, so it should be a simple operation to organize the syntax.

Along with labeling and purposeful (even if redundant) coercion of object variable structure, a set of simple R-based actions can easily be used to recode object variables, or variables Pain.df$F1 and Pain.df$F2 in this lesson:

- Even though pain is viewed as a ranked (i.e., ordinal-type) datum, change the structure of Pain.df$Bed, Pain.df$Standing, and Pain.df$Walking from integer to numeric, to allow the full set of math-oriented actions if needed.
- Transform (i.e., recode) the object variables Pain.df$F1 and Pain.df$F2 into new object variables, to have a better understanding of the data other than the codes found in the original dataset.
- Be sure that object variables Pain.df$F1 and Pain.df$F2 remain in factor-type structure.
- Label the newly created object variables (object variable Pain.df$F1.recode and object variable Pain.df$F2.recode) using the epicalc::label.var() function.
- Use appropriate R-based functions to confirm all restructuring and creation of recoded object variables.

After all of these planned actions, the dataset should be in final form and ready for diagnostic testing and later analyses.

```
str(Pain.df, digits.d=6)   # digits.d argument for WeightLb
# Structure before transformations (Bed, Standing, Walking)
# and recoding (F1 to F1.recode and F2 to F2.recode)

Pain.df$ID          <- as.factor(Pain.df$ID)          # Redundant
Pain.df$F1          <- as.factor(Pain.df$F1)          # Redundant
Pain.df$F2          <- as.factor(Pain.df$F2)          # Redundant
Pain.df$WeightLb    <- as.numeric(Pain.df$WeightLb)   # Redundant
```

```
Pain.df$Bed         <- as.numeric(Pain.df$Bed)        # New
Pain.df$Standing    <- as.numeric(Pain.df$Standing)   # New
Pain.df$Walking     <- as.numeric(Pain.df$Walking)    # New
Pain.df$F1.recode   <- factor(Pain.df$F1,             # Recode
  labels=c("Female", "Male"))
Pain.df$F2.recode   <- factor(Pain.df$F2,             # Recode
  labels=c("Protocol A", "Protocol B", "Protocol C",
           "Protocol D", "Protocol E"))
# Note the use of factor and not as.factor for the object
# variables Pain.df$F1.recode and Pain.df$F2.recode

epicalc::label.var(F1.recode, "F1.recode", dataFrame=Pain.df)
epicalc::label.var(F2.recode, "F2.recode", dataFrame=Pain.df)

epicalc::des(Pain.df)
# Labels, now including labels for the two recoded factor
# object variables, Pain.df$F1.recode and Pain.df$F2.recode
```

```
 No. of observations =  200
  Variable      Class          Description
1 ID            factor         Subject ID
2 F1            factor         Gender
3 F2            factor         Protocol
4 WeightLb      numeric        Weight - Pounds
5 Bed           numeric        Pain - Bed Rest
6 Standing      numeric        Pain - Standing
7 Walking       numeric        Pain - Walking
8 F1.recode     factor         F1.recode
9 F2.recode     factor         F2.recode
```

```
str(Pain.df, digits.d=6)   # digits.d argument for WeightLb
# Structure after transformations (Bed, Standing, Walking)
# and recoding (F1 to F1.recode and F2 to F2.recode)
```

```
'data.frame':   200 obs. of  9 variables:
 $ ID        : Factor w/ 200 levels "Subject_001",..: 1 2 3 4 5
 $ F1        : Factor w/ 2 levels "F1_1","F1_2": 1 1 1 1 1 1 1
 $ F2        : Factor w/ 5 levels "F2_1","F2_2",..: 1 1 1 1 1 1
 $ WeightLb : num  165.14 168.1 167.77 175.04 169.21 176.65
 $ Bed       : num  52 78 61 57 54 61 59 72 NA 70 ...
 $ Standing : num  72 72 69 68 68 72 68 66 61 73 ...
 $ Walking  : num  70 81 77 78 77 82 84 84 79 84 ...
 $ F1.recode: Factor w/ 2 levels "Female","Male": 1 1 1 1 1 1 1
 $ F2.recode: Factor w/ 5 levels "Protocol A","Protocol B",..:
 - attr(*, "var.labels")= chr  "Subject ID" "Gender" "Protocol"
                                "Weight - Pounds" ...
```

If needed, review the help pages for the as.numeric() function and the as.integer() function to see the differences between these two R functions and when it may be best to use each. The same applies to the factor() function and the as.factor() function.

```
attach(Pain.df)    # Redundant, just to confirm all data are
attached
```

A confirming set of functions may not be necessary, but with the attach() function used again, a redundant check of the entire dataframe is always helpful to provide assurance that data in the current R session are correct prior to actual use of the data.

```
epicalc::des(Pain.df)
str(Pain.df, digits.d=6)    # digits.d argument for WeightLb
```

Equally, use the head(), tail(), and summary() functions against the object Pain.df, once again, to gain a continued sense of the data.

```
head(Pain.df)
tail(Pain.df)
summary(Pain.df) # Quality assurance data check

print(Pain.df)
  # Observe what part of the dataset shows on the screen when
  # the print() function is used with a large dataset.

str(Pain.df)
ls.str(Pain.df)
# Note the subtle difference in output between use of the str()
# function, use of the ls.str() function, and use of these two
# functions with no accompanying arguments
```

Be sure to recall the nature of what was recoded in the dataset Pain.df and how two new object variables were created:

- Factor object variable F1 was recoded to F1.recode and the F1_1 and F1_2 values in F1 now show as Female and Male in F1.recode
- Factor object variable F2 was recoded to F2.recode and the F2_1, F2_2, F2_3, F2_4, and F2_5 values in F2 now show as Protocol A, Protocol B, Protocol C, Protocol D, and Protocol E in F2.recode.

```
print(Pain.df$F1.recode)
summary(Pain.df$F1.recode)    # Confirm recode actions

print(Pain.df$F2.recode)
summary(Pain.df$F2.recode)    # Confirm recode actions
```

Note the formal nomenclature used in this recode and the use of DataFrame $ObjectName when working with object variables. Note also how the $ symbol is used to separate the name of the dataframe from the name of the Object: DataframeName$ObjectName.

Once again, these many actions may be somewhat redundant, but this initial work is worth the effort in view of quality assurance. Every effort must be made to be sure that the data are in correct and desired format—before analyses begin. Merely glancing at the dataset, either in an external spreadsheet or by using the print() function, is simply insufficient to meet quality assurance requirements. Never work with unchallenged data. For a researcher, there are few things worse than investing hours of work and placing professional reputation on a dataset that is later found out to have errors—errors that could have easily been corrected at the beginning of a project, largely by using these many quality assurance actions.

8.4 Conduct a Visual Data Check

A constant reminder throughout this lesson is that experienced researchers always check their data and never assume that everything is in good order simply because the data were casually reviewed when first imported in the work session. The use of simple graphics is an excellent way to review data for correctness, completeness, and the possible presence of outliers.

Of the thousands of contributed packages associated with R, there are three main packages in regular use for generating graphics:

1. The graphics package is typically the first choice for beginning students since it is automatically obtained when R is first downloaded. The many functions in the graphics package are generally fairly easy to use, but eventually there are a few limits on presentation capabilities supported by functions in the graphics package. To learn more about the graphics package when using R, key the string expression `help(package=graphics)` at the R prompt to see a complete index of the many capabilities of the graphics package. As a brief note on how functions associated with the graphics package are used in this lesson, imagine that there were a desire to use the graphics-based hist() function against the object variable X. In this lesson, the expression hist(X) is used whereas for functions associated with external packages, the more formal nomenclature `package_name::function_name()` is used to implement a package-based function.
2. The lattice package is often the next choice for generating more detailed figures when the graphics package can no longer easily meet demands for visual detail and clarity. The lattice package supports Trellis graphics for R and this package is especially helpful when it is necessary to present multivariate data and relationships between, and among, object variables.[3] To learn more about the lattice

[3]Trellis graphics was originally developed for S, the precursor to R. As a concept, Trellis graphics provides visualization of complex and multivariate data in an easy to understand fashion. The term *Trellis* graphics is used because the output is often presented in a rectangular set of plots, supposedly resembling a garden trellis.

package when using R, key the string expression `help(package=lattice)` at the R prompt to see a complete index of the many capabilities of the lattice package.

3. The ggplot2 package is now another popular choice for generating detailed figures when using R (the gg of ggplot2 stands for *Grammar of Graphics*). To learn more about the ggplot2 package when using R, key the string expression `help(package=ggplot2)` at the R prompt to see a complete index of the many capabilities of the ggplot2 package. There are two general plotting functions in the ggplot2 package:
   - The qplot() function (quick plot) is generally easy to use and to a degree follows along with capabilities and structure of the graphics package but has eventual limitations.
   - The ggplot() function is somewhat complex and challenging to learn but in turn supports the production of exceptionally detailed and high-quality figures.

8.4.1 Use of the Graphics Package

Although the emphasis in this lesson is on Spearman's rho, a simple throwaway graphic will be prepared for each variable, largely as a quality assurance check against the entire dataset. Note below how par(ask=TRUE) is used to freeze the screen so that figures can be seen one at a time.

```
names(Pain.df)       # Confirm all object variables.

par(ask=TRUE); plot(sort(Pain.df$ID), main="ID")
par(ask=TRUE); plot(sort(Pain.df$F1), main="F1")
par(ask=TRUE); plot(sort(Pain.df$F2), main="F2")
par(ask=TRUE); plot(sort(Pain.df$WeightLb), main="Weight")
par(ask=TRUE); plot(sort(Pain.df$Bed), main="Bed")
par(ask=TRUE); plot(sort(Pain.df$Standing), main="Standing")
par(ask=TRUE); plot(sort(Pain.df$Walking), main="Walking")
par(ask=TRUE); plot(sort(Pain.df$F1.recode), main="F1.recode")
par(ask=TRUE); plot(sort(Pain.df$F2.recode), main="F2.recode")
  # Sorting makes it easier to look for extreme values
```

By using the `;` character in the above examples, two operations (use of the par() function and use of the plot() function) could be placed on the same line. The sort() function provides a useful way of ordering data, again to look for data that may be either illogical or out-of-range.

The graphical images serve a purpose for review but they would never be acceptable for public presentation. Consider them as diagnostic throwaway graphics. However, they have great value since they provide an additional quality assurance check of the data. Among the many ways data are reviewed, a graphical presentation of the data is a main part of the quality assurance process.

A few more simple graphical images would help, however, to learn more about the data and general trends of, between, and among the different object variables of direct importance. Look at the following way color is used to enhance the figures.

Visual Presentation of Factor-Type Object Variables

Bar charts may be simple, but they are always a first choice for displaying general trends for factor-type object variables.

```
table(Pain.df$F1)                              # Table format
par(ask=TRUE); barplot(table(Pain.df$F1))      # Graphical format

table(Pain.df$F1.recode)                       # Table format
par(ask=TRUE)
barplot(table(Pain.df$F1.recode),
  col=c("pink","blue"))                        # Add color

par(ask=TRUE)
barplot(table(Pain.df$F1.recode),
  col=rainbow(length(table(Pain.df$F1.recode))))
  # Add color using rainbow

par(ask=TRUE)
barplot(table(Pain.df$F1.recode),
  col=1:2)
  # Add color using palette default selections
palette()      # Key help(palette)

table(Pain.df$F2)                              # Table format
par(ask=TRUE); barplot(table(Pain.df$F2))      # Graphical format

table(Pain.df$F2.recode)                       # Table format
par(ask=TRUE)
barplot(table(Pain.df$F2.recode),
  col=c("red","green", "blue", "cyan", "black"))
  # Add color forcing color selection

par(ask=TRUE)
barplot(table(Pain.df$F2.recode),
  col=rainbow(length(table(Pain.df$F2.recode))))
  # Add color using rainbow

par(ask=TRUE)
barplot(table(Pain.df$F2.recode),
  col=1:5)
  # Add color using palette default selections
palette()      # Key help(palette)
```

Visual Presentation of Numeric-Type Object Variables

The histogram is a common graphical tool to display distributions of data. A set of simple throwaway histograms are provided below, with other graphics showing more detail and with more appealing presentation.

```
par(ask=TRUE);
hist(Pain.df$WeightLb, main="Weight", col="red", breaks=20)

par(ask=TRUE);
hist(Pain.df$Bed, main="Bed", col="red", breaks=20)

par(ask=TRUE);
hist(Pain.df$Standing, main="Standing", col="red", breaks=20)

par(ask=TRUE);
hist(Pain.df$Walking, main="Walking", col="red", breaks=20)
```

After viewing these throwaway diagnostic histograms, observe how there has been no attempt to embellish either the X axis or the Y axis, possibly by placing a more descriptive label on either axis and making axis labels show in either bold or a contrasting color. There has equally been no attempt to adjust the scale shown on the X axis. Instead, R-based defaults were accepted. These embellishments will be attempted in later figures.

The density plot is very useful to look for a general display of the data. The density plot visualizes distribution patterns and adherence to any semblance of normal distribution, which is a critical concern regarding the decision to view data from a nonparametric perspective or a parametric perspective.

```
par(ask=TRUE)
plot(density(Pain.df$WeightLb,
  na.rm=TRUE),    # Required for the density() function
  main="Density Plot of Weight", lwd=6,
  col="red", font.axis=2, font.lab=2, xlim=c(-10,300))

par(ask=TRUE)
plot(density(Pain.df$Bed,
  na.rm=TRUE),    # Required for the density() function
  main="Density Plot of Pain During Bed Rest", lwd=6,
  col="red", font.axis=2, font.lab=2, xlim=c(-10,110))

par(ask=TRUE)
plot(density(Pain.df$Standing,
  na.rm=TRUE),    # Required for the density() function
  main="Density Plot of Pain When Standing", lwd=6,
  col="red", font.axis=2, font.lab=2, xlim=c(-10,110))

par(ask=TRUE)
plot(density(Pain.df$Walking,
  na.rm=TRUE),    # Required for the density() function
  main="Density Plot of Pain When Walking", lwd=6,
  col="red", font.axis=2, font.lab=2, xlim=c(-10,110))
```

Note how the values for xlim are used to accommodate presentation of the full range of values on the X axis when shown in graphical format.

The boxplot (i.e., box-and-whisker plot) is a traditional tool for viewing the distribution of data, with an emphasis on standard descriptive statistics. See help pages for the fivenum() function and the boxplot.stats() function, along with the boxplot() function, to learn more about this visual tool.

```
par(ask=TRUE)
boxplot(Pain.df$WeightLb,
  main="Boxplot of Weight",
  col="red", lwd=2, cex.axis=1.25,
  ylab="Weight (Pounds)", cex.lab=1.25,
  ylim=c(0,300))           # Note the scale used for the Y axis

par(ask=TRUE)
boxplot(Pain.df$Bed,
  main="Boxplot of Pain at Bed Rest",
  col="red", lwd=2, cex.axis=1.25,
  ylab="Pain (0 to 100)", cex.lab=1.25,
  ylim=c(-5,105))          # Note the scale used for the Y axis

par(ask=TRUE)
boxplot(Pain.df$Standing,
  main="Boxplot of Pain When Standing",
  col="red", lwd=2, cex.axis=1.25,
  ylab="Pain (0 to 100)", cex.lab=1.25,
  ylim=c(-5,105))          # Note the scale used for the Y axis

par(ask=TRUE)
boxplot(Pain.df$Walking,
  main="Boxplot of Pain When Walking",
  col="red", lwd=2, cex.axis=1.25,
  ylab="Pain (0 to 100)", cex.lab=1.25,
  ylim=c(-5,105))          # Note the scale used for the Y axis
```

The three boxplots of pain (i.e., Bed, Standing, Walking) are interesting, and they give a sense that pain increases with increased mobility. Yet, the three boxplots are in separate graphics. The procedure used below will place all three boxplots in the same figure.

- Use the names() function to see the names for each object variable in the dataframe, and then give attention to the sequential ordering of each object variable.
- Note how Pain.df$Bed is the 5th object variable, Pain.df$Standing is the 6th object variable, and Pain.df$Walking is the 7th object variable.
- Use the `[, Starting_Column_Number:Ending_Column_Number]` naming scheme shown below to include all three object variables in the same figure, generating boxplots in this example.

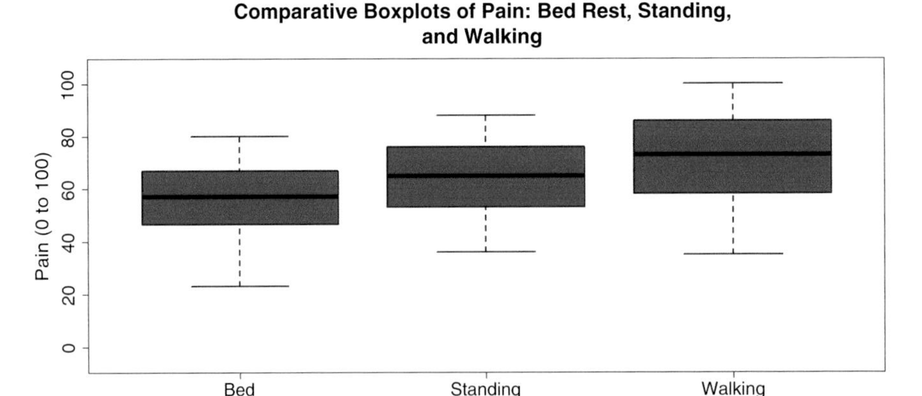

Fig. 8.1 Comparative box plots of separate object variables

```
names(Pain.df)

par(ask=TRUE)
boxplot(Pain.df[, 5:7],                    # Variables 5 to 7
  main="Comparative Boxplots of Pain:  Bed Rest, Standing,
  and Walking",
  col="red", lwd=2, cex.axis=1.25,
  ylab="Pain (0 to 100)", cex.lab=1.25,
  ylim=c(-5,105))          # Note the scale used for the Y axis
```

This side-by-side presentation of boxplots for all three object variables (Bed, Standing, Walking), for comparative purposes, is far more useful than three separate boxplots. Support for these multiple comparisons is an advantage for R (Fig. 8.1).

This lesson is focused on correlation (i.e., association) and the desire to see if there is an association between Variable X and Variable Y. Specifically, this lesson is focused on the use of Spearman's rho to accommodate correlation calculations, since it is judged that the pain-specific data (Pain.df$Bed, Pain.df$Standing, Pain.df$Walking) are ordinal and not interval. Recall, also, how there is a concern about data distribution and the possible impact that this construct may have on acceptance or rejection of nonparametric v parametric approaches to data analysis.

The plot() function will be used to generate basic scatter plots to show the correlation or degree of association between Variable X and Variable Y:

- WeightLb:Bed, WeightLb:Standing, WeightLb:Walking
- Bed:Standing, Bed:Walking
- Standing:Walking

Simple scatter plots will be produced first. A few embellishments will be added to make the figures both more appealing and more descriptive.

```
par(ask=TRUE)
par(mfrow=c(1,3))        # 1 Row by 3 Columns
plot(Pain.df$WeightLb, Pain.df$Bed,
  main="Weight by Bed",
  xlim=c(0,300), ylim=c(0,100))
plot(Pain.df$WeightLb, Pain.df$Standing,
  main="Weight by Standing",
  xlim=c(0,300), ylim=c(0,100))
plot(Pain.df$WeightLb, Pain.df$Walking,
  main="Weight by Walking",
  xlim=c(0,300), ylim=c(0,100))

par(ask=TRUE)
par(mfrow=c(1,2))        # 1 Row by 2 Columns
plot(Pain.df$Bed, Pain.df$Standing,
  main="Bed by Standing",
  xlim=c(0,100), ylim=c(0,100))
plot(Pain.df$Bed, Pain.df$Walking,
  main="Bed by Walking",
  xlim=c(0,100), ylim=c(0,100))

par(ask=TRUE)
plot(Pain.df$Standing, Pain.df$Walking,
  main="Standing by Walking",
  xlim=c(0,100), ylim=c(0,100))
```

Notice in these simple throwaway scatter plots how the figures were organized so that there would be no redundant comparisons. Is a scatter plot of Variable X by Variable Y equal to a scatter plot of Variable Y by Variable X, where only the X axis and Y axis are exchanged?

Now, embellish the scatter plots, offering more appeal and detail. Improve the presentation of the axis, add color, enlarge the symbol used for points in the plot, and add an abline (i.e., regression line), highlighting the intercept and slope.

Note: When viewing these embellished scatter plots, give attention to the abline, also known as a regression line. There are those who suggest that an abline should not be presented for scatter plots that are based on the use of nonparametric data. The figures below include ablines, but consider this caution when determining their appropriate use. Of course, the abline could be easily eliminated, either by eliminating the syntax for this addition to the scatter plot or merely by placing a # character in front of the abline-specific syntax, to *comment-out* the syntax (Fig. 8.2).

```
par(ask=TRUE)
par(mfrow=c(1,3))                          # 1 Row by 3 Columns
plot(Pain.df$WeightLb, Pain.df$Bed,          # X axis by Y axis
  xlab="Weight (Pounds)", ylab="Pain at Bed Rest",
  main="Scatter Plot of Weight by Pain at Best Rest
  With Regression Line",
  pch=23, lwd=4, col="red", cex.axis=1.25, cex.lab=1.25,
  font=2, xlim=c(0,300), ylim=c(-010,110))
abline(lm(Pain.df$Bed ~ Pain.df$WeightLb),
```

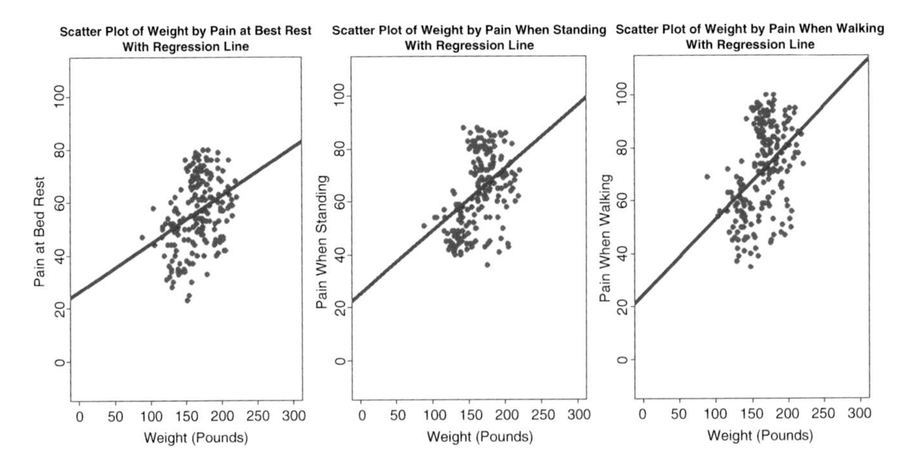

Fig. 8.2 Multiple scatter plots of separate object variables placed into one graphical figure

```
  lwd=6, col="blue")                     # Note abline(lm(Y ~ X))
plot(Pain.df$WeightLb, Pain.df$Standing,     # X axis by Y axis
  xlab="Weight (Pounds)", ylab="Pain When Standing",
  main="Scatter Plot of Weight by Pain When Standing
  With Regression Line",
  pch=23, lwd=4, col="red", cex.axis=1.25, cex.lab=1.25,
  font=2, xlim=c(0,300), ylim=c(-010,110))
abline(lm(Pain.df$Standing ~ Pain.df$WeightLb),
  lwd=6, col="blue")                     # Note abline(lm(Y ~ X))
plot(Pain.df$WeightLb, Pain.df$Walking,      # X axis by Y axis
  xlab="Weight (Pounds)", ylab="Pain When Walking",
  main="Scatter Plot of Weight by Pain When Walking
  With Regression Line",
  pch=23, lwd=4, col="red", cex.axis=1.25, cex.lab=1.25,
  font=2, xlim=c(0,300), ylim=c(-010,110))
abline(lm(Pain.df$Walking ~ Pain.df$WeightLb),
  lwd=6, col="blue")                     # Note abline(lm(Y ~ X))
```

```
par(ask=TRUE)
par(mfrow=c(1,2))                          # 1 Row by 2 Columns
plot(Pain.df$Bed, Pain.df$Standing,          # X axis by Y axis
  xlab="Pain at Bed Rest", ylab="Pain When Standing",
  main="Scatter Plot of Pain at Bed Rest by
  Pain When Standing With Regression Line",
  pch=23, lwd=4, col="red", cex.axis=1.25, cex.lab=1.25,
  font=2, xlim=c(-010,110), ylim=c(-010,110))
abline(lm(Pain.df$Standing ~ Pain.df$Bed),
  lwd=6, col="blue")                     # Note abline(lm(Y ~ X))
plot(Pain.df$Bed, Pain.df$Walking,           # X axis by Y axis
  xlab="Pain at Bed Rest", ylab="Pain When Walking",
  main="Scatter Plot of Pain at Bed Rest by
  Pain When Walking With Regression Line",
  pch=23, lwd=4, col="red", cex.axis=1.25, cex.lab=1.25,
```

```
  font=2, xlim=c(-010,110), ylim=c(-010,110))
abline(lm(Pain.df$Walking ~ Pain.df$Bed),
  lwd=6, col="blue")                   # Note abline(lm(Y ~ X))

plot(Pain.df$Standing, Pain.df$Walking,     # X axis by Y axis
  xlab="Pain When Standing", ylab="Pain When Walking",
  main="Scatter Plot pf Pain When Standing by
  Pain When Walking With Regression Line",
  pch=23, lwd=4, col="red", cex.axis=1.25, cex.lab=1.25,
  font=2, xlim=c(-010,110), ylim=c(-010,110))
abline(lm(Pain.df$Walking ~ Pain.df$Standing),
  lwd=6, col="blue")                   # Note abline(lm(Y ~ X))
```

The purpose of these initial scatter plots is to gain a general sense of the data, individually and with the possible association between different object variables. It was also useful to use these scatter plots to look for outliers. In an attempt to look for outliers, notice how the xlim values and ylim values were extended beyond what is found in the Code Book. Extreme values may or may not be outliers, but they are certainly interesting and demand attention, to determine if they represent a mistake with data entry or if they are valid data, but data that were totally unexpected.

8.4.2 *Use of the Lattice Package*

The lattice package supports a wide variety of functions that are used to show relationships between, and among, data. The lattice::densityplot() function is often a good first choice to better understand measured data. With additional practice, the lattice package can be used to display density plots by breakout groups—Gender and Protocol in this lesson.

```
install.packages("lattice")
library(lattice)              # Load the lattice package.
help(package=lattice)         # Show the information page.
sessionInfo()                 # Confirm all attached packages.
# Select the most local mirror site using Set CRAN mirror.

par(ask=TRUE)
lattice::densityplot(~ WeightLb, data=Pain.df,
  plot.points=TRUE, auto.key=TRUE,
  par.settings=simpleTheme(lwd=4),
  par.strip.text=list(cex=1.15, font=2),
  scales=list(cex=1.15),
  main="Density Plot of Weight",
  xlab=list("Weight (Pounds)", cex=1.15, font=2),
  xlim=c(0,300), # Note the range.
  ylab=list("Density", cex=1.15, font=2),
  aspect=1, breaks=10)
```

By using the above syntax, but with only a few minor changes, the lattice::densityplot() function can be used to display density plots for the other measured object variables used in this lesson.

The lattice::bwplot() function is used to generate boxplots by breakout groups, which in turn provide a simple way to compare distribution patterns for an individual object variable, allowing focus on overall distribution and attention to extreme values (i.e., outliers), if any.

Note below the 2 Columns by 1 Row figure used to show Gender by Protocol boxplot comparisons for Pain at Bed Rest. The 5 Columns by 1 Row figure shows Protocol by Gender boxplot comparisons for Pain at Bed Rest. Again, the other measured variables used in this lesson can be compared by the factor-type variables, all by changing only a few lines of syntax (i.e., code), but space does not allow syntax for every possible comparison (Fig. 8.3).

```
par(ask=TRUE)                                  # 2 Columns by 1 Row
lattice::bwplot(F2.recode ~ Bed | F1.recode,
  data=Pain.df,
  plot.points=TRUE, auto.key=TRUE,
  par.settings=simpleTheme(lwd=2),
  par.strip.text=list(cex=1.15, font=2),
  scales=list(cex=1.15),
  main="Boxplot of Pain at Bed Rest by Gender
  and by Protocol",
  xlab=list("Pain (0 to 100)", cex=1.15, font=2),
  xlim=c(-015,115), # Note the range.
  ylab=list("Protocol", cex=1.15, font=2),
  aspect=1, breaks=10,
  layout = c(2,1))                             # 2 Columns by 1 Row
```

```
par(ask=TRUE)                                  # 5 Columns by 1 Row
lattice::bwplot(F1.recode ~ Bed | F2.recode,
  data=Pain.df,
  plot.points=TRUE, auto.key=TRUE,
  par.settings=simpleTheme(lwd=2),
  par.strip.text=list(cex=1.15, font=2),
  scales=list(cex=1.15),
  main="Boxplot of Pain at Bed Rest by Protocol
  and by Gender",
  xlab=list("Pain (0 to 100)", cex=1.15, font=2),
  xlim=c(-015,115), # Note the range.
  ylab=list("Gender", cex=1.15, font=2),
  aspect=1, breaks=10,
  layout = c(5,1))                             # 5 Columns by 1 Row
```

This lesson is focused on correlation (i.e., association). Review how the lattice package can be used to provide side-by-side scatter plots of X and Y by factor-type breakout object variables.

```
par(ask=TRUE)                                  # 2 Columns by 1 Row
lattice::xyplot(Standing ~ Bed | F1.recode,
```

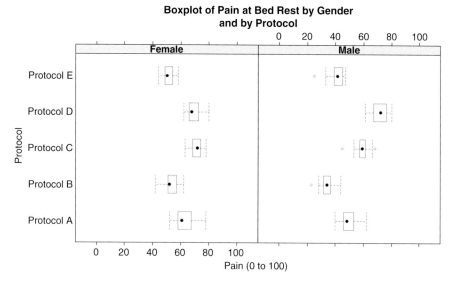

Fig. 8.3 Box plots of two breakout groups using the lattice::bwplot() function

```
  data=Pain.df,
  plot.points=TRUE, auto.key=TRUE,
  par.settings=simpleTheme(lwd=2),
  par.strip.text=list(cex=1.15, font=2),
  scales=list(cex=1.15),
  main="Scatterplot of Pain at Bed Rest
  and Pain When Standing by Gender",
  xlab=list("Pain at Bed Rest", cex=1.15, font=2),
  xlim=c(-015,115), # Note the range.
  ylab=list("Pain When Standing", cex=1.15, font=2),
  aspect=1, breaks=10,
  layout = c(2,1))                       # 2 Columns by 1 Row

par(ask=TRUE)                            # 5 Columns by 1 Row
lattice::xyplot(Walking ~ Bed | F2.recode,
  data=Pain.df,
  plot.points=TRUE, auto.key=TRUE,
  par.settings=simpleTheme(lwd=2),
  par.strip.text=list(cex=1.15, font=2),
  scales=list(cex=1.15),
  main="Scatterplot of Pain at Bed Rest
  and Pain When Walking by Protocol",
  xlab=list("Pain at Bed Rest", cex=1.15, font=2),
  xlim=c(-015,115), # Note the range.
  ylab=list("Pain When Walking", cex=1.15, font=2),
  aspect=1, breaks=10,
  layout = c(5,1))                       # 5 Columns by 1 Row
```

Many other graphically-focused functions are supported by the lattice package. As time permits, read more about the lattice package and why it should be considered when simple graphics are no longer sufficient for presentation.

8.4.3 Use of the ggplot2 Package

The figures presented above are all based on either functions available when R is first downloaded or functions available through the lattice package (which is one of thousands of other R-based packages available as an external package). However, the ggplot2 (again, the term gg stands for *Grammar of Graphics*) package has gained wide acceptance in the R community. A few figures based on use of the ggplot2 package are presented below. There are those who would suggest that the syntax associated with the ggplot2 package may be a bit more challenging than most beginning students need to consider, but the gaining popularity of this package calls for some level of presentation in this lesson.

```
install.packages("ggplot2")
library(ggplot2)                  # Load the ggplot2 package.
help(package=ggplot2)             # Show the information page.
sessionInfo()                     # Confirm all attached packages.
# Select the most local mirror site using Set CRAN mirror.
```

As with nearly all R-based syntax, there are many ways to structure a graphical presentation. Experimentation and practice are needed to gain full advantage of the many capabilities available through use of the ggplot2 package and its many functions and layers of complexity.

Again, histograms are a good starting point for visual displays of measured object variables, even if the data are considered ordinal and not interval.

```
Pain.Standing <- ggplot2::ggplot(data=Pain.df, aes(x=Standing))
  # There are no layers in this object and it will not
  # generate a graphic, by itself.  Instead, other syntax is
  # needed to make graphical images with the ggplot2::ggplot()
  # function.
summary(Pain.Standing)
```

```
data: ID, F1, F2, WeightLb, Bed, Standing, Walking, F1.recode,
      F2.recode [200x9]
mapping:  x = Standing
faceting: facet_null()
```

```
par(ask=TRUE)
Pain.Standing + geom_histogram(fill="red") +
  labs(title="Pain When Standing:  All Subjects") +
  labs(x="Pain (0 to 100) When Standing") +
  labs(y="Frequency") +
```

```
  theme_bw(base_family="sans", base_size=14)
  # Use theme_bw() to generate an easy-to-read white
  # background with contrasting black grid lines.

par(ask=TRUE)
Pain.Standing + geom_histogram(fill="red", color="darkblue") +
  labs(title="Pain When Standing:  All Subjects") +
  labs(x="Pain (0 to 100) When Standing") +
  labs(y="Frequency") +
  theme_bw(base_family="sans", base_size=20) +
  theme(axis.title.y = element_text(color="red", face="bold"),
        axis.title.x = element_text(color="red", face="bold"),
        axis.text.x  = element_text(size=18, face="bold"),
        axis.text.y  = element_text(size=18, face="bold")) +
        xlim(0, 100) + ylim(0, 30)
  # In this graphic, note how limits have been set for both the
  # X axis (0 to 100) and Y axis (0 to 30).

par(ask=TRUE)
Pain.Standing + geom_histogram(fill="red", color="darkblue") +
  labs(title="Pain When Standing by Gender") +
  labs(x="Pain (0 to 100) When Standing") +
  labs(y="Frequency") +
  theme_bw(base_family="sans", base_size=20) +
  theme(axis.title.y = element_text(color="red", face="bold"),
        axis.title.x = element_text(color="red", face="bold"),
        axis.text.x  = element_text(size=16, face="bold"),
        axis.text.y  = element_text(size=18, face="bold"))  +
        facet_wrap(~ F1.recode) +
        xlim(0, 100) + ylim(0, 15)
  # By including + facet_wrap(~ F1.recode) breakouts for the
  # measured variable Standing are now provided for each Gender
  # (Female and Male).

par(ask=TRUE)
Pain.Standing + geom_histogram(fill="red", color="darkblue") +
  labs(title="Pain When Standing by Protocol") +
  labs(x="Pain (0 to 100) When Standing") +
  labs(y="Frequency") +
  theme_bw(base_family="sans", base_size=20) +
  theme(axis.title.y = element_text(color="red", face="bold"),
        axis.title.x = element_text(color="red", face="bold"),
        axis.text.x  = element_text(size=16, face="bold"),
        axis.text.y  = element_text(size=18, face="bold"))  +
        facet_wrap(~ F2.recode) +
        xlim(0, 100) + ylim(0, 15)
  # By including + facet_wrap(~ F2.recode) breakouts for the
  # measured variable Standing are now provided for each
  # Protocol (Protocol A to Protocol E).
```

Along with histograms, the ggplot2 package supports functions used to generate an exceptionally wide variety of figures. Figures generated using ggplot2 can focus on individual object variables, but it is also possible to generate figures that provide information about measured object variables (i.e., Weight, Pain at Bed Rest, Pain When Standing, Pain When Walking) at the level of the many breakout groups of factor-type object variables (i.e., Gender, Protocol).

The ggplot2::ggplot() function will be used to demonstrate correlation (i.e., association), given the focus of this lesson. Notice how the first few scatter plots are very simple with few embellishments. Only the last scatter plot approaches publishable quality.

```
par(ask=TRUE)
ggplot2::ggplot(Pain.df, aes(x=Bed, y=Standing)) +
    geom_point(shape=1)       # Use hollow circles

par(ask=TRUE)
ggplot2::ggplot(Pain.df, aes(x=Bed, y=Standing)) +
    geom_point(shape=1) +     # Use hollow circles
    geom_smooth(method=lm)    # Add linear regression line

par(ask=TRUE)
ggplot2::ggplot(Pain.df, aes(x=Bed, y=Standing)) +
    geom_point(shape=1) +     # Use hollow circles
    geom_smooth(method=lm,    # Add linear regression line
                se=FALSE)     # Avoid a shaded confidence region

par(ask=TRUE)
ggplot2::ggplot(Pain.df, aes(x=Bed, y=Standing)) +
    geom_point(shape=1) +     # Use hollow circles
    geom_smooth()             # Show a loess smoothed fit curve
                              # with confidence region

par(ask=TRUE)
ggplot2::ggplot(Pain.df, aes(x=Bed, y=Standing)) +
  geom_point(shape=21, color = "red", size=4, fill="blue") +
  labs(title="Pain at Bed Rest v Pain When Standing") +
  scale_y_continuous(limits=c(0,100)) +
  scale_x_continuous(limits=c(0,100)) +
  geom_smooth(method=lm, se=TRUE) +
  theme_bw(base_family="sans", base_size=15) +
  theme(axis.title.y = element_text(color="red", face="bold"),
        axis.title.x = element_text(color="red", face="bold"),
        axis.text.x  = element_text(size=14, face="bold"),
        axis.text.y  = element_text(size=14, face="bold"))
  # This graphic generates a single scatterplot of Pain.df$Bed
  # (X Axis) by Pain.df$Standing (Y Axis).  Although it is
  # embellished, it is only a good beginning.  A full set of
  # ggplot2 features could be used to make it publishable.
```

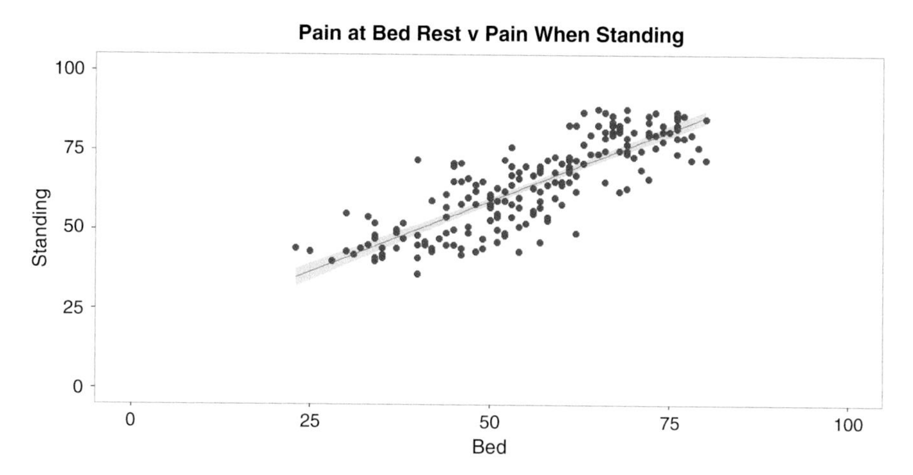

Fig. 8.4 Scatter plot of two continuous object variables using the ggplot2::ggplot() function

The ggplot2 package has may features and it is increasingly popular, but it takes some time to learn the many complexities of this package and how syntax is structured. Experiment with this package and explore its many possibilities after the basics of R graphics are mastered (Fig. 8.4).

8.5 Descriptive Analysis of the Data

Missing data, ideally, should always be avoided. However, missing data are only too common, and experienced researchers must come to grips with the reality of how missing data impact syntax and expected processes for data analysis and graphical presentations. Look at the syntax throughout this text and notice how more than a few functions use the na.rm=TRUE argument to accommodate missing data.

The dataframe associated with this lesson was fairly small (N = 200). If desired, the data could be reviewed line-by-line against field notes, but that of course could never be meaningfully attempted for a large collection of data with thousands of subjects. Saying that, it is often helpful to first check for missing data by using the is.na() function and the complete.cases() function against the entire dataset. Both functions return a TRUE or FALSE response, depending on the function and the outcome of whether data are missing or not.

```
is.na(Pain.df)             # Check for missing data
complete.cases(Pain.df)    # Check for complete cases
```

For the dataset Pain.df, note how there is one missing datum for each measured object variable (i.e., WeightLb, Bed, Standing, Walking). As a first selection on how missing data are approached, the summary() function may be all that is necessary to gain a sense of the data. As typically used, the summary() function is applied against the entire dataset, thus yielding information about all object variables, including the object variable Subject.

```
summary(Pain.df)
```

Give attention to the listing of NAs, if any, for those object variables with missing data. Again, the summary() function is very useful, and it should always be a first selection when preparing descriptive analyses.

Measures of Central Tendency of the Numeric Object Variables
By reviewing the previously created graphical images and studying output from the summary() function, it seems that the data in Pain.df are generally in good form. With this initial level of assurance about the data, and to also supplement the statistics associated with the summary() function, a fairly comprehensive set of R-based functions will be used to expand understanding of the data, especially the data that represent some type of measure: WeightLb, Bed, Standing, and Walking.

To achieve this aim, a few functions found in external packages (asbio::Mode and Zelig::Mode) will be used to expand on those functions immediately available when R is first downloaded. To save space for what would otherwise be an unwieldy display of syntax, the many descriptive statistics will be presented only for Pain.df$WeightLb and Pain.df$Walking.

```
install.packages("asbio")
library(asbio)                # Load the asbio package.
help(package=asbio)           # Show the information page.
sessionInfo()                 # Confirm all attached packages.
# Select the most local mirror site using Set CRAN mirror.

install.packages("Zelig")
library(Zelig)                # Load the Zelig package.
help(package=Zelig)           # Show the information page.
sessionInfo()                 # Confirm all attached packages.
# Select the most local mirror site using Set CRAN mirror.
```

With these external packages brought into this R session, prepare descriptive statistics of selected variables in the Pain.df dataset.

```
median(Pain.df$WeightLb, na.rm=TRUE)    # Median
```

```
[1] 165.64
```

```
mean(Pain.df$WeightLb, na.rm=TRUE)      # Mean
```

```
[1] 164.7947
```

```
sd(Pain.df$WeightLb, na.rm=TRUE)        # Standard Deviation
```

```
[1] 25.6055
```

```
asbio::Mode(Pain.df$WeightLb)              # Mode
```

```
[1] NA
Warning message:
In asbio::Mode(Pain.df$WeightLb) : NAs introduced by coercion
```

```
Zelig::Mode(Pain.df$WeightLb)              # Mode
```

```
[1] 185.75
```

```
range(Pain.df$WeightLb, na.rm=TRUE)        # Range
```

```
[1]  88.62 220.77
```

Notice how the output of each function shows on the next line: Median of Pain.df$WeightLb = 165.64, Mean of Pain.df$WeightLb = 164.7947, Standard Deviation of Pain.df$WeightLb = 25.6055, etc. The one exception is output for the asbio::Mode() function, which provides sufficient information to know that this function, as expressed in this example, cannot accommodate missing data of this type. Fortunately, the Zelig::Mode() function can accommodate missing data and a modal value is provided. Later, review package documentation and note how Mode is expressed for the asbio::Mode() function and the Zelig::Mode() function when there are missing data and/or multiple modes. As a sidebar comment, the way Mode is accommodated by these two functions is an example of why it is always a good idea to use multiple approaches for data analysis, largely to confirm outcomes and to look for consistency. Redundancy is not necessarily wasteful when reviewing data and eventual output.

Using this process, view appropriate descriptive statistics (e.g., Median, Mean, SD, Mode, Range) for the remaining measured object variables, as needed:

```
median(Pain.df$Bed, na.rm=TRUE)            # Median
mean(Pain.df$Bed, na.rm=TRUE)              # Mean
sd(Pain.df$Bed, na.rm=TRUE)                # Standard Deviation
Zelig::Mode(Pain.df$Bed)                   # Mode
range(Pain.df$Bed, na.rm=TRUE)             # Range

median(Pain.df$Standing, na.rm=TRUE)       # Median
mean(Pain.df$Standing, na.rm=TRUE)         # Mean
sd(Pain.df$Standing, na.rm=TRUE)           # Standard Deviation
Zelig::Mode(Pain.df$Standing)              # Mode
range(Pain.df$Standing, na.rm=TRUE)        # Range
```

```
median(Pain.df$Walking, na.rm=TRUE)        # Median
```

```
[1] 73
```

```
mean(Pain.df$Walking, na.rm=TRUE)        # Mean
```

```
[1] 71.58291
```

```
sd(Pain.df$Walking, na.rm=TRUE)          # Standard Deviation
```

```
[1] 16.81425
```

```
Zelig::Mode(Pain.df$Walking)             # Mode
```

```
[1] 84
```

```
range(Pain.df$Walking, na.rm=TRUE)       # Range
```

```
[1]  35 100
```

These one-by-one calculations of descriptive statistics help, but there are other functions that provide (in one simple operation) a composite of all needed descriptive statistics. For this lesson, look at use of the fBasics::basicStats() function and the pastecs::stat.desc() function. Each function provides the same general level of information about the selected variables, so selection is largely a matter of preference. There are many other packages and functions that could also be selected to show multiple descriptive statistics, but these two should meet immediate needs.

```
names(Pain.df)
str(Pain.df, digits.d=6)    # digits.d argument for WeightLb

install.packages("fBasics")
library(fBasics)                # Load the fBasics package.
help(package=fBasics)           # Show the information page.
sessionInfo()                   # Confirm all attached packages.
# Select the most local mirror site using Set CRAN mirror.

options(scipen=80, digits=4)
# Prevent scientific notation and keep printouts to a
# reasonable width

fBasics::basicStats(Pain.df[, 4:7], ci = 0.95)
# Calculate basic statistics against columns 4 to
# 7 in the dataframe Pain.df:
# Column 4 - WeightLb           Weight (Pounds)
# Column 5 - Bed                Pain at Bed Rest
# Column 6 - Standing           Pain When Standing
# Column 7 - Walking            Pain When Walking
# Use a confidence interval of 0.95
```

```
              WeightLb         Bed      Standing      Walking
nobs          200.0000    200.0000    200.00000    200.0000
NAs             1.0000      1.0000      1.00000      1.0000
Minimum        88.6200     23.0000     36.00000     35.0000
Maximum       220.7700     80.0000     88.00000    100.0000
1. Quartile   147.0650     46.5000     53.00000     58.0000
3. Quartile   180.1150     67.0000     76.00000     86.0000
Mean          164.7947     56.1055     64.44221     71.5829
Median        165.6400     57.0000     65.00000     73.0000
Sum         32794.1500  11165.0000  12824.00000  14245.0000
SE Mean         1.8151      0.9391      0.99457      1.1919
LCL Mean      161.2153     54.2536     62.48091     69.2324
UCL Mean      168.3742     57.9575     66.40352     73.9334
Variance      655.6414    175.5090    196.84387    282.7191
Stdev          25.6055     13.2480     14.03011     16.8143
Skewness       -0.1203     -0.2006     -0.08548     -0.1983
Kurtosis       -0.4051     -0.7819     -1.18861     -1.1204
```

Compare the detail and presentation of output from use of the fBasics::basicStats() function to use of the pastecs::stat.desc() function. In many cases, these functions are redundant and selection is largely a matter of preference.

```
install.packages("pastecs")
library(pastecs)              # Load the lessR package.
help(package=pastecs)         # Show the information page.
sessionInfo()                 # Confirm all attached packages.
# Select the most local mirror site using Set CRAN mirror.
```

Notice, again, how selection is only for object variables 4–7, or WeightLb, Bed, Standing, and Walking.

```
options(scipen=80, digits=2)
# Prevent scientific notation and keep printouts to a reasonable
  width

pastecs::stat.desc(Pain.df[,4:7], basic=TRUE, desc=TRUE,
  norm=TRUE, p=0.95)
```

```
              WeightLb         Bed       Standing        Walking
nbr.val         199.00    199.0000     199.000000     199.000000
nbr.null          0.00      0.0000       0.000000       0.000000
nbr.na            1.00      1.0000       1.000000       1.000000
min              88.62     23.0000      36.000000      35.000000
max             220.77     80.0000      88.000000     100.000000
range           132.15     57.0000      52.000000      65.000000
sum           32794.15  11165.0000   12824.000000   14245.000000
median          165.64     57.0000      65.000000      73.000000
mean            164.79     56.1055      64.442211      71.582915
SE.mean           1.82      0.9391       0.994568       1.191931
CI.mean.0.95      3.58      1.8520       1.961305       2.350508
var             655.64    175.5090     196.843866     282.719101
```

```
std.dev          25.61     13.2480     14.030106     16.814253
coef.var          0.16      0.2361      0.217716      0.234892
skewness         -0.12     -0.2006     -0.085480     -0.198348
skew.2SE         -0.35     -0.5819     -0.247985     -0.575424
kurtosis         -0.41     -0.7819     -1.188615     -1.120377
kurt.2SE         -0.59     -1.1397     -1.732470     -1.633009
normtest.W        0.99      0.9788      0.954819      0.958306
normtest.p        0.22      0.0042      0.000006      0.000014
```

Regarding descriptive statistics by breakout groups, the tapply() function can also be applied against measured object variables, serving as one more in a possibly long list of potential functions used to gain a better sense of the data and descriptive statistics. Given interest in nonparametric issues for this lesson, focus on the median.

A full set of descriptive statistics is presented below by breakout groups, by using the tapply() function and using summary as a function argument. Be sure to focus on Median. To save space, a printout of output is shown only for Pain.df$Walking by the five protocol breakouts found in object variable F2.recode.

```
tapply(WeightLb, F1.recode, summary, na.rm=TRUE, data=Pain.df)
tapply(WeightLb, F2.recode, summary, na.rm=TRUE, data=Pain.df)

tapply(Bed,      F1.recode, summary, na.rm=TRUE, data=Pain.df)
tapply(Bed,      F2.recode, summary, na.rm=TRUE, data=Pain.df)

tapply(Standing, F1.recode, summary, na.rm=TRUE, data=Pain.df)
tapply(Standing, F2.recode, summary, na.rm=TRUE, data=Pain.df)

tapply(Walking,  F1.recode, summary, na.rm=TRUE, data=Pain.df)
tapply(Walking,  F2.recode, summary, na.rm=TRUE, data=Pain.df)
```

```
$`Protocol A`
   Min. 1st Qu.  Median    Mean 3rd Qu.    Max.
     58      70      74      74      78      84

$`Protocol B`
   Min. 1st Qu.  Median    Mean 3rd Qu.    Max.
     37      46      52      53      60      75

$`Protocol C`
   Min. 1st Qu.  Median    Mean 3rd Qu.    Max.
     71      81      88      86      92      96

$`Protocol D`
   Min. 1st Qu.  Median    Mean 3rd Qu.    Max.    NA's
     75      86      89      90      95     100       1

$`Protocol E`
   Min. 1st Qu.  Median    Mean 3rd Qu.    Max.
     35      51      56      56      60      72
```

Application of the Anderson-Darling Test

Graphical images and descriptive statistics are needed to understand the data. It is also best to apply selected statistical tests to serve as an additional support for decision-making on acceptance of nonparametric or parametric views toward the data. To that end, consider application of the Anderson-Darling Test, the Lilliefors (KS) Test, and the Shapiro-Wilk Test. It should be mentioned that these tests may be influenced by sample size and that they provide one view, but not the only view, on the nature of distribution patterns. Experience, needs, and practical judgment, supported by careful review of graphical images, descriptive statistics, and statistical tests, should be used when deciding if variables from a dataset are best viewed from a nonparametric or parametric perspective.

```
install.packages("nortest")
library(nortest)              # Load the nortest package.
help(package=nortest)         # Show the information page.
sessionInfo()                 # Confirm all attached packages.
# Select the most local mirror site using Set CRAN mirror.
```

For this lesson, it is sufficient to only apply the Anderson-Darling Test. The Null Hypothesis for the Anderson-Darling Test is structured to examine whether the data follow a specified distribution:

Anderson-Darling Null Hypothesis: The data follow the normal distribution.

```
nortest::ad.test(Pain.df$WeightLb)     # Anderson-Darling Test
```

```
        Anderson-Darling normality test

data:  Pain.df$WeightLb
A = 0.53, p-value = 0.1697
```

```
nortest::ad.test(Pain.df$Bed)          # Anderson-Darling Test
```

```
        Anderson-Darling normality test

data:  Pain.df$Bed
A = 0.93, p-value = 0.01828
```

```
nortest::ad.test(Pain.df$Standing)     # Anderson-Darling Test
```

```
        Anderson-Darling normality test

data:  Pain.df$Standing
A = 2.3, p-value = 0.000008517
```

```
nortest::ad.test(Pain.df$Walking)      # Anderson-Darling Test
```

```
        Anderson-Darling normality test

data:  Pain.df$Walking
A = 2.4, p-value = 0.000004758
```

The calculated Anderson-Darling Test for normality p-value for weight (Paind.f$WeightLb), which is a measured variable, exceeded 0.05 which supports the view that weight follows normal distribution. For weight, the Null Hypothesis is accepted and it judged that the data follow the normal distribution.

The calculated Anderson-Darling Test for normality p-values for all three measures of pain (Pain.df$Bed, Pain.df$Standing, and Pain.df$Walking) which are self-rated values, were less than 0.05 which supports the view that pain does not follow normal distribution. For all three measures of pain, the Null Hypothesis is rejected and it judged that the data do not follow the normal distribution.

Given these p-values, it is appropriate to approach measures of association from a nonparametric view. A QQ plot may help reinforce the distribution patterns and demonstrate that pain-specific data do not display normal distribution.

```
par(ask=TRUE)
par(mfrow=c(2,2))                          # 2 Columns by 2 Rows
qqnorm(Pain.df$WeightLb, col="red", font=2, font.lab=2,
  cex.axis=1.5, main="QQPlot of Pain.df$WeightLb")
qqline(Pain.df$WeightLb, lwd=4, col="darkblue")
qqnorm(Pain.df$Bed, col="red", font=2, font.lab=2,
  cex.axis=1.5, main="QQPlot of Pain.df$Bed")
qqline(Pain.df$Bed, lwd=4, col="darkblue")
qqnorm(Pain.df$Standing, col="red", font=2, font.lab=2,
  cex.axis=1.5, main="QQPlot of Pain.df$Standing")
qqline(Pain.df$Standing, lwd=4, col="darkblue")
qqnorm(Pain.df$Walking, col="red", font=2, font.lab=2,
  cex.axis=1.5, main="QQPlot of Pain.df$Walking")
qqline(Pain.df$Walking, lwd=4, col="darkblue")
```

The QQ plot (i.e., normal probability plot) provides additional confirmation that the data, overall, are best viewed from a nonparametric perspective. Look especially at the tails to see pain-specific data deviating away from the qqline (Fig. 8.5).

8.6 Conduct the Statistical Analysis

The many graphical images and descriptive statistics provide excellent background on the data of direct interest: Weight, Pain at Bed Rest, Pain When Standing, and Pain When Walking. A first attempt has also been made to look at breakouts by Gender and by Protocol.

However, the task for this lesson is correlation and, specifically, correlation with the view that the object variables Pain.df$Bed, Pain.df$Standing, and Pain.df$Walking represent ordinal data therefore requiring a nonparametric approach for data analysis. Consider the tasks needed to determine the correlation between the (generic) variables X and Y, of which there are multiple X:Y combinations in this dataset.

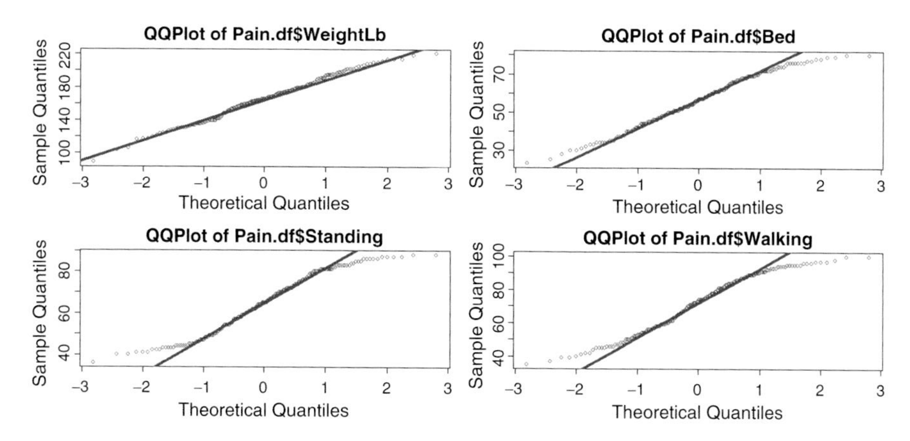

Fig. 8.5 Multiple QQ plots in one graphic, to compare distribution patterns

By using R, there are many ways to determine Spearman's rho. From the perspective of brute force, look at the way multiple individual correlations are prepared below. View this approach as a declining cascade of comparisons between X:Y, recognizing that an initial comparison of X:Y equates to a later comparison of Y:X (i.e, calculation of Spearman's rho coefficient of correlation between X and Y results in the same statistic as calculation of Spearman's rho coefficient of correlation between Y and X).

```
options(scipen=80, digits=8)
# Adjust digits in output to the screen

cor(Pain.df$WeightLb, Pain.df$Bed,
  use="pairwise.complete.obs", method="spearman")
```

```
[1] 0.35223058
```

```
cor(Pain.df$WeightLb, Pain.df$Standing,
  use="pairwise.complete.obs", method="spearman")
```

```
[1] 0.43271092
```

```
cor(Pain.df$WeightLb, Pain.df$Walking,
  use="pairwise.complete.obs", method="spearman")
```

```
[1] 0.42324437
```

```
cor(Pain.df$Bed, Pain.df$Standing,
  use="pairwise.complete.obs", method="spearman")
```

```
[1] 0.84038098
```

```
cor(Pain.df$Bed, Pain.df$Walking,
  use="pairwise.complete.obs", method="spearman")
```

```
[1] 0.86685276
```

```
cor(Pain.df$Standing, Pain.df$Walking,
  use="pairwise.complete.obs", method="spearman")
```

```
[1] 0.89624247
```

These different individual Spearman's rho calculations of correlation can be more easily put into one unified presentation, again using the previously shown Pain.df[, 4:7] nomenclature for declaring desired object variables.

```
cor(Pain.df[, 4:7],   use="pairwise.complete.obs",
  method="spearman")
```

```
           WeightLb        Bed   Standing    Walking
WeightLb 1.00000000 0.35223058 0.43271092 0.42324437
Bed      0.35223058 1.00000000 0.84038098 0.86685276
Standing 0.43271092 0.84038098 1.00000000 0.89624247
Walking  0.42324437 0.86685276 0.89624247 1.00000000
```

With Spearman's rho statistics of 0.35–0.43, it can be stated that there is a general level of correlation (i.e., association) between WeightLb (Weight) and Bed (Pain at Bed Rest), WeightLb (Weight) and Standing (Pain When Standing), and WeightLb (Weight) and Walking (Pain When Walking). A caution is offered, however, that WeightLb may be an inappropriate object variable given the absence of any information about height and Body Mass Index (BMI) since those data are not provided in this lesson. Even with this limitation, it can be stated with some degree of assurance that as weight increases there is an overall post-procedure increase in pain, too.

The Spearman's rho statistics for comparisons of pain, alone, are far more telling. Note how the association between Pain at Bed Rest compared to Pain When Standing, Pain at Bed Rest compared to Pain When Walking, and Pain When Standing compared to Pain When Walking all produced Spearman's rho statistics of about 0.85. A Spearman's rho coefficient of correlation of approximately 0.85 indicated that there is a fairly strong degree of association between the variables in question.[4]

These numerical calculations are all interesting and they certainly provide evidence that there is an association involving weight and pain and that there is an even greater association between pain at various stages of mobility (i.e., bed rest,

[4]Correlation coefficients range from −1.00 to +1.00. A correlation coefficient of 0.85 is considered a very strong measure of association.

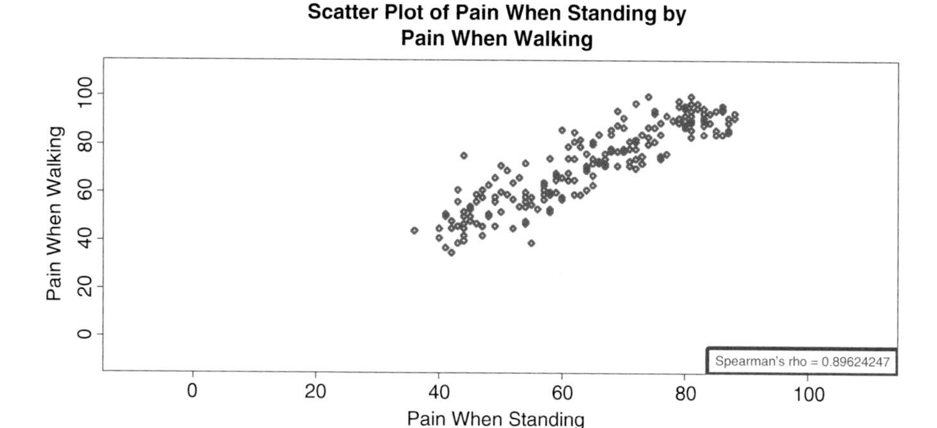

Fig. 8.6 Scatter plot of two continuous object variables with a legend showing Spearman's rho statistic

standing, walking). Review the previous scatter plots again, but this time with the abline removed (in deference to those who object to an abline for nonparametric data). Instead, a legend will be placed in the lower right corner, identifying the numerical value of Spearman's rho (Fig. 8.6).

```
par(ask=TRUE)
plot(Pain.df$WeightLb, Pain.df$Bed,          # X axis by Y axis
  xlab="Weight (Pounds)", ylab="Pain at Bed Rest",
  main="Scatter Plot of Weight by Pain at Best Rest",
  pch=23, lwd=4, col="red", cex.axis=1.25, cex.lab=1.25,
  font=2, xlim=c(0,300), ylim=c(-010,110))
legend("bottomright",
  xjust=1, bty="y", box.lwd=6, box.col="darkblue",
  text.col="darkblue", text.font=2,
  "        Spearman's rho = 0.35223058  ")

par(ask=TRUE)
plot(Pain.df$WeightLb, Pain.df$Standing,     # X axis by Y axis
  xlab="Weight (Pounds)", ylab="Pain When Standing",
  main="Scatter Plot of Weight by Pain When Standing",
  pch=23, lwd=4, col="red", cex.axis=1.25, cex.lab=1.25,
  font=2, xlim=c(0,300), ylim=c(-010,110))
legend("bottomright",
  xjust=1, bty="y", box.lwd=6, box.col="darkblue",
  text.col="darkblue", text.font=2,
  "        Spearman's rho = 0.43271092  ")

par(ask=TRUE)
plot(Pain.df$WeightLb, Pain.df$Walking,      # X axis by Y axis
  xlab="Weight (Pounds)", ylab="Pain When Walking",
  main="Scatter Plot of Weight by Pain When Walking",
  pch=23, lwd=4, col="red", cex.axis=1.25, cex.lab=1.25,
```

```
  font=2, xlim=c(0,300), ylim=c(-010,110))
legend("bottomright",
  xjust=1, bty="y", box.lwd=6, box.col="darkblue",
  text.col="darkblue", text.font=2,
  "       Spearman's rho = 0.42324437  ")

par(ask=TRUE)
plot(Pain.df$Bed, Pain.df$Standing,        # X axis by Y axis
  xlab="Pain at Bed Rest", ylab="Pain When Standing",
  main="Scatter Plot of Pain at Bed Rest by
  Pain When Standing",
  pch=23, lwd=4, col="red", cex.axis=1.25, cex.lab=1.25,
  font=2, xlim=c(-010,110), ylim=c(-010,110))
legend("bottomright",
  xjust=1, bty="y", box.lwd=6, box.col="darkblue",
  text.col="darkblue", text.font=2,
  "       Spearman's rho = 0.84038098  ")

par(ask=TRUE)
plot(Pain.df$Bed, Pain.df$Walking,         # X axis by Y axis
  xlab="Pain at Bed Rest", ylab="Pain When Walking",
  main="Scatter Plot at Pain at Bed Rest by
  Pain When Walking",
  pch=23, lwd=4, col="red", cex.axis=1.25, cex.lab=1.25,
  font=2, xlim=c(-010,110), ylim=c(-010,110))
legend("bottomright",
  xjust=1, bty="y", box.lwd=6, box.col="darkblue",
  text.col="darkblue", text.font=2,
  "       Spearman's rho = 0.86685276  ")

plot(Pain.df$Standing, Pain.df$Walking,    # X axis by Y axis
  xlab="Pain When Standing", ylab="Pain When Walking",
  main="Scatter Plot of Pain When Standing by
  Pain When Walking",
  pch=23, lwd=4, col="red", cex.axis=1.25, cex.lab=1.25,
  font=2, xlim=c(-010,110), ylim=c(-010,110))
legend("bottomright",
  xjust=1, bty="y", box.lwd=6, box.col="darkblue",
  text.col="darkblue", text.font=2,
  "       Spearman's rho = 0.89624247  ")
```

As useful as the plot() function may be, it is by no means the only R-based function used to visualize the association between two variables. Going back to a constant theme in these lessons on the use of R for biostatistics, visual presentations are perhaps the best way to gain attention of the typical reader. Consider a few tools shown below on how to present multiple correlation comparisons in one convenient image, using the pairs() function, lattice::splom() function, psych::pairs.panels() function, car::scatterplotMatrix() function, and the psych::cor.plot() function. The same general theme and subsequent output are addressed with each function, but presentation is slightly different, allowing a variety of selections for final presentation based on preferences and needs.

The pairs() function is likely the first choice for production of a visual correlation matrix. Of course, the visual representation of X:Y is very helpful as an adjunct to the otherwise static Spearman's rho coefficient statistics.

```
par(ask=TRUE)
pairs(~WeightLb+Bed+Standing+Walking, data=Pain.df, col="red",
  main="Scatter Plot Matrix (SPLOM) of Weight and
  Post-Procedure Pain at Different Levels of Mobility")
```

If it is difficult to visualize in the same output the scatter plot for X:Y and Y:X, then merely use the upper.panel=NULL argument to generate an easier-to-visualize output of the associations.

```
par(ask=TRUE)
pairs(~WeightLb+Bed+Standing+Walking, data=Pain.df,
  col="black", pch=23, bg="red",                # Adjust points
  upper.panel=NULL,                          # Easy-to-Read Output
  main="Scatter Plot Matrix (SPLOM) of Weight and
  Post-Procedure Pain at Different Levels of Mobility")
```

The lattice::splom() function is also a good choice to show association, but be sure to see how the presentation improves as the number of comparisons is set to a limited number, or in the examples below as the number of comparisons is reduced from six to three (Fig. 8.7).

```
par(ask=TRUE)
lattice::splom(~Pain.df[4:7], font=2, col="red",
   main="Scatter Plot Matrix (SPLOM) of Weight and
   Post-Procedure Pain at Different Levels of Mobility")
   # Scatter plots for variables 4, 5, 6, and 7 only
```

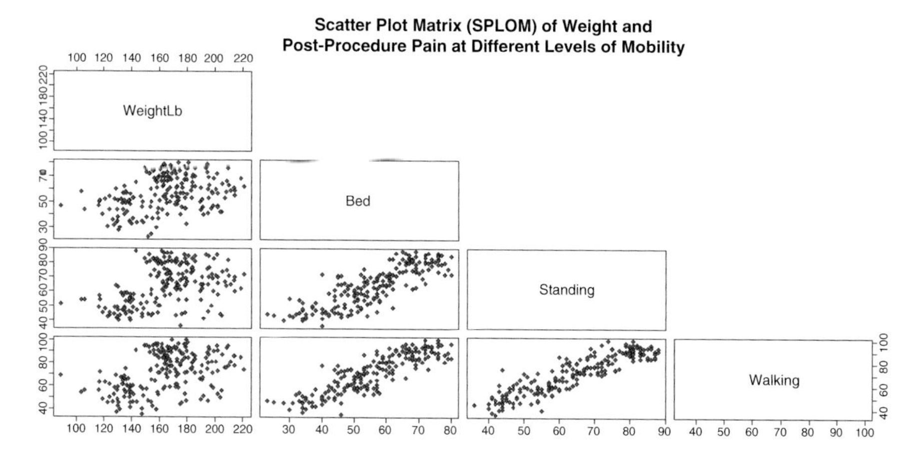

Fig. 8.7 Scatter plot matrix (SPLOM) showing only the lower panel

Following along with the different ways R supports the creation of a scatter plot matrix (SPLOM), consider use of the psych::pairs.panels() function. The output is as appealing as the other SPLOM-type functions, and it may be easier to read. The output includes a histogram and density plot of each individual variable and then a scatter plot of each X:Y comparison.

```
install.packages("psych")
library(psych)                    # Load the psych package.
help(package=psych)               # Show the information page.
sessionInfo()                     # Confirm all attached packages.
# Select the most local mirror site using Set CRAN mirror.

par(ask=TRUE)
psych::pairs.panels(Pain.df[4:7],
  method="spearman", rug=TRUE, hist.col="red", cex.cor=0.5,
  main="Scatter Plot Matrix (SPLOM) (Lower Diagonal) and
  Spearman's rho (Upper Diagonal) of Weight and Pain")
```

The car::scatterplotMatrix() function provides another view of a scatter plot matrix. Again, there are many options and eventually individual preferences often determine selected functions.

```
install.packages("car")
library(car)                      # Load the car package.
help(package=car)                 # Show the information page.
sessionInfo()                     # Confirm all attached packages.
# Select the most local mirror site using Set CRAN mirror.

car::scatterplotMatrix(~ WeightLb+Bed+Standing+Walking,
  main="Scatterplot Matrix (SPLOM) of Weight and
  Post-Procedure Pain at Different Levels of Mobility",
  transform=TRUE, data=Pain.df, smoother=loessLine,
  legend.plot=TRUE, row1attop=TRUE)
```

As an interesting change from the traditional SPLOM, look at output from the psych::cor.plot() function and how color gradients are used to signify the degree of correlation (-1.0 to $+1.0$) and, subsequently, Spearman's rho ranging from -1.0 (Dark Red) to 0.00 (White) to +1.00 (Dark Blue).

```
par(ask=TRUE)
psych::cor.plot(cor(Pain.df[4:7],
  use="complete.obs", method="spearman"),
  main="Color-Gradient Correlation Plot of Weight and
  Post-Procedure Pain: Dark Red for Spearman's rho = -1.0
  to Dark Blue for Spearman's rho = +1.0",
  font.lab=2, font.axis=2)
```

From among the many R-based functions shown above, as well as other functions that could have been presented, the X:Y scatter plot is well-established and there are many ways to prepare and present a scatter plot. A fairly new approach, however, is to use the bagplot to show the degree of association between two separate variables,

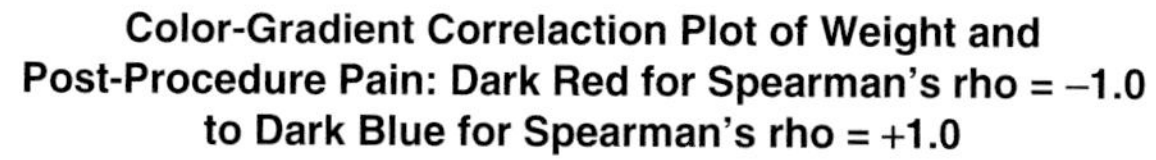

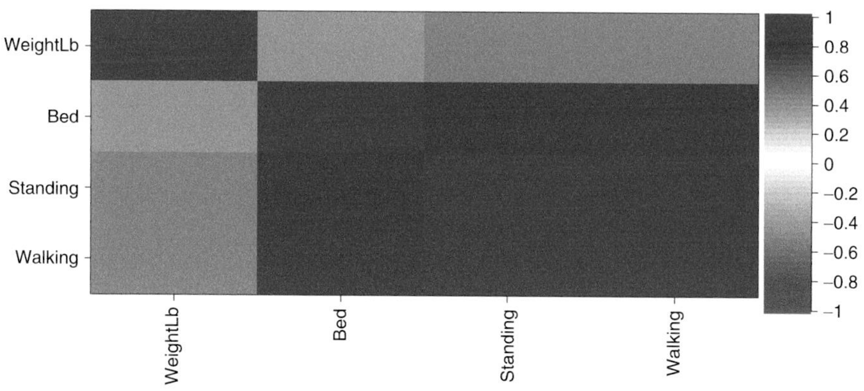

Fig. 8.8 Color-gradient correlation plot of four continuous object variables using the psych::cor.plot() function

X:Y. The bagplot is a bivariate boxplot, where 50 % of all points are contained in the central bag. A fence surrounds the bag and from this fence the remaining points radiate out, giving a view of distribution points and consequently extreme values, if there are any (Fig. 8.8).

Compare the visualization of the association between Pain.df$Bed (X axis) by Pain.df$Walking (Y axis) in a bagplot (below) as compared to the more traditional X:Y scatter plot. If desired, this syntax could then be reused for the other variables, largely just by altering variable names.

Give special notice to the way values for the X axis and Y axis are set. For this set of graphics, xlim=range(Minimum:Maximum) was used instead of xlim=c(Minimum, Maximum) with the same scheme used for the ylim. With R, there are usually many ways to achieve the same aim, and this example provides another way of setting axis limits, at least for this function.

```
install.packages("aplpack")
library(aplpack)              # Load the aplpack package.
help(package=aplpack)         # Show the information page.
sessionInfo()                 # Confirm all attached packages.
# Select the most local mirror site using Set CRAN mirror.

savelwd      <- par(lwd=2)         # Heavy line
savefont     <- par(font=2)        # Bold
savecex.lab  <- par(cex.lab=1.25)  # Label
savecex.axis <- par(cex.axis=1.25) # Axis
par(ask=TRUE)
aplpack::bagplot(Pain.df$Bed, Pain.df$Walking,          # X by Y
  main="Bagplot of Pain at Bed Rest (X) by Pain When Walking (Y)
  With Central Bag, Fence, and Distribution Points",
  na.rm=TRUE,                 # Accommodate missing data
```

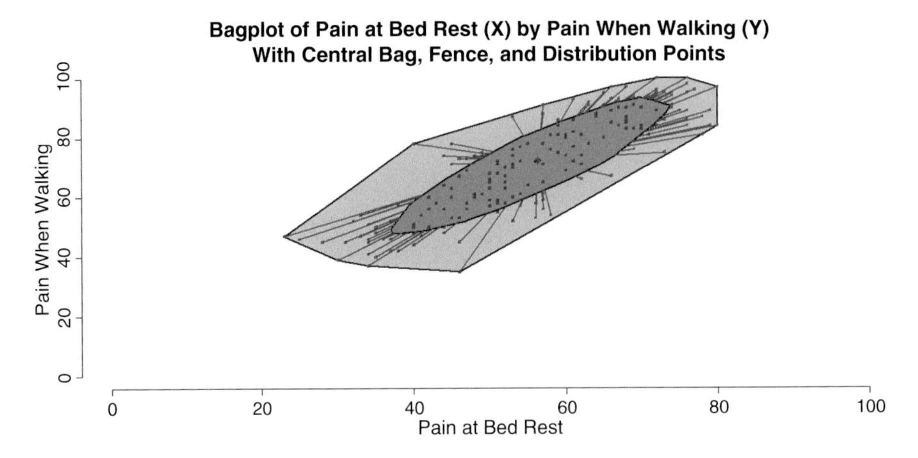

Fig. 8.9 Bagplot of two continuous object variables using the aplpack::bagplot() function

```
  xlim=range(0:100), ylim=range(0:100),   # Range for each axis
  xlab="Pain at Bed Rest", ylab="Pain When Walking",
  show.outlier=TRUE,            # At the R prompt, key
  show.whiskers=TRUE,           # help(bagplot) to see details for
  show.looppoints=TRUE,         # each argument, show.outlier,
  show.bagpoints=TRUE,          # show.whiskers,etc.  Then, decide
  show.loophull=TRUE,           # which arguments meet individual
  show.baghull=TRUE,            # needs.
  pch=c(22))                    # Filled square red symbol
par(savelwd); par(savefont); par(savecex.lab)
par(savecex.axis)
```

Although it is useful to view Spearman's rho correlation coefficients and the many graphics shown in this lesson, as well as general themes for viewing correlation (i.e., association), it is still unknown if there are statistically significant (`p <= 0.05`) correlations for these different comparisons. To investigate statistical significance, one method is to use the cor.test() function, with method="spearman" as the selected argument for what type of correlation test to use (Fig. 8.9).

```
cor.test(WeightLb, Bed, method="spearman", data=Pain.df)
```

```
        Spearman's rank correlation rho

data:  WeightLb and Bed
S = 838018.65, p-value = 0.00000036
alternative hypothesis: true rho is not equal to 0
sample estimates:
       rho
0.35223058
```

```
cor.test(WeightLb, Standing, method="spearman", data=Pain.df)
```

```
        Spearman's rank correlation rho

data:  WeightLb and Standing
S = 733901.32, p-value = 0.0000000001934
alternative hypothesis: true rho is not equal to 0
sample estimates:
       rho
0.43271092
```

```
cor.test(WeightLb, Walking, method="spearman", data=Pain.df)
```

```
        Spearman's rank correlation rho

data:  WeightLb and Walking
S = 746148.19, p-value = 0.0000000005221
alternative hypothesis: true rho is not equal to 0
sample estimates:
       rho
0.42324437
```

```
cor.test(Bed, Standing, method="spearman", data=Pain.df)
```

```
        Spearman's rank correlation rho

data:  Bed and Standing
S = 206498.96, p-value < 0.00000000000000022
alternative hypothesis: true rho is not equal to 0
sample estimates:
       rho
0.84038098
```

```
cor.test(Bed, Walking, method="spearman", data=Pain.df)
```

```
        Spearman's rank correlation rho

data:  Bed and Walking
S = 172252.46, p-value < 0.00000000000000022
alternative hypothesis: true rho is not equal to 0
sample estimates:
       rho
0.86685276
```

```
cor.test(Standing, Walking, method="spearman", data=Pain.df)
```

```
        Spearman's rank correlation rho

data:  Standing and Walking
S = 134231.01, p-value < 0.00000000000000022
alternative hypothesis: true rho is not equal to 0
sample estimates:
       rho
0.89624247
```

Each correlation has a calculated p-value of <= 0.05. As such, all comparisons in this lesson exhibit statistically significant correlations (p <= 0.05).

Although the cor.test() function may be all that is needed to calculate Spearman's rho, explore the use of other functions, to look for consistency in outcomes and whether the output is possibly more useful or easier to understand. The pspearman::spearman.test() function, the fBasics::spearmanTest() function, and the Hmisc::rcorr() function serve the same purpose of the cor.test() function, but observe how format for the output is different for each function.

Ideally, the statistics in question (i.e., Spearman's rho for this lesson) should be equivalent, or at least in close parity for each function, typically depending on how missing values are accommodated. To save space, the output of only a few samples is shown below but the full set of syntax and data can be used to recreate all analyses and figures.

```
install.packages("pspearman")
library(pspearman)            # Load the pspearman package.
help(package=pspearman)       # Show the information page.
sessionInfo()                 # Confirm all attached packages.
# Select the most local mirror site using Set CRAN mirror.

pspearman::spearman.test(Pain.df$WeightLb, Pain.df$Bed)
pspearman::spearman.test(Pain.df$WeightLb, Pain.df$Standing)
pspearman::spearman.test(Pain.df$WeightLb, Pain.df$Walking)

pspearman::spearman.test(Pain.df$Bed, Pain.df$Standing)
pspearman::spearman.test(Pain.df$Bed, Pain.df$Walking)

pspearman::spearman.test(Pain.df$Standing, Pain.df$Walking)
```

```
        Spearman's rank correlation rho

data:  Pain.df$Standing and Pain.df$Walking
S = 134231.01, p-value < 0.00000000000000022
alternative hypothesis: true rho is not equal to 0
sample estimates:
       rho
0.89624247

Warning message:
In pspearman::spearman.test(Pain.df$Standing, Pain.df$Walking):
  Cannot compute exact p-values with ties
```

```
fBasics::spearmanTest(Pain.df$Weight, Pain.df$Bed,
  title = "Spearman's rho for Pain.df:  Weight v Bed Rest")
fBasics::spearmanTest(Pain.df$Weight, Pain.df$Standing,
  title = "Spearman's rho for Pain.df:  Weight v Standing")
fBasics::spearmanTest(Pain.df$Weight, Pain.df$Walking,
  title = "Spearman's rho for Pain.df:  Weight v Walking")

fBasics::spearmanTest(Pain.df$Bed, Pain.df$Standing,
  title = "Spearman's rho for Pain.df:  Bed Rest v Standing")
fBasics::spearmanTest(Pain.df$Bed, Pain.df$Walking,
  title = "Spearman's rho for Pain.df:  Bed Rest v Walking")

fBasics::spearmanTest(Pain.df$Standing, Pain.df$Walking,
  title = "Spearman's rho for Pain.df:  Standing v Walking")
```

```
Title:
 Spearman's rho for Pain.df:  Standing v Walking

Test Results:
  SAMPLE ESTIMATES:
    rho: 0.8962
  STATISTIC:
    S: 134231.0103
  P VALUE:
    Alternative Two-Sided: < 0.00000000000000022
    Alternative      Less: 1
    Alternative   Greater: < 0.00000000000000022
  Cannot compute exact p-value with ties
```

Look at output from use of the Hmisc::rcorr() function. This function is quite information rich, and it generates three types of output: (1) Spearman's rho values for each comparison of X:Y, (2) N for each X:Y comparison with missing values taken out of the comparisons, and (3) X:Y p-values.

```
install.packages("Hmisc")
library(Hmisc)                # Load the Hmisc package.
help(package=Hmisc)           # Show the information page.
sessionInfo()                 # Confirm all attached packages
# Select the most local mirror site using Set CRAN mirror.
```

When viewing the syntax immediately below, be sure to review how the dataframe must be accommodated as a matrix for the Hmisc::rcorr() function to work. This requirement is easily accommodated by wrapping the as.matrix() function around the dataframe name, as shown below.

```
Hmisc::rcorr(as.matrix(Pain.df[, 4:7], type=spearman))
```

```
          WeightLb  Bed Standing Walking
WeightLb      1.00 0.35     0.43    0.44
Bed           0.35 1.00     0.84    0.87
Standing      0.43 0.84     1.00    0.90
Walking       0.44 0.87     0.90    1.00

n
         WeightLb Bed Standing Walking
WeightLb      199 198      198     198
Bed           198 199      198     198
Standing      198 198      199     198
Walking       198 198      198     199

P
         WeightLb Bed Standing Walking
WeightLb           0   0        0
Bed      0             0        0
Standing 0         0            0
Walking  0         0   0
```

Output from the Hmisc::rcorr() function is somewhat brief, but that can be viewed as an advantage when faced with overly-detailed output which is the case with some R functions.

8.7 Summary

This lesson was focused on measures of association, specifically using data from a health setting. Subject weights were available, as well as post-procedure self-ratings of pain at three levels of movement on a continuum of mobility: bed rest, standing immediately after bed rest, and walking after standing.

Various R-based functions were used and the general outcome of how weight and pain by continuum of mobility are associated with each other is best presented in a correlation matrix, based on Spearman's rho since the data were viewed from a nonparametric perspective:

```
           WeightLb        Bed   Standing    Walking
WeightLb 1.00000000 0.35223058 0.43271092 0.42324437
Bed      0.35223058 1.00000000 0.84038098 0.86685276
Standing 0.43271092 0.84038098 1.00000000 0.89624247
Walking  0.42324437 0.86685276 0.89624247 1.00000000
```

Based on this correlation matrix and using general terms related to correlation, it can be said that there is a moderate association between weight and self-rating of pain along a continuum of mobility. Spearman's rho coefficients of correlation for weight and pain were approximately in the rho = 0.40 range, which is viewed as a moderate measure of correlation.

The same correlation matrix provided evidence that there was a strong measure of association for pain along the continuum of mobility. Spearman's rho coefficients of correlation for the different times when pain was self-rated were approximately in the rho = 0.85 range, which is viewed as a strong measure of correlation.

Further use of R-based functions provided confirmation that there was a statistically significant (`p <= 0.05`) correlation for all X:Y comparisons. The graphics and statistics provided a great deal of basic information. However, attention should be given to outcomes of the many X:Y correlations (based on Spearman's rho) to gain a sense of association. When considering any general trends be careful to recall the constant reminder that correlation or association does not equate to causation. X may be associated with Y, but by no means does that mean that X causes Y.

For those with continued interest in applications of the dataset used in this lesson, give attention to analyses by gender (Female v Male) and by Protocol (A, B, C, D, and E):

- Are there differences in self-ratings of pain by the two genders?
- Are there differences in self-ratings of pain by protocol?

Going beyond this broad level of comparison, those who wish to examine the data may want to see if outcomes are consistent for all breakout comparisons. As an example, imagine that it is determined that there is a statistically significant difference (`p <= 0.05`) in the self-rating of pain at bed rest by the two genders.

- What is the practical significance of this finding?
- Is it then necessary to determine if there are differences between the two genders for pain when standing, for pain when walking?
- Then, to examine outcomes with even more detail, are any observed differences by gender consistent across all five protocols or are there differences here, too?

These additional questions are all interesting, although beyond the immediate purpose of this lesson. Yet, these questions demonstrate how research in the biological sciences tends to lead to new questions that need attention.

8.8 Addendum: Kendall's Tau

Spearman's rho is well established and it is generally the first choice for investigations into correlation or association for nonparametric data. However, Kendall's tau is another test that should also receive some degree of attention.

In the brief demonstration of Kendall's tau, note especially the warning about tied parings and the difficulty of calculating exact p values when there are tied pairs (e.g., a subject that has the same value for both Bed and Standing).

Consider the output for comparisons of WeightLb, Bed, Standing, and Walking from the perspective of both Spearman's rho and Kendall's tau, using the cor() function but with different arguments for the cor() function: (1) method="spearman" and (2) method="kendall".

```
cor(Pain.df[, 4:7], use="pairwise.complete.obs",
  method="spearman")
```

```
          WeightLb        Bed   Standing    Walking
WeightLb 1.00000000 0.35223058 0.43271092 0.42324437
Bed      0.35223058 1.00000000 0.84038098 0.86685276
Standing 0.43271092 0.84038098 1.00000000 0.89624247
Walking  0.42324437 0.86685276 0.89624247 1.00000000
```

```
cor(Pain.df[, 4:7], use="pairwise.complete.obs",
  method="kendall")
```

```
          WeightLb        Bed   Standing    Walking
WeightLb 1.00000000 0.22551955 0.27805696 0.26886907
Bed      0.22551955 1.00000000 0.64429919 0.67910798
Standing 0.27805696 0.64429919 1.00000000 0.71752596
Walking  0.26886907 0.67910798 0.71752596 1.00000000
```

Spearman's rho and Kendall's tau are both nonparametric (i.e., the focus is on ranks) tests that address correlation (i.e, association). Correlation coefficients range from −1.0 (perfect negative correlation) to +1.0 (perfect positive correlation). When correlation coefficients are generated by the two tests, Kendall's tau correlation coefficients are usually in parity, but of lesser value, than Spearman's rho correlation coefficients.

It is beyond the purpose of this lesson discuss the algorithms associated with the two tests and when one should be selected over the other. For now, know that Spearman's rho is usually the first choice for correlation analyses involving nonparametric data.

As one last view on the use of Kendall's tau, use the psych::corr.test() function, but now with method set to kendall instead of method set to spearman.

```
psych::corr.test(Pain.df[, 4:7], use="pairwise",
  method="kendall", alpha=.05)
```

```
Correlation matrix
         WeightLb  Bed Standing Walking
WeightLb     1.00 0.23     0.28    0.27
Bed          0.23 1.00     0.64    0.68
Standing     0.28 0.64     1.00    0.72
Walking      0.27 0.68     0.72    1.00
Sample Size

         WeightLb Bed Standing Walking
WeightLb      199 198      198     198
Bed           198 199      198     198
Standing      198 198      199     198
Walking       198 198      198     199

Probability values
```

```
         WeightLb Bed Standing Walking
WeightLb        0   0        0       0
Bed             0   0        0       0
Standing        0   0        0       0
Walking         0   0        0       0
```

Notice how the correlation matrix parallels what was generated using the cor() function, subject only to rounding. The probability values are all shown as 0, again confirming that all correlations are statistically significant (`p <= 0.05`).

8.9 Prepare to Exit, Save, and Later Retrieve This R Session

```
getwd()               # Identify the current working directory.
ls()                  # List all objects in the working
                      # directory.
ls.str()              # List all objects, with finite detail.
list.files()          # List files at the PC directory.

save.image("R_Lesson_Spearman.rdata")

getwd()               # Identify the current working directory.
ls()                  # List all objects in the working
                      # directory.
ls.str()              # List all objects, with finite detail.
list.files()          # List files at the PC directory.

alarm()               # Alarm, notice of upcoming action.
q()                   # Quit this session.
                      # Prepare for Save workspace image? query.
```

Use the R Graphical User Interface (GUI) to load the saved rdata file: File -> Load Workspace. Otherwise, use the load() function, keying the full pathname, to load the .rdata file and retrieve the session.

Recall, however, that it may be just as useful to simply use the .R script file (typically saved is a .txt ASCII-type file) and recreate the analyses and graphics, provided the data files remain available.

Chapter 9
Other Nonparametric Tests for the Biological Sciences

Abstract The purpose of this lesson is to highlight a few other nonparametric tests that may be of interest to those who work in the biological sciences. These additional nonparametric tests range in complexity and use. The Binomial Test can be fairly simple in structure and application. Other nonparametric tests, such as Binomial Logistic Regression, can become quite complex both in the way data are organized and in the way results are interpreted. This lesson ends with the reminder that nonparamteric tests are by no means less desirable than tests associated with parametric analyses. Quite the opposite, nonparametric tests have a valuable role in the use, analysis, and interpretation of real-world data—data that do not always meet the conditions needed for parametric analyses but data that still have value.

Keywords Analysis of variance (ANOVA) • Association • Bar plot (stacked, side-by-side) • Beta values • Binomial logistic regression • Binomial probability • Binomial test • Box plot • Code book • Comma-separated values (.csv) • Conditional density • Continuous scale • Correlation • Correlation coefficient • Cumulative probability • Density plot • Descriptive statistics • Distribution -free • Factor • Frequency distribution • Histogram • Interval • Kolmogorov-Smirnov (K-S) two-sample test • Mean • Median • Mode • Nominal • Nonparametric • Normal distribution • Null hypothesis • Odds • Odds ratio • Ordinal • Parametric • Percentile • Predictor variable • Probability (p-value) • Quantile-Quantile (QQ, Q-Q) • STEAM (Science, Technology, Engineering, Art + Design, and Mathematics) • STEM (Science, Technology, Engineering, and Mathematics) • Scatter plot • Statistical significance • Walsh test for two related samples

A few different nonparametric tests are briefly covered in this concluding lesson. The tests range in complexity from fairly simple to more than complex. Final thoughts on future applications of nonparametric statistics are then offered. This lesson ends with contact information for the two authors and pointers on where to find the many .csv datasets used in this text.

Electronic supplementary material The online version of this chapter (doi: 10.1007/978-3-319-30634-6_9) contains supplementary material, which is available to authorized users.

T.W. MacFarland, J.M. Yates, *Introduction to Nonparametric Statistics for the Biological Sciences Using R*, DOI 10.1007/978-3-319-30634-6_9

9.1 Binomial Test

Background: The data for this lesson on the Binomial Test come from a feeding experiment with 50 cattle. The subjects were temporarily confined in separate holding pens during feeding, largely to limit distractions from other cattle.

As the test was organized, the 50 confined cattle were given a choice of two formulated feeds. The two feeds were judged to be in general parity in terms of nutritional value, appearance, and palatability:

- Feed A was a standard feed mixture that met all nutritional needs but Feed A also had an added supplement. As the supplement was formulated, it was suspected that Feed A would have a better smell and taste and would be more appealing to the cattle.
- Feed B was also a standard feed mixture that met all nutritional needs. However, Feed B did not have an added supplement.

While in individual temporary holding pens, the 50 cattle were offered the two feeds in two separate stations, one station holding Feed A and the other station holding Feed B. To further differentiate between the two choices, the two feeding stations were at opposite ends of the holding pen, so that subjects had to purposely move to either of the two separate stations and could not eat from both stations at the same time.

The cattle were then observed to see which of the two feeds they completed first, Feed A or Feed B. The assumption here is that the feed that is completed first is the preferred feed. For the purpose of this experiment, it is assumed that each feed had an equal chance of being eaten first, given that the cattle had a binary choice of finishing Feed A first or Feed B first.

Data: After the experiment, it was observed that 38 subjects out of 50 completed Feed A first and 12 subjects out of 50 completed Feed B first. Using terms (i.e., success, trial(s), probability of success) associated with the Binomial Test:

- 38 is the number of successes (i.e., cattle that finished the experimental Feed A first)
- 50 is the number of trials
- `p <= 0.5` is the hypothesized or theoretical probability of success

Note how the term *success* should be viewed as a reserved term in this binomial (e.g., Go/Stop, Live/Die, Success/Failure, True/False, Yes/No, etc.) scenario and the term success is nominal.

Null Hypothesis (Ho): Given two choices for preferred feeding selection, Feed A or Feed B, there is no statistically significant difference (`p <= 0.05`) in the number of confined cattle that finished Feed A (a feed that has an added supplement with ostensibly improved smell and taste) first and the number of confined cattle that finished Feed B (a feed that does not have an added supplement) first.

As this binomial feeding experiment is structured, cattle have *free choice* and they can either finish Feed A first or they can finish Feed B first, resulting in a theoretical 50/50 view toward selection of the two choices. For this experiment:

- 38 cattle finished Feed A first
- 12 cattle finished Feed B first

Before any data are used, it is best to be sure that all directories and files are organized and placed where desired. This action will apply to all analyses in this lesson.

Start a new R session and then attend to beginning actions such as removing unwanted files from prior work, declaring the working directory, etc.

```
###############################################################
# Housekeeping                            Use for All Analyses   #
###############################################################
date()              # Current system time and date.
R.version.string    # R version and version release date.
ls()                # List all objects in the working
                    # directory.
rm(list = ls())     # CAUTION: Remove all files in the working
                    # directory. If this action is not desired,
                    # use the rm() function one-by-one to remove
                    # the objects that are not needed.
ls.str()            # List all objects, with finite detail.
getwd()             # Identify the current working directory.
setwd("F:/R_Nonparametric")
                    # Set to a new working directory.
                    # Note the single forward slash and double
                    # quotes.
                    # This new directory should be the directory
                    # where the data file is located, otherwise
                    # the data file will not be found.
getwd()             # Confirm the working directory.
list.files()        # List files at the PC directory.
###############################################################
```

Visualize the Data: Use the barplot() function to show where 38 (success) of 50 (trials) shows as probability under the Null Hypothesis:

```
trials <- 50                             # N or number of trials
prob   <- 0.5                            # Declared probability
x      <- seq(0, trials)                 # sequence, to trials
y      <- dbinom(x, size=trials, p=prob)# y vector of heights

par(ask=TRUE)
barplot(height=y, names.arg=x,
  main="Probability of Success in a Binomial Scenario:
  Feed A Selected First",
  xlab="Ate Feed A First",
  ylab="Probability",
  cex.lab=1.25, col="red", font=2)
```

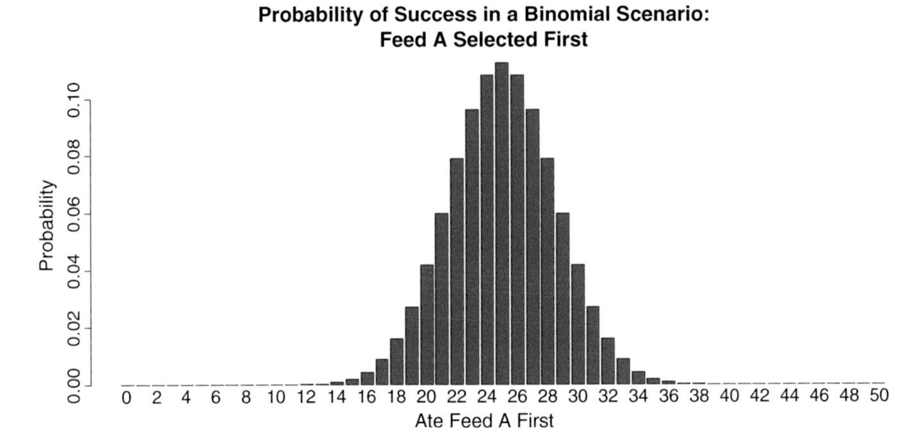

Fig. 9.1 Histogram of binomial probability

Statistical Analysis: The binom.test() function should be sufficient to meet the needs of this study. The arguments (and their values) that go along with the binom.test() function are (Fig. 9.1):

- x (38) - number of successes
- n (50) - number of trials
- p (0.5) - hypothesized or theoretical probability of success
- alternative - selection for the alternative hypothesis: "two.sided", "greater" or "less"
- conf.level - confidence level

```
binom.test(x=38, n=50, p=0.5, alternative="two.sided",
  conf.level=0.95)
```

```
        Exact binomial test

data:  38 and 50
number of successes = 38, number of trials = 50,
  p-value = 0.0003059
alternative hypothesis: true probability of success is
  not equal to 0.5
95 percent confidence interval:
 0.6183093 0.8693901
sample estimates:
probability of success
                  0.76
```

Summary: The calculated p-value is 0.0003059 which is certainly less than the criterion p-value of `p <= 0.05`. The Null Hypothesis is rejected.[1]

Based on this finding, there is a statistically significant difference (`p <= 0.05`) in the number of cattle kept in confinement that finished first a feed that had an added supplement that may improve smell and taste (Feed A) as compared to the number of cattle kept in confinement that finished first a feed that did not have an added supplement (Feed B).

- Finished Feed A first = 38/50 = 76 percent selection
- Finished Feed B first = 12/50 = 24 percent selection

Given a 50/50 (i.e., 50 % theoretical or hypothesized probability for this binomial scenario) view toward selection, the Binomial Test confirms that cattle finished Feed A first at a statistically significant higher rate of selection over Feed B.

There was a statistically significant (`p <= 0.05`) preference for Feed A over Feed B. The importance of applying the Binomial Test is that there is now initial empirical confirmation that the addition of the supplement (i.e., Feed A) was appealing, and, with proper management practices, it may increase the preference for cattle to eat their feed more readily and in turn help meet management goals for weight gain while avoiding feed waste and spoilage. Because the Binomial Test is a fairly simple test, far more research would be needed before expensive changes would ever be implemented in this livestock management scenario.

9.2 Walsh Test for Two Related Samples of Interval Data

Background: The Walsh Test for Two Related Samples of Interval Data (i.e. Walsh Test) is a nonparametric test used to examine whether there is a difference between two possibly related samples, typically organized as matched-pairs (i.e., related samples). The Walsh Test uses differences (d) between paired data, where:

- It is assumed that the measured data are interval.
- It is assumed that the data exhibit symmetrical distribution, such that the mean and the median accurately represent central tendency.

With the Walsh Test, unlike Student's t-Test for Matched Pairs, the differences between x and y (or, for this lesson, between Pretest and Posttest) do not have to be from normal populations. And, unlike the nonparametric Wilcoxon Matched-Pairs Signed Ranks Test which is based on the use of ordinal data, the Walsh Test is dependent on interval data. Consider these requirements when recalling how researchers must know the nature of their data before any statistical analyses are attempted.

---

[1] It is not uncommon to see the expression *The Null Hypothesis is not accepted* instead of the expression *The Null Hypothesis is rejected*. Although there may be no practical difference between these two expressions, it is important to those who have a keen interest in the heuristics of statistics.

Data and Codebook: For this lesson assume that the data come from 15 separate subjects (Subject A to Subject O). Each subject undertakes a pretest, receives some type of treatment, and then undertakes a posttest. Because the data are from 15 subjects only, the difference (d) between pretest results and posttest results (Pr-Po=d) are easily hand-calculated, if needed.

For the purpose of this lesson, is not necessary to know the nature of the biological organism representing the subjects, pretest, treatment, or posttest. It is only necessary to know that the data are considered interval and that the data are distributed in a symmetrical manner. However, because normal distribution is not assumed, the nonparametric Walsh Test is selected using difference scores with a focus on the median, which should ostensibly be in parity with the mean.

Create an object called Change.df. The object Change.df will be a dataframe, as indicated by the enumerated .df extension to the object name. This object will represent the output of applying the read.table() function against the comma-separated values file called Change.csv. Note the arguments used with the read.table() function, showing that there is a header with descriptive variable names (header = TRUE) and that the separator between fields is a comma (sep = ",").

```
Change.df <- read.table (file =
  "Change.csv",
  header = TRUE,
  sep = ",")                          # Import the .csv file

getwd()                               # Identify the working directory
ls()                                  # List objects
attach(Change.df)                     # Attach the data, for later use
str(Change.df)                        # Identify structure
nrow(Change.df)                       # List the number of rows
ncol(Change.df)                       # List the number of columns
dim(Change.df)                        # Dimensions of the dataframe
names(Change.df)                      # Identify names
colnames(Change.df)                   # Show column names
rownames(Change.df)                   # Show row names
head(Change.df)                       # Show the head
tail(Change.df)                       # Show the tail
Change.df                             # Show the entire dataframe
summary(Change.df)                    # Summary statistics

Change.df$S  <- as.factor(Change.df$S)
Change.df$Pr <- as.numeric(Change.df$Pr)
Change.df$Po <- as.numeric(Change.df$Po)
Change.df$d  <- as.numeric(Change.df$d)

attach(Change.df)
Change.df
str(Change.df)
```

```
'data.frame':    15 obs. of  4 variables:
 $ S : Factor w/ 15 levels "A","B","C","D",..: 1 2 3 4 5 6
 $ Pr: num  4 4 3 5 2 4 2 2 4 4 ...
 $ Po: num  2 2 1 3 3 2 3 1 2 3 ...
 $ d : num  2 2 2 2 -1 2 -1 1 2 1 ...
```

```
############################################################
# Code Book for Change.df                                  #
#                                                          #
# S   Subject ............................ Factor  A to O #
#                                                          #
# Pr  Pretest ........................... Numeric  0 to 5 #
#                                                          #
# Po  Posttest .......................... Numeric  0 to 5 #
#                                                          #
# d   Difference .... Numeric Difference between Pr and Po #
############################################################
```

Null Hypothesis (Ho): The median difference between the Pretest and Posttest is zero. That is to say, subjects will perform on the pretest and posttest equally well (p <= 0.05).

Visualize the Data: Display a density plot for Change.df$Pr (Pretest) and Change.df$Po (Posttest) in the same figure, to gain a sense of data distribution for each. To achieve this aim, create an object that represents density statistics for the Pretest (Pr) and another object that represents density statistics for the Posttest (Po). These new objects of density-type statistics will be used to prepare a density plot figure for both object variables, Pr and Po.

```
Pr_density <- density(Pr)
# Prepare an object of density() function statistics
Pr_density
```

```
Call:
        density.default(x = Pr)

Data: Pr (15 obs.);     Bandwidth 'bw' = 0.6818

       x                 y
 Min.   :-1.0453   Min.   :0.0008807
 1st Qu.: 0.9773   1st Qu.:0.0262478
 Median : 3.0000   Median :0.1268527
 Mean   : 3.0000   Mean   :0.1234355
 3rd Qu.: 5.0227   3rd Qu.:0.2058566
 Max.   : 7.0453   Max.   :0.2661030
```

```
Po_density <- density(Po)
# Prepare an object of density() function statistics
Po_density
```

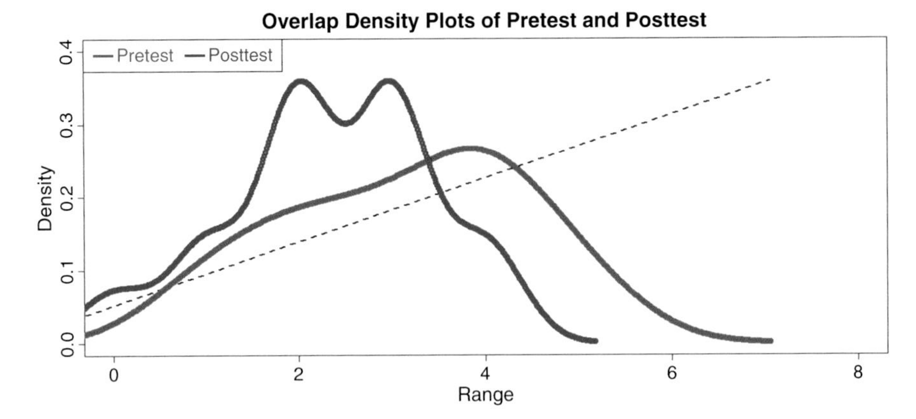

Fig. 9.2 Comparative density plots with color-coded legend

```
Call:
        density.default(x = Po)

Data: Po (15 obs.);     Bandwidth 'bw' = 0.3908

       x                  y
 Min.   :-1.1723   Min.   :0.000766
 1st Qu.: 0.4138   1st Qu.:0.056858
 Median : 2.0000   Median :0.142094
 Mean   : 2.0000   Mean   :0.157419
 3rd Qu.: 3.5862   3rd Qu.:0.283889
 Max.   : 5.1723   Max.   :0.359178
```

```
par(ask=TRUE)
plot(range(Pr_density$x, Po_density$x),
  range(Pr_density$y, Po_density$y),
  main="Overlap Density Plots of Pretest and Posttest",
  xlab="Range", ylab="Density",
  cex.axis=1.25, cex.lab=1.25, font=2,
  xlim=c(0,8), ylim=c(0.0,0.40),
  type="l", lty=2, lwd=2)
points(Pr_density, col="red", lwd=4)
points(Po_density, col="blue", lwd=4)
legend("topleft",
  legend=c("Pretest", "Posttest"),
  col=c("red", "blue"),
  ncol=2, cex=1.25, lwd=4,
  text.font=2, text.col=c("red", "blue"))
  # Use the previously established density statistics
  # to construct the two density plots in this figure.
```

Descriptive Statistics: Given that this lesson is based on two simple sets of data, organized as Pretest scores and Posttest scores, the needed descriptive statistics are generally simple and it is not necessary to go into extensive detail (Fig. 9.2).

```
median(Change.df$Pr)
```

```
[1] 3
```

```
mean(Change.df$Pr); sd(Change.df$Pr); length(Change.df$Pr)
```

```
[1] 3.133333
[1] 1.302013
[1] 15
```

```
median(Change.df$Po)
```

```
[1] 2
```

```
mean(Change.df$Po); sd(Change.df$Po); length(Change.df$Po)
```

```
[1] 2.333333
[1] 1.112697
[1] 15
```

Statistical Analysis: The Walsh Test for Two Related Samples of Interval Data was purposely selected for this lesson to show one of the challenges of computer-mediated statistical analyses. That is to say, the Walsh Test is only infrequently used and there are no known R-based functions currently existing in any packages for implementation of this test. Reacting to this issue, it may be best to substitute both the nonparametric wilcox.test() function and the parametric t.test() function, both for paired data, to examine trends and outcomes, with the alternate being hand-calculation of the Walsh Test:

```
wilcox.test(Change.df$Pr, Change.df$Po, paired=TRUE)
  # Use wilcox.test() as a substitute for the Walsh Test
```

```
        Wilcoxon signed rank test with continuity correction

data:  Change.df$Pr and Change.df$Po
V = 97.5, p-value = 0.03051
alternative hypothesis: true location shift is not equal to 0
```

```
t.test(Change.df$Pr, Change.df$Po, paired=TRUE)
  # Use t.test() as a substitute for the Walsh Test
```

```
        Paired t-test

data:  Change.df$Pr and Change.df$Po
t = 2.2563, df = 14, p-value = 0.04057
alternative hypothesis: true difference in means is not equal
to 0
```

Summary: By applying the nonparametric wilcox.test() function and the parametric t.test() function against the data, as substitutes for the Walsh Test, the same general trend was observed in that there is a statistically significant difference (`p <= 0.05`) between the Pretest and the Posttest:

- p-value = 0.03051 using the wilcox.test() function, which is less than `p <= 0.05`.
- p-value = 0.04057 using the t.test() function, which is less than `p <= 0.05`.[2]

These tests in many ways go along with simple observation of the descriptive statistics, where the Pretest median was 3 and the Posttest median was 2. Using all available graphical images, statistical resources, and related outcomes, it can be said with a fair degree of assurance that Pretest scores are greater than Posttest scores and that the difference is due to true difference and not due to chance.

It can also be said that there is a need for a R-based Walsh Test function. Hopefully a function meeting this need will soon be available, due to the open-source nature of R.

9.3 Kolmogorov-Smirnov (K-S) Two-Sample Test

Background: The Kolmogorov-Smirnov (K-S) Two-Sample Test is a nonparametric test used to determine if two independent samples are taken from either the same population or from two populations that have the same distribution pattern. The K-S Test is sensitive to distribution differences, either differences in central tendency or dispersion. The focus here is on two separate sets of data.

Ordinal data are used with the K-S Two-Sample Test and this test is especially useful with small samples, such as when there are fewer than 40 subjects in each of the two samples. The K-S Test is especially useful for when possible differences exist between the two sets of data due more to dispersion than differences in central tendency. That is to say, two sets of data can have the same median and mean, but because of differences in distribution patterns the K-S Test will help discern if there are statistically significant differences between the two datasets.

Data and Codebook: This lesson is related to an experiment on a colostrum substitute, largely to determine if there is a difference in the weight of 3-month-old female dairy calves between those calves that received colostrum soon after birth and counterpart calves that instead received a colostrum substitute. There is a known concern for calves that do not receive colostrum soon after birth and their risk for infections, possibly placing a future limit on vigor and weight gain. It is

---

[2]For these two tests, there is a statistically significant difference at `p <= 0.05`, but does this finding apply to `p <= 0.01`, given how p-values or 0.03 and 0.04 are less than 0.05 but more than 0.01? This example serves as a reminder on why it is important to provide calculated p-values. It is insufficient to only state that there is (or is not) a statistically significant difference.

valuable to the dairy industry to have an effective substitute for colostrum-deprived calves and this analysis begins to addresses that concern.

Subjects: There are 30 calves in this experiment and all calves are of the same breed. All 30 calves have different mothers. All 30 calves in this experiment have the same father, which is made possible through artificial insemination (AI). These two actions (i.e., same breed for mother and father and same father for all calves) may limit, to some degree, possible differences in subject weights due to genetic variability.

Methods: The control group (WeightLb3MonthCalfColostrum, N = 15 calves) received colostrum from their mothers. The experimental group (WeightLb3MonthCalfSubstitute, N = 15 calves) were denied feeding access to their mothers immediately after birth and were instead provided a colostrum substitute. Otherwise, the 30 calves were all housed in proximity to each other, experienced the same feeding regime, and experienced the same set of management practices and environmental factors.

Data Collection: Ear tags were used for identification purposes and approximately 90 days after birth all calves were weighed, which was recorded using pounds (Lbs) as the measuring unit. Although the scale was calibrated, it is known that the exact weight of excited and moving calves is difficult to obtain, and, in turn, the weights were viewed as ordinal, not interval, data—due to fluctuations during the weighing process. Further, it was noticed that there may be concerns about parity in distribution patterns for weights of the two groups of calves.

Given concerns about the ordinal nature of the data and uncertain data distribution patterns, it is best to use the Kolmogorov-Smirnov (K-S) Two-Sample Test to determine if there are statistically significant (`p <= 0.05`) differences between the control group (received colostrum) and the experimental group (received a colostrum substitute). Weight (pounds, Lbs) at 3 months or approximately 90 days after birth is the measured datum for comparative purposes.

```
WeightLbColostrum   <- c(301, 308, 318, 325, 305, 311, 315,
  320, 299, 319, 313, 305, 307, 317, 296)
summary(WeightLbColostrum)
```

```
   Min. 1st Qu.  Median    Mean 3rd Qu.    Max.
    296     305     311     311     318     325
```

```
WeightLbSubstitute  <- c(287, 299, 286, 297, 298, 279, 281,
  309, 286, 276, 279, 294, 302, 292, 300)
summary(WeightLbSubstitute)
```

```
   Min. 1st Qu.  Median    Mean 3rd Qu.    Max.
    276     284     292     291     298     309
```

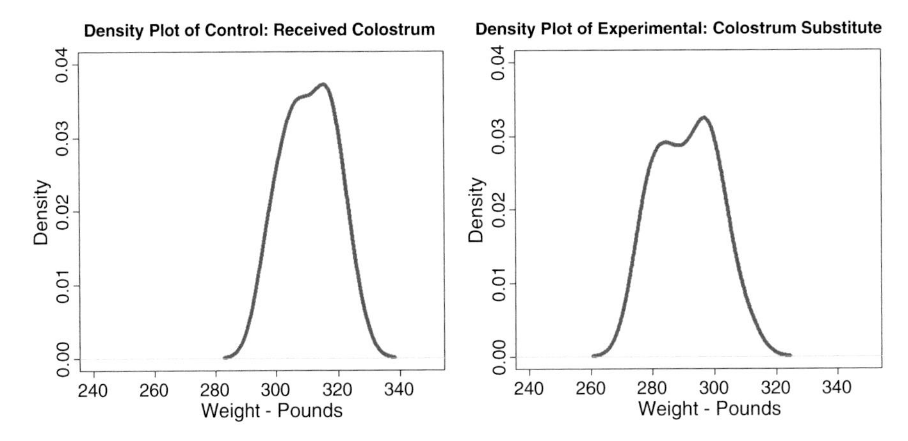

Fig. 9.3 Simple comparison of two side-by-side density plots

```
#################################################################
# Code Book for Calves.df                                       #
#                                                               #
# WeightLb3MonthCalfColostrum .................... Ordinal #
#             Weight (Lbs) of calf that received colostrum #
#                                                               #
# WeightLb3MonthCalfSubstitute ................... Ordinal #
#             Weight (Lbs) of calf that received substitute #
#################################################################
```

Null Hypothesis (Ho): There is no statistically significant difference (`p <= 0.05`) in weight at 3 months between calves that received colostrum soon after birth and counterpart calves that instead received a colostrum substitute soon after birth.

Visualize the Data: A side-by-side density curve of the two variables is perhaps the best way to both visualize and compare the data, calf weights at 90 days after birth.

```
par(ask=TRUE)
par(mfrow=c(1,2))        # 1 Row by 2 Columns
plot(density(WeightLbColostrum, na.rm=TRUE),
  xlim=c(240,350), ylim=c(0,0.04),
  main="Density Plot of Control:  Received Colostrum",
  xlab="Weight - Pounds",
  lwd=6, col="red", font.axis=2, font.lab=2)
plot(density(WeightLbSubstitute, na.rm=TRUE),
  xlim=c(240,350), ylim=c(0,0.04),
  main="Density Plot of Experimental:  Colostrum Substitute",
  xlab="Weight - Pounds",
  lwd=6, col="red", font.axis=2, font.lab=2)
```

Descriptive Statistics: The data for this lesson are currently found in two separate variables, and they are not part of a common object. Combine the two variables into one common object, as a dataframe, and then apply the pastecs::stat.desc() function to produce a detailed, but easy-to-read, output of descriptive statistics (Fig. 9.3).

```
Calves.df <- data.frame(cbind(
  WeightLbColostrum, WeightLbSubstitute))
  # Wrap the data.frame() function around the cbind() function
  # to put the two separate object variables into one common
  # object---organized as a dataframe.

Calves.df

install.packages("pastecs")
library(pastecs)              # Load the pastecs package.
help(package=pastecs)         # Show the information page.
sessionInfo()                 # Confirm all attached packages.
# Select the most local mirror site using Set CRAN mirror.

options(scipen=80, digits=4)
# Prevent scientific notation and keep printouts to a
# reasonable width

pastecs::stat.desc(Calves.df)
```

```
             WeightLbColostrum WeightLbSubstitute
nbr.val               15.00000           15.00000
nbr.null               0.00000            0.00000
nbr.na                 0.00000            0.00000
min                  296.00000          276.00000
max                  325.00000          309.00000
range                 29.00000           33.00000
sum                 4659.00000         4365.00000
median               311.00000          292.00000
mean                 310.60000          291.00000
SE.mean                2.19263            2.54858
CI.mean.0.95           4.70272            5.46615
var                   72.11429           97.42857
std.dev                8.49201            9.87059
coef.var               0.02734            0.03392
```

Statistical Analysis: A brief review of the previously shown density plots as well as the descriptive statistics provides a sense that there may be a difference in weight at 3 months between those calves that received colostrum and those calves that instead received a colostrum substitute. Of course, an appropriate statistical analysis is needed to provide assurance that these casual observations are indeed the case. For this lesson, the Kolmogorov-Smirnov (K-S) Two-Sample Test is judged the most appropriate test, as applied by use of the ks.test() function.

```
ks.test(Calves.df$WeightLbColostrum,
  Calves.df$WeightLbSubstitute,
  alternative="two.sided", exact=TRUE)
```

```
        Two-sample Kolmogorov-Smirnov test

data:  Calves.df$WeightLbColostrum and
       Calves.df$WeightLbSubstitute
D = 0.7333, p-value = 0.0006277
alternative hypothesis: two-sided
```

Summary: Regarding weights for the two sets of calves, the calculated p-value is 0.0006277, suggesting statistical difference (`p <= 0.05`):

- Median weight = 311 pounds—Colostrum
- Median weight = 292 pounds—Colostrum Substitute

There is a statistically significant difference in weights for the two sets of calves. The calculated p-value was 0.0006277 which is less than the criterion p-value of <= 0.05.

For this one-time study, it was evident that calves that received colostrum soon after birth weighed more at 3 months than those calves that did not receive colostrum soon after birth. Given the economics of a dairy operation and within the limits of this one-time study, it is suggested that colostrum is associated with increased weights after calving and based on prior experience, increased weights early-on are associated with heightened profits. The colostrum substitute for this study did not result in weight gains in parity with natural access to colostrum soon after birth.

9.4 Binomial Logistic Regression

Background: Binomial (i.e., Binary) Logistic Regression is presented in this lesson as a nonparametric test in that the variable of immediate attention is nominal, with a binary set of outcomes:

- Absent/Present
- Correct/Incorrect
- Dead/Alive
- Fail/Pass
- False/True
- No/Yes
- Off/On

A binary outcome is not measured on any type of continuum, neither as an ordinal value nor as an interval value.

Past behavior is the best predictor of future behavior. This statement applies to the biological sciences as well as the social sciences. Regression is used with existing data to make predictions of the future. The unique nature of Binomial Logistic Regression is that it can be used to determine the odds ratio of a future binary outcome.

Data and Codebook: This lesson is focused on a chemical application trial, where an agricultural crop grown in a greenhouse was subjected to the application of an experimental chemical. The term Subject represents an individual plant growing in an individual pot, with all Subjects growing in the same greenhouse:

- Overcrowding is not an issue since the plants (i.e., Subjects) will only be monitored for a few weeks and there is sufficient space in the greenhouse.
- All plants are of the same variety and strain, limiting genetic variability.
- All plants are grown in the same greenhouse under controlled conditions, limiting environmental (e.g., sunlight, temperature, nutrients, water availability, humidity, etc.) variability.

A few days prior to the start of this study, a team of greenhouse workers prepared 3,500 pots with a dry growing media and placed the pots on raised beds in a greenhouse. Early in the morning on the 1st day of the study a team of greenhouse workers placed one seed of the type associated with the study in each pot. By noon planting had been completed and overhead sprinklers were used to wet the pots and begin germination. Favorable growing conditions were maintained throughout the study.

On the 17th day of the study the few pots where the seed did not germinate were culled and removed from the greenhouse. It was observed that germination was above 90 %, which was judged acceptable for this study.

On the 18th day of the study, a team of research assistants, under the lead of the principal investigator, made two measurements of the live plants:

- M1 (i.e., Measure 1) is based on a 100–200 scale.
- M2 (i.e., Measure 2) is based on a 2.00–4.00 scale, with precision stated to two places to the right of the decimal point.

Due to rigorous training of the research assistants and prior estimates of reliability and validity by the principal investigator, the scales and processes for M1 and M2 measurements support the view that the data for these two variables are interval and not ordinal.

At the beginning of the 19th day of the study, the entire collection of plants in the greenhouse was subjected to an otherwise unidentified chemical treatment. Favorable growing conditions were continued. On the 22nd day of the study, the principal investigator and the team of research assistants went back to the greenhouse, and, based on prior training, judged whether individual plants had died or survived.

- If the plant in an individual pot was dead, then the Subject received a numerical code of 0, or Dead.

- If the plant in an individual pot was alive, then the Subject received a numerical code of 1, or Survive.

Note how the was no continuum of measurement for Dead or Survive. It was judged that the team of research assistants had received sufficient training and instead of a continuum, a binary nominal classification was used, expressed in numerical format for quick data entry: 0 (i.e., Dead) or 1 (i.e., Survive).

```
#####################################################
# Code Book for DeadSurvive.df                      #
#                                                   #
# Subject .. Nominal    S_1 to S_3276               #
#            Approximately 6% did not germinate     #
#                                                   #
# M1 ....... Interval   100 to 200                  #
#                                                   #
# M2 ....... Interval   2.00 to 4.00                #
#                                                   #
# Status ... Nominal    0 (Dead) or 1 (Survive)     #
#                                                   #
# Outcome .. Nominal    Dead or Survive             #
#####################################################
```

Among the many possible approaches toward data analysis for this rich dataset, it will be interesting to see if there is any relationship between M1, M2, and the variable of primary interest to see if an individual plant (i.e., Subject) is either dead or alive after application of the chemical treatment.

Create an object called DeadSurvive.df. The object DeadSurvive.df will be a dataframe, as indicated by the enumerated .df extension to the object name. This object will represent the output of applying the read.table() function against the comma-separated values file called DeadSurvive.csv. Note the arguments used with the read.table() function, showing that there is a header with descriptive variable names (header = TRUE) and that the separator between fields is a comma (sep = ",").

```
DeadSurvive.df <- read.table (file =
  "DeadSurvive.csv",
  header = TRUE,
  sep = ",")                 # Import the .csv file

getwd()                      # Identify the working directory
ls()                         # List objects
attach(DeadSurvive.df)       # Attach the data, for later use
str(DeadSurvive.df)          # Identify structure
nrow(DeadSurvive.df)         # List the number of rows
ncol(DeadSurvive.df)         # List the number of columns
dim(DeadSurvive.df)          # Dimensions of the dataframe
names(DeadSurvive.df)        # Identify names
colnames(DeadSurvive.df)     # Show column names
rownames(DeadSurvive.df)     # Show row names
```

```
head(DeadSurvive.df, n=10)    # Show the head
tail(DeadSurvive.df, n=10)    # Show the tail
DeadSurvive.df                # Show the entire dataframe
summary(DeadSurvive.df)       # Summary statistics

str(DeadSurvive.df)

DeadSurvive.df$Subject       <- as.factor(DeadSurvive.df$Subject
DeadSurvive.df$M1            <- as.numeric(DeadSurvive.df$M1)
DeadSurvive.df$M2            <- as.numeric(DeadSurvive.df$M2)
DeadSurvive.df$Status.recode <- factor(DeadSurvive.df$Status,
  labels=c("Dead", "Survive"))
  # Use factor() and not as.factor().
DeadSurvive.df$Outcome       <- as.factor(DeadSurvive.df$Outcome

str(DeadSurvive.df)
```

```
'data.frame':   3276 obs. of  6 variables:
 $ Subject      : Factor w/ 3276 levels "S_1","S_10","S_100"
 $ M1           : num  129 133 134 135 136 138 138 138 139
 $ M2           : num  2.34 2.4 2.19 2.39 2.39 2.21 2.33
 $ Status       : int  0 0 0 1 0 0 0 0 0 ...
 $ Outcome      : Factor w/ 2 levels "Dead","Survive": 1 1 1
 $ Status.recode: Factor w/ 2 levels "Dead","Survive": 1 1 1
```

When reviewing the data in original format, note how the data were sorted by M1. It is beyond the purpose of this lesson to go into any great detail on the sort() function, but this may be a function that deserves further review to use R to best advantage.

Visualize the Data: The data for this lesson support a variety of graphical presentations. Some will be fairly simple throwaway graphics, used only for casual quality assurance (QA) purposes. Some figures will be quite detailed and could be used with confidence in a group presentation or in a publication (Figs. 9.4 and 9.5).

```
par(ask=TRUE)
plot(DeadSurvive.df$Subject,
  main="Frequency Distribution of Subject")
  # Due to the many subjects, it is not possible to
  # identify individual subjects using this QA tool

par(ask=TRUE)
plot(DeadSurvive.df$Status.recode,
  main="Frequency Distribution of Status:  Dead or Survive",
  lwd=6, col="red", font.axis=2, font.lab=2)

par(ask=TRUE)
plot(DeadSurvive.df$Outcome,
  main="Frequency Distribution of Outcome:  Dead or Survive",
  lwd=6, col="red", font.axis=2, font.lab=2)
```

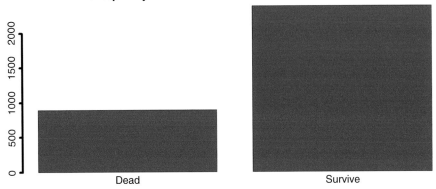

Fig. 9.4 Simple frequency distribution of two breakout groups

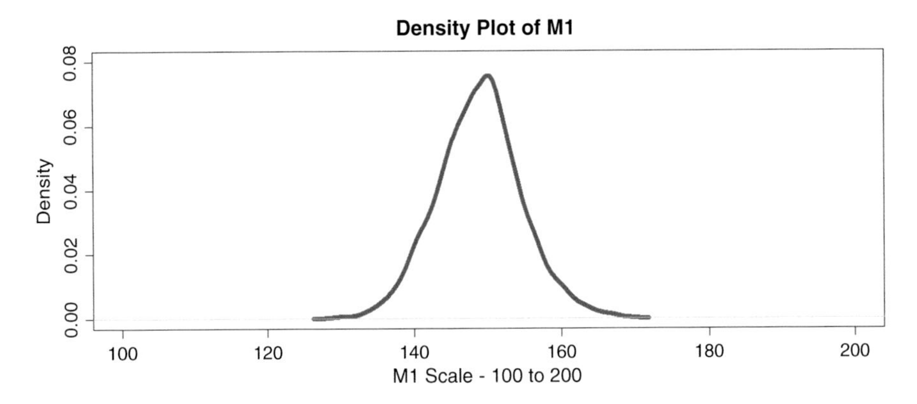

Fig. 9.5 Density plot of M1: original scale 100–200

```
par(ask=TRUE)
plot(density(DeadSurvive.df$M1, na.rm=TRUE),
  xlim=c(100,200), ylim=c(0,0.08),
  main="Density Plot of M1",
  xlab="M1 Scale - 100 to 200",
  lwd=6, col="red", font.axis=2, font.lab=2)
```

```
par(ask=TRUE)
plot(density(DeadSurvive.df$M2, na.rm=TRUE),
  xlim=c(2,4), ylim=c(0,1),
  main="Density Plot of M2",
  xlab="M2 Scale - 2.00 to 4.00",
  lwd=6, col="red", font.axis=2, font.lab=2)
```

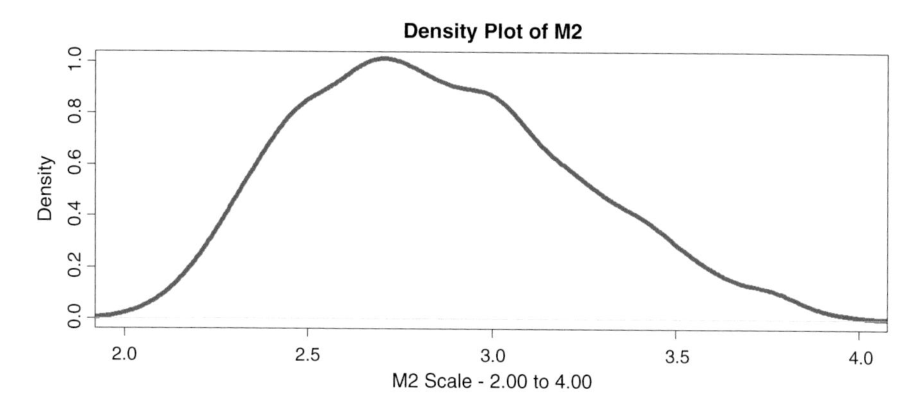

Fig. 9.6 Density plot of M2: original scale 2.00–4.00

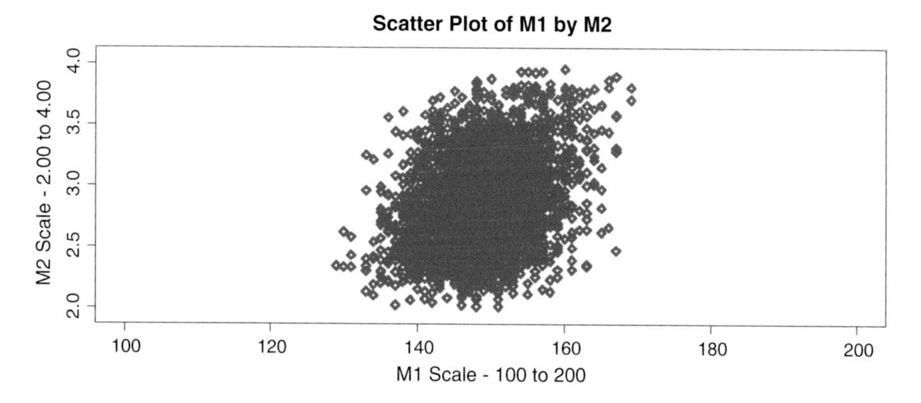

Fig. 9.7 Scatter plot of M1 and M2

The prior figures are all useful for review purposes, to gain a better understanding of the data. However, regression is about relationships between, and among, variables and ultimately, the prediction of future outcomes. The figures below begin to address these relationships (Figs. 9.6, 9.7, 9.8, 9.9, 9.10).

```
par(ask=TRUE)
plot(DeadSurvive.df$M1, DeadSurvive.df$M2,            # X by Y
  xlab="M1 Scale - 100 to 200",
  ylab="M2 Scale - 2.00 to 4.00",
  main="Scatter Plot of M1 by M2",
  pch=23, lwd=4, col="red", cex.axis=1.25, cex.lab=1.25,
  font=2, xlim=c(100,200), ylim=c(1.95,4.05))
  # Note how xlim and ylim scales are declared, to allow for
  # full presentation of outcomes with adequate white space
```

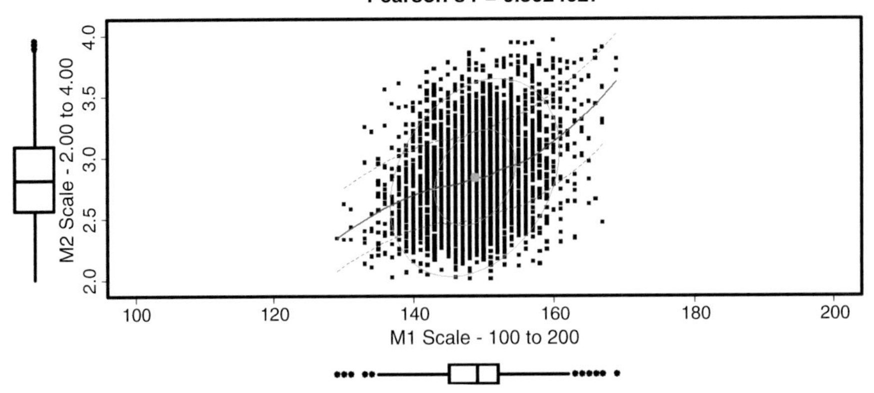

Fig. 9.8 Scatter plot with box plots on X axis and Y axis using the car::scatterplot() function

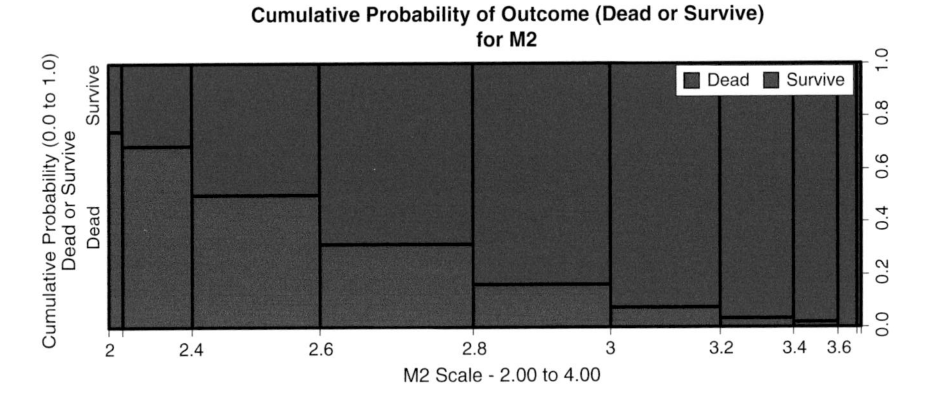

Fig. 9.9 Cumulative probability (0.0–1.0) plot

```
install.packages("car")
library(car)                    # Load the car package.
help(package=car)               # Show the information page.
sessionInfo()                   # Confirm all attached packages.
# Select the most local mirror site using Set CRAN mirror.

cor(DeadSurvive.df$M1, DeadSurvive.df$M2, method="pearson")
# Calculate Pearson's r for correlation
```

```
[1] 0.3025
```

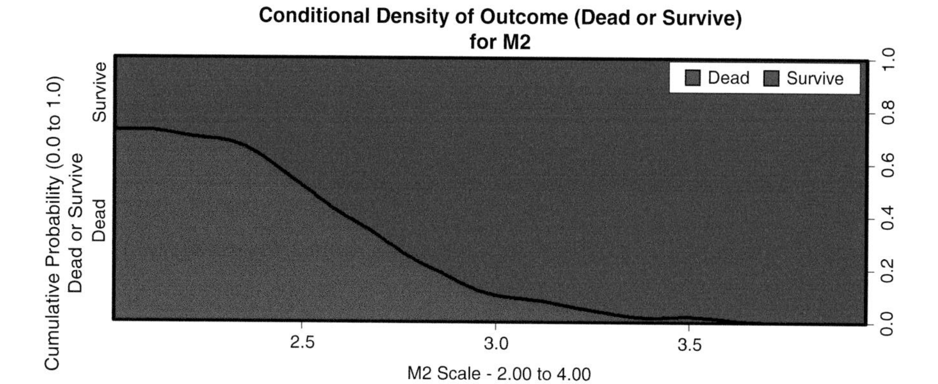

Fig. 9.10 Conditional density plot

```
savelwd      <- par(lwd=4)          # Heavy line
savefont     <- par(font=2)         # Bold
savecex.lab  <- par(cex.lab=1.5)    # Label
savecex.axis <- par(cex.axis=1.5)   # Axis
par(ask=TRUE)
car::scatterplot(M2 ~ M1,                                 # Y ~ X
  data=DeadSurvive.df,
  xlab="M1 Scale - 100 to 200",
  ylab="M2 Scale - 2.00 to 4.00",
  main="Scatter Plot of M1 by M2 With Loess Line and Ellipse
  Pearson's r = 0.3024627",
  smooth=TRUE, reg.line=TRUE, boxplots="xy",
  grid=FALSE, pch=15, font.lab=2, font.axis=2, lty=1,
  cex.main=1.5, xlim=c(100,200), ylim=c(1.95,4.05),
  ellipse=TRUE, robust=TRUE )
  # Show data-concentration ellipse and center of ellipse
  # If smooth=TRUE then loessLine is generated
par(savelwd); par(savefont); par(savecex.lab)
par(savecex.axis)
```

```
saveaxis     <- par(cex.axis=1.25)   # Axis - Large
savefont     <- par(font=2)          # Font - Bold
savelab      <- par(cex.lab=1.25)    # Label - Large
savelwd      <- par(lwd=4)           # Line - Thick
par(ask=TRUE)
plot(DeadSurvive.df$Outcome ~ DeadSurvive.df$M1,
  main="Cumulative Probability of Outcome (Dead or Survive)
  for M1",
  xlab="M1 Scale - 100 to 200",
  ylab="Cumulative Probability (0.0 to 1.0) Dead or Survive",
  xlim=c(0, 1), col=c("red", "blue"))
legend("topright",
  levels(DeadSurvive.df$Outcome),
  fill=c("red", "blue"), bg=c("white"), bty="y",
```

```
  inset=0.01, box.lwd=1, xjust=0, ncol=2)
par(saveaxis); par(savefont); par(savelab); par(savelwd)

saveaxis     <- par(cex.axis=1.25)  # Axis - Large
savefont     <- par(font=2)         # Font - Bold
savelab      <- par(cex.lab=1.25)   # Label - Large
savelwd      <- par(lwd=4)          # Line - Thick
par(ask=TRUE)
plot(DeadSurvive.df$Outcome ~ DeadSurvive.df$M2,
  main="Cumulative Probability of Outcome (Dead or Survive)
  for M2",
  xlab="M2 Scale - 2.00 to 4.00",
  ylab="Cumulative Probability (0.0 to 1.0) Dead or Survive",
  xlim=c(0, 1), col=c("red", "blue"))
legend("topright",
  levels(DeadSurvive.df$Outcome),
  fill=c("red", "blue"), bg=c("white"), bty="y",
  inset=0.01, box.lwd=1, xjust=0, ncol=2)
par(saveaxis); par(savefont); par(savelab); par(savelwd)
```

```
summary(DeadSurvive.df$M1) # Focus on minimum and maximum

par(ask=TRUE)
saveaxis     <- par(cex.axis=1.25)  # Axis - Large
savefont     <- par(font=2)         # Font - Bold
savelab      <- par(cex.lab=1.25)   # Label - Large
savelwd      <- par(lwd=4)          # Line - Thick
par(ask=TRUE)
cdplot(Outcome ~ M1,  data=DeadSurvive.df,
  main="Conditional Density of Outcome (Dead or Survive)
  for M1",
  xlab="M1 Scale - 100 to 200",
  ylab="Cumulative Probability (0.0 to 1.0) Dead or Survive",
  xlim=c(129, 169), col=c("red", "blue"))
legend("topright",
  levels(DeadSurvive.df$Outcome),
  fill=c("red", "blue"), bg=c("white"), bty="y",
  inset=0.01, box.lwd=1, xjust=0, ncol=2)
par(saveaxis); par(savefont); par(savelab); par(savelwd)
  # Note use of the cdplot() function and how the produced
  # graphic is different from use of the plot() function

summary(DeadSurvive.df$M2) # Focus on minimum and maximum

par(ask=TRUE)
saveaxis     <- par(cex.axis=1.25)  # Axis - Large
savefont     <- par(font=2)         # Font - Bold
savelab      <- par(cex.lab=1.25)   # Label - Large
savelwd      <- par(lwd=4)          # Line - Thick
par(ask=TRUE)
cdplot(Outcome ~ M2,  data=DeadSurvive.df,
  main="Conditional Density of Outcome (Dead or Survive)
  for M2",
```

```
  xlab="M2 Scale - 2.00 to 4.00",
  ylab="Cumulative Probability (0.0 to 1.0) Dead or Survive",
  xlim=c(2.01, 3.96), col=c("red", "blue"))
legend("topright",
  levels(DeadSurvive.df$Outcome),
  fill=c("red", "blue"), bg=c("white"), bty="y",
  inset=0.01, box.lwd=1, xjust=0, ncol=2)
par(saveaxis); par(savefont); par(savelab); par(savelwd)
```

Descriptive Statistics: Although there are many functions available in R for descriptive statistics, the summary() function applied against the DeadSurvive.df dataframe may be more than sufficient to initially understand the data. The summary() function provides basic information (e.g., Minimum, 1st Quartile (25th Percentile), Median (50th Percentile), Mean, 3rd Quartile (75th Percentile), and Maximum). Other functions certainly have value, but the summary() function remains a common first choice for descriptive statistics.

```
summary(DeadSurvive.df[, 2:3])
# Apply the summary() function against columns
# 2 to 3 in the dataframe DeadSurvive.df:
# Column 2 - M1
# Column 3 - M2
```

```
       M1              M2
 Min.   :129   Min.   :2.01
 1st Qu.:145   1st Qu.:2.57
 Median :149   Median :2.82
 Mean   :149   Mean   :2.85
 3rd Qu.:152   3rd Qu.:3.10
 Max.   :169   Max.   :3.96
```

```
summary(DeadSurvive.df[, 4:6])
# Apply the summary() function against columns
# 4 to 6 in the dataframe DeadSurvive.df:
# Column 4 - Status
# Column 5 - Outcome
# Column 6 - Status.recode
```

```
     Status           Outcome       Status.recode
 Min.   :0.000   Dead    : 894   Dead    : 894
 1st Qu.:0.000   Survive:2382   Survive:2382
 Median :1.000
 Mean   :0.727
 3rd Qu.:1.000
 Max.   :1.000
```

Statistical Analysis: It is evident that there is some degree of association (Pearson's r = 0.3024627) between the two measured object variables, DeadSurvive.df$M1 and DeadSurvive.df$M2. The two Cumulative Probability of Outcome (Dead or Survive) plots and the two Conditional Density of Outcome

(Dead or Survive) plots equally address association. In these four plots, as scores for both DeadSurvive.df$M1 and DeadSurvive.df$M2 increase, there is a greater observation of plants classified as Survive instead of Dead.

Binomial (i.e., Binary) Logistic Regression will be used in this lesson to provide specifics as to these associations. The glm() function (glm refers to Generalized Linear Models) will be the primary tool to initiate these analyses.

```
options(scipen=80, digits=4)

Plants.glm <- glm(DeadSurvive.df$Outcome ~ DeadSurvive.df$M1 +
  DeadSurvive.df$M2, family=binomial)
  # Prepare an object that represents the outcome of applying
  # glm (Generalized Linear Model) against the relevant
  # variables, giving attention to a binomial perspective to
  # the data.

Plants.glm

summary(Plants.glm)
```

```
Call:
glm(formula = DeadSurvive.df$Outcome ~ DeadSurvive.df$M1 +
  DeadSurvive.df$M2, family = binomial)

Deviance Residuals:
   Min      1Q  Median      3Q     Max
-3.195  -0.657   0.342   0.692   2.320

Coefficients:
                    Std. Error z value              Pr(>|z|)
(Intercept)             1.4237   -16.9 <0.0000000000000002 ***
DeadSurvive.df$M1       0.0091    10.4 <0.0000000000000002 ***
DeadSurvive.df$M2       0.1815    22.4 <0.0000000000000002 ***
---
Signif. codes:  0 '***' 0.001 '**' 0.01 '*' 0.05 '.' 0.1 ' ' 1
```

As is seen with the three `***` symbols showing in this output, there are statistically significant relationships (`p <= 0.001`, as indicated by the asterisks) between the variables.

```
car::Anova(Plants.glm)
# Use ANOVA for a general examination of the data
```

```
Analysis of Deviance Table (Type II tests)

Response: DeadSurvive.df$Outcome
                  LR Chisq Df          Pr(>Chisq)
DeadSurvive.df$M1      116  1 <0.0000000000000002 ***
DeadSurvive.df$M2      750  1 <0.0000000000000002 ***
---
Signif. codes:  0 '***' 0.001 '**' 0.01 '*' 0.05 '.' 0.1 ' ' 1
```

The ANOVA analysis confirms the prior glm analysis that indeed there are statistically significant relationships between the variables.

Now that significance has been confirmed, it is necessary to focus on beta values. Because there are multiple predictor variables (i.e., M1 and M2), recall that beta values serve as an indicator, or measure, of how strongly each predictor variable influences the outcome (i.e., criterion, dependent) variable. It is beyond the purpose of this lesson to go into more detail on the theories and algorithms of regression, but there are many available resources for those with specific interest.

```
Plants.glm.betahat <- Plants.glm$coefficients
# Create an object that holds coefficients from
# the glm-based object

Plants.glm.betahat
```

```
      (Intercept) DeadSurvive.df$M1 DeadSurvive.df$M2
        -24.12172           0.09441           4.06719
```

Then, use the exp() function to compute the exponential function overall and for each individual beta statistic. These statistics are part of the process needed to calculate odds ratios.

```
exp(Plants.glm.betahat)     # Intercept and predictor variables
exp(Plants.glm.betahat[1]) # Intercept
exp(Plants.glm.betahat[2]) # 1st predictor variable
exp(Plants.glm.betahat[3]) # 2nd predictor variable

exp(coef(Plants.glm))       # Odds ratio only
```

```
      (Intercept) DeadSurvive.df$M1 DeadSurvive.df$M2
 0.00000000003343  1.09901133803832 58.39243209491096
```

```
options(scipen=80, digits=1)
# Adjust for output width

exp(cbind(OR = coef(Plants.glm), confint(Plants.glm)))
# Odds ratio and 95% CI for the intercept and both
# predictor variables (M1 and M2) related to the outcome
# of Dead or Survive
```

```
Waiting for profiling to be done...
                              OR           2.5 %         97.5 %
(Intercept)         0.00000000003  0.000000000002  0.0000000005
DeadSurvive.df$M1   1.09901133804  1.079743147202  1.1189627822
DeadSurvive.df$M2 58.39243209491 41.165605267114 83.8618497930
```

The process for this regression analysis is somewhat complex, but follow along with these sequential steps to generate a table that clearly outlines the Odds Ratio (i.e., OR, as seen immediately above) for each predictor variable:

- The Odds Ratio (OR) for DeadSurvive.df$M1 = 1.09901133804.
- The Odds Ratio (OR) for DeadSurvive.df$M2 = 58.39243209491.

Look below to see an interpretation of how to *apply* the outcomes of a Binomial (i.e., Binary) Logistic Regression.

Summary: As time permits, read on the terms odds, probability, and odds ratio. These terms are not synonyms and other resources can be reviewed for a more complete discussion on these terms, where they are similar and where they differ.

Of immediate interest for this lesson, give special attention to the Odds Ratio (i.e., OR) output eventually gained from regression applications against the linear model, as shown above:

- For a one-unit increase in M1, the odds of an individual plant surviving the chemical treatment (versus dying after the chemical treatment) increased by a factor of 1.09 (DeadSurvive.df$M1 OR = 1.09901133804).
- For a one-unit increase in M2, the odds of an individual plant surviving the chemical treatment (versus dying after the chemical treatment) increased by a factor of 58.39 (DeadSurvive.df$M2 OR = 58.39243209491).

It is unknown what M1 and M2 represent, and for the purpose of this lesson it is not necessary to know. What is important, however, is that there are two outcomes to the experiment associated with this lesson: (1) an individual plant was either recorded as Dead after chemical treatment or (2) an individual plant was recorded as Survive after chemical treatment. Although it is evident that a one unit increase in M1 has far less impact on survival than a one unit increase in M2—given the reminder that the scales for M1 and M2 are different, it is unknown what is needed to effect an increase in either scale.

Far more research would be needed before it would ever be financially justified to focus major resources on any specific variable, based on the premise that Survive is a more desirable outcome than Dead. Even so, given the reality of ROI (i.e., Return on Investment), it may be desirable to focus on M2 and how even small changes in this measured variable are associated with desired outcomes (i.e., increased the odds ratio of surviving the chemical treatment).

9.5 Prepare to Exit, Save, and Later Retrieve This R Session

```
getwd()                # Identify the current working directory.
ls()                   # List all objects in the working
                       # directory.
ls.str()               # List all objects, with finite detail.
list.files()           # List files at the PC directory.

save.image("R_Lesson_Future.rdata")

getwd()                # Identify the current working directory.
```

```
ls()                # List all objects in the working
                    # directory.
ls.str()            # List all objects, with finite detail.
list.files()        # List files at the PC directory.

alarm()             # Alarm, notice of upcoming action.
q()                 # Quit this session.
                    # Prepare for Save workspace image? query.
```

Use the R Graphical User Interface (GUI) to load the saved rdata file: File -> Load Workspace. Otherwise, use the load() function, keying the full pathname, to load the .rdata file and retrieve the session.

Recall, however, that it may be just as useful to simply use the .R script file (typically saved is a .txt ASCII-type file) and recreate the analyses and graphics, provided the data files remain available.

9.6 Future Applications of Nonparametric Statistics

STEM (Science, Technology, Engineering, and Mathematics) (and now STEAM, Science, Technology, Engineering, Art + Design, and Mathematics) receives nearly daily notice in the popular press.[3] STEM is also a focus of many preKindergarten to postsecondary educational initiatives. Given our increasingly high-tech world and the emerging IoT (Internet of Things), cloud computing, genetic recombination, smartphones, etc., it is likely that the study of statistics will only increase in importance, as statistics supports decision-making for these areas.

Within statistics and especially the application of statistics to the biological sciences, it is equally likely that nonparametric statistics will gain in importance as more emphasis is placed on quantification of outcomes. Statistical analyses will increasingly be used to justify budgets and direction, but based upon what conditions?

- Our measures may not always be as precise as we wish.
- Data distribution may not always be as normal as we wish.
- Sampling realities may not always allow for subject selection as we wish.

Given these three realities, nonparametric analyses have an important and expanding role as the tenants of statistics are applied to biological organisms—organisms that do not always allow for the luxury of precise measures, perfect distribution, or planned sampling.

[3]The term *STEM Smart* is frequently used by the press to refer to activities that encourage parents, teachers, school administrators, and elected officials to implement educational policies and procedures and allocate human and fiscal resources that emphasize mathematics and the sciences.

On this thought, consider also the role of R in biostatistics. It has recently been reported that R is now among the 10 most frequently used programming languages. As an open-source product with an international user base, it can only be imagined that R will continue to increase in acceptance as a leading platform for biostatistics.

9.7 Contact the Authors

Dr. Thomas W. MacFarland is Senior Research Associate (Office of Institutional Effectiveness) and Associate Professor (College of Engineering and Computing), Nova Southeastern University, Fort Lauderdale, Florida, USA, `tommac@nova.edu`. Dr. Jan M. Yates is Associate Professor (Abraham S. Fischler College of Education), Nova Southeastern University, Fort Lauderdale, Florida, USA, `yates@nova.edu`. Both authors first used S on a UNIX-based host computer in the 1980s, prior to R, when S was then freely available to educational institutions.

The many accompanying .csv (comma-separated values) datasets are available on the publisher's Web page associated with this text. Contact the authors if there are any questions about the use of this text, details on the accompanying .csv datasets, or if additional pointers on R for biostatistics are needed. Questions, comments, and feedback are always appreciated. When sending e-mail to the authors, use a meaningful and descriptive term in the subject header so that the message does not get sent to a rarely monitored SPAM folder or is otherwise ignored.

Index

T.W. MacFarland, J.M. Yates, *Introduction to Nonparametric Statistics for the Biological Sciences Using R*, DOI 10.1007/978-3-319-30634-6